Data Integrity in Pharmaceutical and Medical Devices Regulation Operations

Best Practices Guide to Electronic Records Compliance

Data Integrity in Pharmaceutical and Medical Devices Regulation Operations

Best Practices Guide to Electronic Records Compliance

Orlando Lopez

CRC Press
Taylor & Francis Group
Boca Raton London New York

CRC Press is an imprint of the
Taylor & Francis Group, an **informa** business
A PRODUCTIVITY PRESS BOOK

CRC Press
Taylor & Francis Group
6000 Broken Sound Parkway NW, Suite 300
Boca Raton, FL 33487-2742

First issued in paperback 2022

ISBN-13: 978-1-498-77324-9 (hbk)
ISBN-13: 978-1-03-233988-7 (pbk)
DOI: 10.1201/9781315367095

Publisher's Note

The publisher has gone to great lengths to ensure the quality of this reprint but points out that some imperfections in the original copies may be apparent.

Library of Congress Cataloging-in-Publication Data

Names: Lâopez, Orlando, author.
Title: Data integrity in pharmaceutical and medical devices regulation operations : best practices guide to electronic records compliance / Orlando Lopez.
Description: Boca Raton : CRC Press/Taylor & Francis, 2017. | Includes bibliographical references and index.
Identifiers: LCCN 2016035531 | ISBN 9781498773249 (hard back : alk. paper)
Subjects: | MESH: Information Storage and Retrieval--methods | Electronic Health Records--organization & administration | Computer Security--standards | Practice Guideline
Classification: LCC R858 | NLM W 26.55.I4 | DDC 610.285--dc23
LC record available at https://lccn.loc.gov/2016035531

Visit the Taylor & Francis Web site at
http://www.taylorandfrancis.com

and the CRC Press Web site at
http://www.crcpress.com

For Lizette,

Mikhail Sr., István, Christian, and

Mikhail Jr. who make the journey of life worth while.

Contents

Foreword ... xiii

Preface ... xv

Authors ... xix

Contributors ... xxi

1 **Introduction** ... 1
Additional Readings ... 4

2 **Inspection Trends** ... 5
Additional Readings ... 37

3 **Electronic Records Life Cycle** ... 39
Introduction ... 39
Creation ... 40
Access, Use, and Reuse ... 40
Migration ... 42
Transformation ... 42
Physical Deletion ... 43
E-Records and Computer Systems Life Cycles ... 44
Additional Readings ... 45

4 **Electronic Records Related Definitions** ... 47
Introduction ... 47
Data Terminology ... 48
Introduction to Automated Manufacturing System ... 51
How Are MHRA Definitions Applicable? ... 53
Primary Records ... 55
Records Retention on Raw Data ... 55
Summary ... 56
Additional Readings ... 57

5 Electronic Records Handling: 21 CFR Part 211 59
Introduction 59
Access Authorization Principles 60
Data Input/Output Principles 61
Data Storage and Backup Principles 61
Accuracy Check 62
Additional Readings 62

6 Electronic Records Handling: EMA Annex 11 63
Introduction 63
Creation 64
Access, Use, and Reuse 65
Physical Deletion 69
Controls Based on System Life Cycle 69
Additional Readings 75

7 Relevant Worldwide GMP Regulations and Guidelines 77
Introduction 77
API 78
GMP 86
Additional Reading 99

8 Trustworthy Computer Systems 101
Introduction to Trustworthy Computer Systems 102
Computer Systems Suited to Performing Their Intended Functions 103
ISO 9000-3 105
US FDA 105
European Medicines Agency (EMA) Annex 11, Therapeutic Goods Administration (TGA), and China's SFDA 106
PIC/S PI-011-3, Association of Southeast Asian Nations (ASEAN), and Canadian HPFBI 106
International Conference on Harmonization of Technical Requirements for Registration of Pharmaceuticals for Human Use (ICH) 107
World Health Organization (WHO) 107
Japanese MHLW 107
Brazil ANVISA 107
Provide a Reasonably Reliable Level of Availability, Reliability, and Correct Operation 107
ISO 9000-3 109

US FDA 109
EMA and TGA 109
PIC/S PI-011-3, ASEAN, and Canadian HPFBI 110
ICH 110
WHO 110
China SFDA 110
Brazil ANVISA 111
Secure from Intrusion and Misuse 111
ISO 9000-3 112
US FDA 112
EMA, TGA, and China SFDA 112
PIC/S PI-011-3, ASEAN, and Canadian HPFBI 112
ICH 113
WHO 113
Brazil ANVISA 113
Adhere to Generally Accepted Security Principles 114
Trustworthy Computer Systems Infrastructure 116
Computer System Procedures 118
Summary 118
Additional Readings 119

9 MHRA Guidance 121
Introduction 121
Data Governance 123
Computer Systems Validation 124
Requirements 125
Risk Assessment 126
Data Migration and Computer Systems Release to Operations 129
Operations 130
Computer System Retirement: E-Records Migration 131
E-Records Archiving 132
E-Records Destruction 132
Additional Reading 132

10 Electronic Records Governance 133
Introduction 133
E-Records Integrity Strategy 135
E-Records Integrity Policy 136
E-Records Integrity Plan 136
E-Records Integrity Procedural Controls 138

E-Records Integrity Guidelines 138
Organization 138
E-Records Repository Inventory 139
Training 139
Enforcement 140
Additional Reading 141

11 Procedural Controls for Handling E-Records 143
Introduction 143
E-Records Integrity Procedural Controls 144
Other Related Procedural Controls: Operational Activities 147
Archiving 148
Backups 148
Business Continuity 149
E-Records Quality Control 149
E-records Storage 150
Infrastructure Maintenance 150
Problem Reporting 151
Problem Management 151
Retirement 151
Restore 152
Risk Management 152
Security 152
Training 153
Other Related Procedural Controls: Maintenance Activities 153
Verification and Revalidation 153
Change Control 154
Checks 154
Additional Readings 155

12 Electronic Record Controls: Supporting Processes 157
Business Continuity 157
Incident Management 158
Periodic Reviews 158
Personnel 159
Requirements Document 159
Risk Management 160
Security 162
Suppliers and Service Providers 166

Timestamping Controls 166
Additional Readings 167

13 **Electronic Records Controls: Records Retained by Computer Storage 169**
Introduction 169
E-Records Archiving 170
E-Records Migration 172
E-Records Storage 173
File Integrity Checking 175
E-Records Handling 176
Additional Readings 177

14 **Electronic Record Controls: During Processing 179**
Archiving 179
Audit Trails 179
Built-In Checks 181
Electronic Signature 181
Operational Checks 181
Printouts/Reports 182
Security 184

15 **Electronic Record Controls: While in Transit 185**
Qualification of IT Infrastructure 185
Built-In Checks 186
Accuracy Checks 188

16 **Electronic Records and Contract Manufacturers 189**
Additional Readings 191

17 **Electronic Records and Cloud Computing 193**
Additional Readings 199

18 **Self-Inspections 201**
Introduction 201
E-Records Self-Inspections 202
E-Records Remediation 204
Additional Reading 205

19 **Electronic Records Remediation Project 207**
Evaluate E-Records Controls 208
Corrective Action Planning 209

Remediation....210
Interpretation....211
Training....211
Remediation Execution....211
New Applications and Application Upgrade Assessments....212
Suppliers Qualification Program....212
Remediation Project Report....212
Additional Reading....212

20 Summary....213

Appendix I....219

Appendix II....251

Appendix III....255

Appendix IV....273

Appendix V....289

Appendix VI....299
R.D. McDOWALL, DIRECTOR, R.D. McDOWALL LTD.

Appendix VII....321
M. ROEMER, MANAGING DIRECTOR, COMES COMPLIANCE SERVICES

Appendix VIII....341

Appendix IX....353

Appendix X....357

Index....365

Foreword

Data integrity is one of the most pressing current concerns for GMP-regulated (Good Manufacturing Practices) companies worldwide. Regulators and health agencies have increasingly stressed the importance of the topic in guidance, citations, and public comments.

Good documentation, recordkeeping, and data integrity are an essential part of the pharmaceutical quality assurance system and vital to operating in compliance with GMP requirements and also, even more importantly, in protecting the quality of the product and the safety of the patient and the public.

Regulated companies must maintain and ensure the accuracy and consistency of data and records over their entire life cycle. A lack of acceptable data integrity practices has led to serious regulatory and financial consequences for many companies.

To all involved in the design, implementation, operation, or maintenance of computerized systems that collect, process, or archive GMP data, clear guidance on the regulatory requirements is invaluable.

Orlando Lopez has over 25 years of experience working with GMP-regulated systems, and has gathered great experience and knowledge during this time. He has published many books, articles, and papers, and has worked with many companies to achieve compliance and solve problems in a practical way.

For many years he has diligently collated, assessed, and compared international regulatory requirements for computerized system compliance and data integrity. He has been active in discussing and promoting the understanding of these regulations.

In this book he shares his valuable experience and knowledge with the industry as it struggles with this most important topic.

Sion Wyn
Conformity Limited, United Kingdom

Preface

The increased use of computer systems with both production systems and quality control systems relevant to medicines' manufacturing requires the understanding and application of the expectations of the regulatory agencies or competent authority on these systems.

> *When operating under a quality system, manufacturers develop and document control procedures to complete, secure, protect, and archive records, including data, which provide evidence of operational and quality system activities.*
>
> **US FDA Guidance for Industry Quality Systems Approach to Pharmaceutical CGMP Regulations**
>
> *September 2006*

One of the expectations applicable to computer systems performing production-related regulated functions is that the integrity in their electronic records* (e-records) takes the highest priority in any Worldwide Health Agency good manufacturing practices (GMPs). E-records integrity is the foundation of GMPs. Properly recorded electronic information is the basis for manufacturers to ensure product identity, strength, purity, and safety.† E-records also demonstrate that the manufacturer's process adheres to the GMPs, including instructions.

As a state or condition, e-records integrity is a measure of the validity and fidelity of a data object. E-records integrity is a requirement that information and programs are changed only in a specified and authorized manner. It is

* Electronic record: Information recorded in electronic form that requires a computer system to access or process (SAG, "A Guide to Archiving of Electronic Records", February 2014).

† Wechsler, J., *Data Integrity Key to GMP Compliance, Pharmaceutical Technology*, September 2014.

necessary that e-records be protected against alteration without appropriate permission.

> ***Data Integrity:*** *The property that data have not been altered in an unauthorized manner. Data integrity covers data in storage, during processing, and while in transit.*
>
> **NIST SP 800-33**

Since 2004, worldwide inspection trends have been absent on the integrity of critical e-records.* Of all the drug GMP warning letters issued in 2014 by United States Food and Drug Administration (US FDA) investigators, eight warning letters were related to e-records integrity issues.

By August 2014, European competent authorities issued six Statements of Noncompliance related to data integrity.

The reasons for this increased level of health authority concern include regulatory awareness regarding gaps between industry choices and appropriate and modern control strategies.†

Nevertheless, e-records integrity is not a new regulatory requirement, as basic e-records integrity principles are already described in any Worldwide Health Agency Good Manufacturing Practices (GMP) regulation and/or guidance. As an example, the US FDA 211.68(b) (1978 revision) and European Medicines Agency (EMA) Annex 11‡ (1992 revision) delimited the basic requirements for e-records integrity. The requirements for audits of data integrity during US FDA Pre-Approval inspections have been set in the Compliance Policy Guide (CPG) 7346.832.

E-records integrity controls maintain and ensure the accuracy and dependability of e-records over their entire life cycle, and it is a critical aspect in the design, implementation, and operation of any system that stores, maintains, and retrieves GMP-related records (i.e., regulated records in this book).

Lack of data integrity in critical e-records affects all areas of the Worldwide Health Agency GMP, good clinical practices (GCPs), good laboratory practices (GLPs), and many more.

---

* Critical electronic records: In this book critical e-records are interpreted as meaning e-records with high risk to product quality or patient safety (ISPE GAMP COP Annex 11—Interpretation, Pharmaceutical Engineering, July/August 2011).

† WHO, Guidance on Good Data and Record Management Practices, TRS 996 Annex 5, May 2016.

‡ EU, Good Manufacturing Practice, Annex 11 Computerized Systems, 1992.

This book covers the good e-records integrity practices (GEIPs) relevant to the Worldwide Health Agency GMP. It provides practical information to enable compliance with e-records integrity, while highlighting and efficiently integrating worldwide regulation into the subject. The ideas that are presented in this book are based on many years of experience in the regulated industries in various computer systems development, maintenance, and quality functions. Based on risk assessment principles, a practical approach is presented with the objective of guiding the readers around the technical and design e-records integrity controls recommended in worldwide regulations and guidelines.

Out of the scope of this book are the behavioral aspects of regulated life science industries that knowingly employ unreliable or unlawful activities.

I acknowledge Marcus Roemer and Dr. Bob McDowall for their contributions in this book.

Enjoy the reading. If you have any suggestion for improvement or questions, send them to olopez6102@msn.com.

Orlando López
E-Records Integrity SME

Author

Orlando López is the subject matter expert (SME) for the good automated manufacturing practices (GAMP) Data Integrity special interest group (SIG). He has over 25 years of experience in in the areas of worldwide pharmaceutical validation, Part 11 remediation, and European Medicines Agency (EMA) Annex 11 in the production and quality control systems relevant to the manufacture of medicinal products. He is an SME on electronic records integrity and worldwide regulations applicable to computer compliance. He has had papers published in the International Society for Pharmaceutical Engineering (ISPE'S) *Pharmaceutical Engineering, Pharmaceutical Technology* and *GXP Journal.*

His supplementary understanding includes international computer systems regulatory requirements and guidance including Australian, Japanese, World Health Organization (WHO), Pharmaceutical Inspection Co-Operation Scheme (PIC/S), and International Conference for Harmonization (ICH). He has directly participated in FDA agency remedial action plans, regulatory inspections, response activities, and consent decree remediation related verifications.

His practices include

- Validation/qualification of data warehouses (DW) and business intelligence (BI) environments
- Writing service-level agreements in DW/BI environments
- Computer systems validation and computer infrastructure qualification, and retrospective evaluation
- E-records integrity controls
- Integration of IT departments system life cycle (SLC) and computer systems validation (CSV) methodologies

He is the author of three other books: *21 CFR Part 11—A Complete Guide to International Compliance*, *Computer Infrastructure Qualification for FDA Regulatory Industries*, and *EU Annex 11 Guide to Computer Validation Compliance for the Worldwide Health Agency GMP*.

Disclaimer

The information contained in this book is provided in good faith and reflects the personal views of the GAMP Data Integrity SIG and ISPE. These views do not necessary reflect the perspective of the author's employer. No liability can be accepted in any way. The information provided does not constitute legal advice.

Contributors

R. D. McDowall is an analytical chemist with over 40 years of experience including 6 years as a forensic toxicologist, 15 years working in the pharmaceutical industry, and 24 years as a consultant specializing in process improvement, informatics, computer validation, data integrity, auditing, and interpretation of pharmaceutical regulations. His formal experience of computerized system validation started in 1986, and since then he has written on the topic and presented many short courses both in-house and publicly. Bob edited the first book on laboratory information management system (LIMS) in 1987 and has published extensively on the subject with over 60 published papers. In recognition of his input to the subject and teaching, the LIMS Institute presented him the 1997 LIMS Award. Bob is also the writer of the "Focus on Quality" column in *Spectroscopy* magazine and the "Questions of Quality" column in *LC-GC Europe*. He has written widely on the subject of electronic working and the use of electronic signatures and is also the author of a book, *Validation of Chromatography Data Systems*, published in 2005 and is currently writing a revised second edition due for publication at the end of 2016. He is currently director of R. D. McDowall Ltd, a post he has held since 1998, and was principal of McDowall Consulting (1993–2015) and a visiting research fellow at the University of Surrey, UK, from 1991 to 2001. Bob has contributed to the *GAMP Good Practice Guides on IT Infrastructure Control and Compliance* (2005); *Risk Based Validation of Laboratory Computerized Systems, Second Edition* (2012); and is an industry expert of the GAMP Data Integrity Special Interest Group core group.

Markus Roemer is managing director at Comes Compliance Services, Ravensburg, Germany. He is an auditor and IT validation expert, and manages business management compliance projects and support, the audit service center, and GMP compliance projects,. After studying physics, Markus started his career at Vetter Pharma Fertigung and joined Rockwell Automation Propack Data in 2001. He was Senior Validation Consultant at Invensys Validation Technologies, Montreal, Canada, and after that position then at Systec & Services GmbH and he also headed different local and global GMP Quality Compliance positions. Markus is a frequently invited speaker and trainer by organizations such as PTS (Pharmaceutical Training Services), ISPE and European qualified person (QP) Association at more than 100 events or training. In his current position as Managing Director at Comes Compliance Services, he is in charge of consultancy services for information technologies (IT) and pharmaceutical quality system (PQS) compliance. Since 2008 Markus has also been the ISPE Ambassador of the Deutschland/Österreich/Schweiz (DACH) Affiliate.

Chapter 1

Introduction

Global medicines regulatory systems include guidelines on the use of computer systems to conform to regulations governing medicine manufacturing practices and the applicable controls that must be in place to ensure the integrity of e-records throughout the retention period.

Currently, the integrity of e-records is a major global concern for, among others, the U.S. Food and Drug Administration (FDA), Australia's Therapeutic Goods Administration (TGA), Canada's Health Products and Food Branch Inspectorate, and European Regulatory Agencies. Multiple FDA Warning Letters and EU Good Manufacturing Practice (GMP) Noncompliance Reports (Chapter 2) have emphasized the volume of key e-records integrity failures in regulated life science industries.

Poor e-records integrity by regulated entities is considered to be a serious GMP deficiency. Such deficiencies demonstrate that quality control systems do not adequately ensure the integrity of the records generated and stored by these regulated entities.

In response to deficiencies in preapproval inspections (PAIs) documentation, the US FDA issued CPG 7346.832, which has been in effect since May 2012. CPG Objective 3 covers the authentication of data submitted in the Chemistry, Manufacturing, and Controls (CMC) section of the PAIs application, including audits of laboratory e-records integrity. In August 2014, the US FDA issued Level 2 guidance covering shared computer login authentication.*

* FDA, Questions and answers on current good manufacturing practices, good guidance practices, level 2 guidance: Records and reports, 2015, http://www.fda.gov/Drugs/GuidanceComplianceRegulatoryInformation/Guidances/ucm124787.htm.

In 2011, the European Medicines Agency (EMA) increased the number of clauses relating to e-records integrity in Annex 11 to the EU GMP guide (Chapter 6).

EMA Annex 11 was expanded by the Medicines and Healthcare Products Regulatory Agency (MHRA), Britain's Medicines and Medical Devices Regulatory Agency, to include the expectation that regulated life science industries must review the effectiveness of their governance systems (Chapter 10). The purpose of these reviews is to ensure data integrity and traceability. In March 2015, MHRA issued a second revision of the GMP Data Integrity Definitions and Guidance for Industry (Chapter 9). This guidance document outlines an e-records integrity governance program, and principles for defining quality and e-records integrity in processes and systems. In addition, the guidance document defines terms and provides associated expectations and examples for many of these (Chapter 4). The MHRA guidance document may be used to ensure a common understanding of terms and concepts.

As regulatory agencies and competent authorities tighten up their inspection requirements, it is important that managers, supervisors, and users in regulated entities understand the issues around e-records integrity. Improved governance programs must be implemented to ensure that computer systems performing GMP-regulated functions correctly process e-records.

This book is relevant to production and quality control systems used when manufacturing medicinal products. It provides practical information to enable e-records integrity regulatory requirements compliance, while highlighting best practice for e-records maintenance, associated risk-assessed controls, and e-records management.*

Chapter 2 summarizes examples of e-records integrity issues as documented by US FDA, Europa, Health Canada, and World Health Organization (WHO).

Chapter 3 discusses the e-records life cycle. This life cycle needs to be understood to effectively manage e-records and to ensure their integrity.

Chapter 4 reviews terms introduced by the GMP Data Integrity Definitions and Guidance for Industry, published by MHRA in 2015, in the context of a typical manufacturing environment. Appendices V through VII include examples of e-records for nonclinical laboratories, clinical systems, data warehousing, and business intelligence.

---

* Data handling: The process of ensuring that data is stored, archived, or disposed in a safe and secure manner during the data life cycle.

While GMPs vary globally, the e-records management requirements identified are broadly similar.* Chapters 5 through 7 discuss e-records controls in US FDA 21 CFR Part 211, EMA Annex 11, and other GMP-related regulations and guidelines.

Chapter 8 discusses the controls associated with trustworthy computer systems. To ensure the integrity of e-records, it is essential that the systems managing these e-records must also be trustworthy.

Chapter 9 analyzes MHRA Data Integrity Definitions and Guidance, the first guideline published by a regulatory agency.

Chapter 10 examines e-records integrity governance. This is a key element to effectively managing and maintaining e-records integrity.

The appropriate management of e-records requires a considered implementation of integrated system controls, some procedural (e.g., segregation of duties, standard operating procedures), some physical (e.g., different locations to establish redundancy), and some electronic (e.g., computer security rights and roles). Chapters 11 through 15 cover good data integrity practices (GDIP) to ensure e-records integrity (content, structure, and context). These practices are implemented via technical and procedural controls that are discussed in these chapters.

Chapters 16 and 17 address e-records in contract manufacturing and cloud service environments.

Chapter 18 addresses how internal audits can uncover e-records integrity issues.

Chapter 19 briefly discusses data integrity remediation activities.

Chapter 20 provides a summary of critical e-records integrity issues.

Appendix III contains a tabulated comparison between EMA Annex 11, 21 CFR Parts 11, 211 and 820, and many other global regulations.

To provide additional supporting information, this book references relevant abridged regulations and guidelines.

Rather than developing an industry standard, this book is intended to provide guidance on how the industry can effectively manage e-records and improve basic compliance.

With the exception of the definition of "Data Integrity," this book is consistent with the MHRA's data integrity guidance document.†

---

* GAMP®/ISPE, Risk Assessment for Use of Automated Systems Supporting Manufacturing Process: Risk to Record, *Pharmaceutical Engineering*, Nov/Dec 2002.

† MHRA, *MHRA GMP Data Integrity Definitions and Guidance for the Industry*, March 2015.

The recommendations on implementing controls to avoid issues with e-records integrity described in this book are the author's opinion. They are not intended to serve as official implementation processes as specified by regulatory agencies.

Additional Readings

MHRA, *MHRA expectation regarding self inspection and data integrity*, May 2014.

Sampson, K., *Data integrity*, The Food and Drug Law Institute, 6, 6–10, 2014. http://www.nxtbook.com/ygsreprints/FDLI/g46125_fdli_novdec2014/index.php#/0.

US FDA, FDA PAI *Compliance program guidance*, CPG 7346.832, Compliance *Program manual*, May 2010. http://www.ipqpubs.com/wp-content/uploads/2010/05/FDA_CPGM_7346.832.pdf.

Chapter 2

Inspection Trends*

Since 2004, inspection trends worldwide have focused on issues related to the integrity of e-records with the issue also coming to prominence in the United States since 2007 (Figure 2.1).

Three major cases on e-records integrity were reported in the United States in 2006 and 2007: Able Laboratories (2006), Leiner Healthcare Products (2007), and Actavis Totowa (2007).

The Actavis Totowa case related to inconsistencies between e-records and notebook data. The U.S. Food and Drug Administration (FDA) also recorded that there was no evidence of the manufacturer checking the accuracy of data files.

Based on 2007 inspection findings similar to the aforementioned, the US FDA has refocused on the integrity of e-records and enhanced staff training in this area.†

* López, O., Annex 11 and Electronic Records Integrity, in *EU Annex 11 Guide to Computer Validation Compliance for the Worldwide Health Agency GMP*, 1st edn, CRC Press, 2015, pp. 239–251.

† Budihandojo, R., Coates, R., Huber, L., Matos, J.E., Schmitt, S., David Stokes, D., Tinsley, G., Rios, M., A perspective on computer validation, *Pharmaceutical Technology*, July 2007.

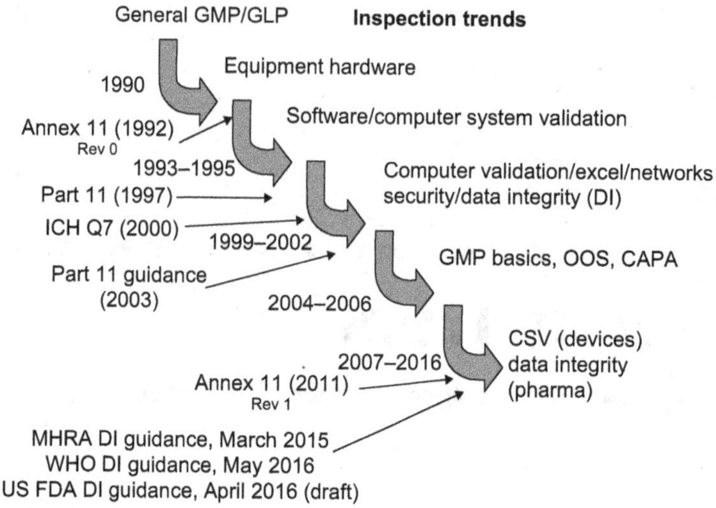

Figure 2.1 Inspection trends.

> *We are looking for integrity of your data, and the way we may check that is to look at audit trails to compare information provided in applications compared to on-site raw data.*
>
> **D. DiGuilio**
>
> *Facility Reviewer, Office of Process and Facilities in US FDA CDER's OPQ. Quality Management Network, 2015, Volume 7, No. 34*

The US FDA considers allegations of poor e-records integrity to be one of the most serious and damaging complaints that can be made against regulated users, as the US FDA needs to have confidence in the records that are provided to their inspectors.* Due to the possible associated public health issues resulting from poor management of e-records integrity, regulatory agencies or competent authorities focus their assessments on the integrity of e-records. Regulatory agencies or competent authorities also focus their interest on e-records integrity as deviations have a potential public health impact. Data integrity issues are central to current good manufacturing practice (CGMP) regulation.

* The Golden Sheet, Data integrity issues highlighted in FY 2007 warning letters, June 2008.

Health Canada considers that any findings that involve fraud, misrepresentation, or falsification of products or data is considered to be a critical observation.*

In 2014, Medicines and Healthcare Products Regulatory Agency (MHRA) and the FDA published separate reports demonstrating that the incidence of data integrity issues is increasing, with some very high profile cases having been detected in the industry in recent years.

Year	EMA	US FDA[a]
2013	Six statements of noncompliance related to data integrity were issued.	Eight of 26 warning letters (WLs) the agency issued to foreign manufacturers cited data integrity.
2014	Six statements of noncompliance (August 2014) related to data integrity were issued.	12 of 13 WLs issued up to July 2014 have found problems with data integrity.
2015 (Fiscal year)	—	13 of 43 drug good manufacturing practice (GMP) WLs have at least one observation related to e-records integrity. 10 of 43 drug GMP WLs were to active pharmaceutical ingredients (API) manufacturers. Two of 43 drug GMPs WLs were related to solid oral dosage forms. One of 43 drug GMPs WLs was related to injectable dosage forms.

[a] *QMN Weekly Bulletin* 6, 29.

In 2015, 10 API manufacturers from India (5), China (2), Canada (1), Thailand (1), and Czech Republic (1) received WLs from the US FDA.

The number of drug GMP warning letters that focus on data integrity has increased from two in 2010 to 13 in 2015. As of the publication of this book in 2016, there have been sixteen Non Compliance Reports posted on the EU site. Of those 16, five of the reports contain data integrity issues.

As a result of this interest by the regulatory agencies, the regulated life science industries were informed that there will be a greater focus on e-records integrity during regular inspections.

Table 2.1 depicts the recent regulatory citations for e-records integrity at the time of publication.

Table 2.1, 2013-16 Cases E-records Integrity, depicts the recent regulatory citations for e-records integrity at the time this book was to the publisher.

* Health Canada, Risk classification of good manufacturing practices (GMP) observations (GUI-0023), November 2012.

Table 2.1 2013–2016 Cases Relating to E-Records Integrity

Company Name	*Date*	*Type of Observation*	*Regulation*	*Note*
Hospira	Mar 2013	483	211.180(d)	Data Integrity. The raw data generated from the semiautomated thickness tester used to measure the thickness of perimeter seals on bags used as container closure systems for injectable drugs can be overwritten with new data without explanation and the original data is erased from the computer's memory when overwritten.
Gilead CA, United States	Apr 2013	483	–	Discrepancies with printed results. This data integrity issue is a repeated issue since July 2012.
Puget Sound Blood Center and Program	Apr 2013	WL	211.68(b)	Lack of I/O verification (data accuracy).
RPG Life Sciences Ltd	May 2013	WL	211.68(b)	The computer system being used for high performance liquid chromatography (HPLC) did not have adequate controls to prevent unrecorded changes to data.
Fresenius Kabi AG	Jul 2013	WL	API*	Unacceptable practices in the management of electronic data.
Aarti Drug Ltd	Jul 2013	WL	API	Failure to implement access controls and audit trails for laboratory computer systems.

Wockhardt Ltd	Jul 2013	Statement of noncompliance with GMPs	2003/94/EC (EU GMPs)	A critical deficiency was identified that compromised the integrity of analytical data produced by the quality control (QC) department. Evidence was seen of data falsification. A significant number of product stability data results reported in the product quality reviews had been fabricated. Neither hard copy nor electronic records were available. In addition, issues were seen with HPLC electronic data indicating unauthorized manipulation of data and incidents of unreported trial runs prior to reported analytical runs. (MHRA)
Wockhardt Ltd	Jul 2013	WL	211.194(a)	Failure to ensure that laboratory records included complete data derived from all tests necessary to ensure compliance with established specifications and standards.
Posh Chemicals Pvt Ltd	Aug 2013	WL	API	Failure to protect computerized data from unauthorized access or changes.
Agila Specialist Private Ltd	Sep 2013	WL	211.68(b)	The computer system being used for HPLC did not have adequate controls to prevent unrecorded changes to data.
Smruthi Organics Ltd	Oct 2013	Statement of noncompliance with GMPs	Article 47 of 2001/83/EEC	The agency observed manipulation and falsification of documents and data in different departments. There was no raw data available in the QC laboratory for the verification of compendial analytical methods. (French Health Products Safety Agency)

(Continued)

Table 2.1 (Continued) 2013–2016 Cases Relating to E-Records Integrity

Company Name	*Date*	*Type of Observation*	*Regulation*	*Note*
Ind-Swift Ltd	Oct 2013	Statement of noncompliance with GMPs	2003/94/EC (EU GMPs)	It was not possible to confirm the validity of stability testing data. Several falsified and inaccurate results had been reported in long-term stability and batch testing. Discrepancies between electronic data and those results formally reported were identified. Established processes to verify data accuracy and integrity had failed and there had been no formal investigation by the company. The company provided commitments to address the data integrity concerns and initiated a wider review of quality critical data. Additional discrepancies were identified in process validation and release data. During ongoing communications with the licensing authority regarding the data review, the company failed to disclose data integrity issues for all products. No satisfactory explanation was given for this discrepancy. (MHRA)
Zeta Analytical Ltd	Nov 2013	Statement of noncompliance with GMPs	European Union's GMP guideline	The computer system being used for HPLC did not have adequate controls to prevent unrecorded changes to data. (MHRA)
Wockhardt Ltd	Nov 2013	Statement of noncompliance with GMPs	Art. 111(7) of Directive 2001/83/EC as amended.	Entries were seen to be made when personnel were not present on site, documentation was seen that was not completed contemporaneously despite appearing to be completed in this manner. (Competent Authority of United Kingdom)

Wockhardt Ltd	Nov 2013	Statement of noncompliance with GMPs	2003/94/EC (EU GMPs)	The deficiency related to data integrity, deleted electronic files with no explanation. (MHRA)
Wockhardt Ltd	Nov 2013	WL	21 CFR Part 211.194(a), Part 211.68(b)	Failure to maintain complete data derived from all laboratory tests (Chikalthana facility). Inadequate control of computer systems (Waluj and Chikalthana facilities). The computer system being used for HPLC did not have adequate controls to prevent unrecorded changes to data.
Seikagaku Corporation	Dec 2013	Statement of noncompliance with GMPs	2003/94/EC (EU GMPs)	The critical deficiency concerns systematic rewriting/manipulation of documents, including QC raw data. The company has not been able to provide acceptable investigations and explanations of the differences seen in official and nonofficial versions of the same documents. (Competent Authority of Sweden)
Smruthi Organics Ltd	Jan 2014	Statement of noncompliance with GMPs	Article 47 of 2001/83/EEC	There was no raw data available in the QC laboratory for the verification of compendial analytical methods. (French Health Products Safety Agency)
Ranbaxy Laboratories, Inc.	Jan 2014	483	211.68(b)	The computer system being used for HPLC did not have adequate controls to prevent unrecorded changes to data.
Punjab Chemicals and Crop Corporation Ltd	Jan 2014	Statement of noncompliance with GMPs	Article 47 of 2001/83/EEC	One individual training file of an employee has been observed to be recently rewritten; the batch manufacturing record was lacking details about manufacturing steps and in-process controls; the sample retention log book for Trimethoprim had falsified entries. (French Health Products Safety Agency)

(*Continued*)

Table 2.1 (Continued) 2013–2016 Cases Relating to E-Records Integrity

Company Name	*Date*	*Type of Observation*	*Regulation*	*Note*
USV Ltd	Feb 2014	WL	211.68(b)	The computer system being used for the QC laboratory did not have adequate controls to prevent unrecorded changes to data.
Canton Laboratories Private Ltd	Feb 2014	WL	API	The computer system being used for the atomic absorption spectrophotometer did not have adequate controls to prevent unrecorded changes to data. Failure to maintain complete data derived from all laboratory tests.
SOMET	Mar 2014	Statement of non compliance with GMPs	Article 47 of 2001/83/EEC Article 51 of 2001/82/EC	Complete records of raw data generated during cleanliness tests by thin layer chromatography are missing. (French Health Products Safety Agency)
Smruthi Organics Ltd	Mar 2014	WL	API	Failure to maintain complete and accurate laboratory test data generated in the course of establishing compliance of your APIs to established specifications and standards.
Colorado Histo-Prep	Mar 2014	WL	58.81(b)(10)	Your firm failed to establish standard operating procedures (SOPs) describing the handling and retrieval of electronic data. Handling of electronic data includes the security (e.g., audit trails) and statistical analysis of raw data.

				Although you provided the US FDA Investigator with SOP H-31, "Server" and "Data Storage and Disaster Recovery," which describes the physical storage of electronic data in a central file server, your SOP lacks details concerning how you ensure the security of data, and how changes to the files are managed and documented. Furthermore, you failed to monitor access and record changes (via an audit trail) of electronic statistical data and statistical analyses. Thus, the quality and integrity of your data and analyses cannot be ensured.
Wockhardt Ltd	Mar 2014	Statement of noncompliance with GMPs	2003/94/EC (EU GMPs) Article 47 of 2001/83/EEC	A critical deficiency was cited with regard to data integrity of GMP records, entries were seen to be made when personnel were not present on site, and documentation was seen that was not completed contemporaneously despite appearing to be completed in this manner. (Competent Authority of United Kingdom)
Steris Corporation	May 2014	WL	820.70(i)	The application is set up to automatically discard any dosimeter absorbance readings outside the set operating range of *(b)(4)* to *(b)(4)* absorbance units.
Sun Pharmaceutical Industries Ltd	May 2014	WL	211.68(b)	Deleted raw data files on computers used for your gas chromatography (GC) instruments in your QC laboratory. Computer systems do not have security controls. As an example, there are several machines with PLC controls and/or man-machine interface (MMI). All equipment access is via use of a password for each of the three levels of access i.e., operator, supervisor, and administrator. A common password is used by several individuals.

(*Continued*)

Table 2.1 (Continued) 2013–2016 Cases Relating to E-Records Integrity

Company Name	*Date*	*Type of Observation*	*Regulation*	*Note*
Wockhardt Ltd Illinois	May 2014	483	211.68(b)	A general login on one computer allows data stored on the hard drives of these instruments to be changed or deleted by any user.
Micro Labs Ltd	May 2014	Notice of Concern (WHO)	WHO references 15.9, 17.3d, 15.1	HPLCs did not have audit trails enabled, some audit trails were missing when peaks were manually integrated, no SOP to describe when manual integration is acceptable. Some instruments had date and time functions unlocked and were not linked to a server, so time stamps could be manipulated. One HPLC had a shared password so actions were not attributable to a particular individual. In some cases, trial injections were carried out but were not included as part of the test record.
Mahendra Chemicals	May 2014	WL	API	Failure to prevent unauthorized access or changes to data, and to provide adequate controls to prevent omission of data. Your laboratory systems lacked access controls to prevent raw data from being deleted or altered. For example a. There is no assurance that you maintain complete electronic raw data for your GC instrument. US FDA investigators observed multiple copies of raw data files in the recycle bin connected to the GC instrument QC-04 even in the presence of "Do Not Delete Any Data" notes posted on two laboratory workstation computer monitors.

				b. Employees were allowed uncontrolled access to operating systems and data acquisition software tracking residual solvent, and test and moisture content. Our investigators noted that there was no password functionality to log into the operating system or the data acquisition software for the GC, or the HPLC instrument QC-17, or the Karl Fischer (KF) Titrator QC-13. c. HPLC SpinChrome and GC Lab Station data acquisition software lacked active audit trail functions to record changes in data, including original results, who made changes, and when. In your response, you state that your laboratory GC, HPLC, and KF systems are now password protected and that you have begun drafting analytical software password procedures for the GC, HPLC, and KF laboratory instruments. However, your response does not state whether every analyst will have their own user identification and password. You also mention plans to install a validated computer system. However, you did not provide a detailed corrective action and preventive action (CAPA) plan or conduct a review of the reliability of your historical data to ensure the quality of your products distributed to the US market.

(*Continued*)

Table 2.1 (Continued) 2013–2016 Cases Relating to E-Records Integrity

Company Name	*Date*	*Type of Observation*	*Regulation*	*Note*
				Inadequate controls of your computerized analytical systems raise questions about the authenticity and reliability of your data and the quality of your APIs. It is essential that your firm implements controls to prevent data omissions or alterations. It is critical that these controls record changes to existing data, such as the name of the individuals making changes, the dates, and the reasons for changes. In response to this letter, provide your comprehensive CAPA plan for ensuring that electronic data generated in your manufacturing operations, including laboratory testing, cannot be deleted or altered. Also identify your QC laboratory equipment and any other manufacturing-related equipment that may be affected by inadequate controls to prevent data manipulation.
Micro Labs Tamil Nadu	Not available	Not available	—	Data Integrity (Regulatory Partners)
Micro Labs Goa	Not available	Not available	—	Data Integrity (Regulatory Partners)
Micro Labs Bangalore	Not available	Not available	—	Data Integrity (Regulatory Partners)
Apotex Inc.	Jun 2014	WL	API	General lack of reliability and accuracy of data generated by your firm's laboratory, which is a serious CGMP deficiency that raises concerns about the integrity of all data generated by your firm.

				Failure to maintain complete data derived from all laboratory tests.
Apotex Pharmachem India Private Ltd (APIPL)	Not available	Not available		Data integrity. (Health Canada/Regulatory Partners)
Apotex Research Private Ltd (ARPL)	Not available	Not available		Data integrity. (Health Canada/Regulatory Partners)
Trifarma S.p.A.	Jul 2014	WL	API	Failure to maintain complete data derived from all laboratory tests. The firm deleted all electronic raw data supporting the company's HPLC testing. Failure to prevent unauthorized access or changes to data. The computer system grants all laboratory personnel full privileges to delete or alter raw data on the laboratory systems. At the time of the inspection, the company's HPLC and GC software had no audit trails to show when raw data was changed and who changed it.
Impax	Jul 2014	483	211.68(b)	The plant has two spectrophotometers that don't have adequate controls to ensure analysts cannot rewrite or delete analytical data. The systems are used for testing raw materials, stability and release.

(Continued)

Table 2.1 (Continued) 2013–2016 Cases Relating to E-Records Integrity

Company Name	*Date*	*Type of Observation*	*Regulation*	*Note*
Renown Pharmaceuticals Pvt Ltd	Aug 2014	Statement of noncompliance with GMPs	2003/94/EC (EU GMPs)	Record integrity and veracity: Some records were made up or altered. Lack of mechanisms to ensure integrity of analytical data. (Spanish Agency of Medicines and Medical Devices)
Hebei Dongfeng Pharmaceutical Co. Ltd	Aug 2014	Statement of noncompliance with GMPs	Article 47 of 2001/83/EEC	Data recording and integrity in the QC laboratory. (Competent Authority of Romania)
Fujian South Pharmaceutical	Sep 2014	Statement of noncompliance with GMPs	Art. 111(7) of Directive 2001/83/EC	The computerized systems in the QC department could not show whether approval of raw materials and final API was based on valid and accurate data. (Italian Medicines Agency)
Taishan City Chemical Pharmaceutical Co. Ltd	Sep 2014	Statement of noncompliance with GMPs	Article 47 of Directive 2001/83/EC	Insufficient securization of the electronic raw data in the QC laboratory (no limitation of access levels, no restriction on the deleting of data, no audit trail, inadequate traceability and archiving practices). (French Health Products Safety Agency)
Cadila Pharmaceuticals Ltd	Oct 2014	WL	API	Failure to prevent unauthorized access or changes to data, and to provide adequate controls to prevent omission of data.
Sharp Global Ltd	Oct 2014	WL	API	Printing batch records from personal computers over which the company lacked adequate controls. GCs didn't prevent the deletion or altering of raw data files, and lacked audit trails that record any changes to data. Sharp management told investigators that the company's practice was to delete raw data files once the chromatograms were printed.

				Failure to prevent unauthorized access or changes to data and to provide adequate controls to prevent omission of data.
Zhejiang Apeloa Kangyu Bio-Pharmaceutical Co. Ltd	Oct 2014	Statement of noncompliance with GMPs	Art. 80(7) of Directive 2001/82/EC	The company failed to establish a procedure to identify and validate GMP-relevant computerized systems in general. Two batch analysis reports for Colistin Sulfate proved to be manipulated. HPLC chromatograms had been copied from previous batches and renamed with different batch and file names. Several electronically stored HPLC runs had not been entered into the equipment logbooks. The origin of this data could not be clearly traced. Neither the individual workstation nor the central server had been adequately protected against uncontrolled deletion or change of data. The transfer of data between workstations and server was incomplete. No audit trail and no consistency checks had been implemented to prevent misuse of data.
Apotex Pharmachem Canada	Nov 2014	483	211.68(b)	Five cases of failure to prevent unauthorized access or changes to data.
Dr. Reddy's Laboratories	Nov 2014	483	211.68(b)	Computerized systems don't have proper controls in place to prevent unauthorized access or changes to data.

(*Continued*)

Table 2.1 (Continued) 2013–2016 Cases Relating to E-Records Integrity

Company Name	*Date*	*Type of Observation*	*Regulation*	*Note*
North China Pharmaceutical Group Semisyntech Co., Ltd	Nov 2014	Statement of noncompliance with GMPs	Article 47 of Directive 2001/83/EC and Article 51 of Directive 2001/82/EC	Manipulation and falsification of GMP documents (rewriting of records with change of content, an inconsistency of signatures, and dates in many records, etc.) were observed in different departments. Lack of data integrity in the QC laboratory (no access control, inadequate traceability and archiving practices, no audit trail, no restriction on the deleting of data, etc.) and falsification of the analytical results for residual solvents. (Competent Authority of France)
North China Pharmaceutical Group Semisyntech Co., Ltd	Not available	Not available	—	Data integrity. (Regulatory Partners)
GVK Biosciences	Dec 2014	—	—	Concerns over the quality of data from clinical trials conducted by GVK regulators in France, Germany, Belgium, and Luxembourg suspended the marketing approval of 25 generic drugs. (http://economictimes.indiatimes.com/industry/healthcare/biotech/pharmaceuticals/france-germany-suspend-some-drug-approvals-over-data-by-gvk-biosciences/articleshow/45392105.cms

				http://economictimes.indiatimes.com/industry/healthcare/biotech/pharmaceuticals/four-european-union-countries-suspend-authorisation-of-25-drugs-studied-at-gvk-biosciences/articleshow/45396530.cms)
Novacyl Wuxi Pharmaceutical Co., Ltd	Dec 2014	WL	API	Failure to manage laboratory systems with sufficient controls to ensure conformance to established specifications and prevent omission of data. Other significant deficiencies noted in your laboratory system include failure to use separate passwords for each analyst's access to the laboratory systems.
Sri Krishna Pharmaceuticals Ltd	Dec 2014	Statement of noncompliance with GMPs	Art. 111(7) of Directive 2001/83/EC as amended.	1. The company did not have a proper system in place to make sure that electronic raw data cannot be adulterated or deleted. Analysts routinely use the PC administrator privileges to set the controlling time and date settings back to overwrite previously collected failing and/or undesirable sample results. This practice is repeated until passing and/or desirable results are achieved. 2. Established laboratory control mechanisms are not followed. Electronic records are used, but they do not meet systems validation requirements to ensure that they are trustworthy, reliable and generally equivalent to paper records. (Italian Medicines Agency)
Sri Krishna Pharmaceuticals Ltd	Not available	Not available		Data integrity. (Source: Health Canada) (Regulatory partners)

(Continued)

Table 2.1 (Continued) 2013–2016 Cases Relating to E-Records Integrity

Company Name	*Date*	*Type of Observation*	*Regulation*	*Note*
North China Pharmaceutical Group Semisyntech Co., Ltd	Jan 2015	Statement of noncompliance with GMPs	Article 47 of Directive 2001/83/EC and Article 51 of Directive 2001/82/EC	No access control, inadequate traceability and archiving practices, no audit trail, and no restriction on the deleting of data. (French National Agency for Medicines and Health Products Safety)
Micro Labs Ltd (Solid oral dosage form)	Jan 2015	WL	21 CFR Part 211.68(b)	Failed to exercise appropriate controls over computer or related systems to ensure that only authorized personnel make changes in master production and control records, or other records.
Apotex Inc. (Solid oral dosage form)	Jan 2015	WL	21 CFR Part 211.68(b)	Inadequate control over computer systems.
Novacyl (Thailand) Ltd	Feb 2015	WL	API	Not retaining complete raw data from testing performed to ensure the quality of your APIs. Lack of proper controls in place to prevent the unauthorized manipulation of your laboratory's raw electronic data. The GC computer software lacked password protection allowing uncontrolled full access to all employees.

Cadila Pharmaceuticals Ltd	Feb 2015	WL	API	Failure to prevent unauthorized access or changes to data and to provide adequate controls to prevent omission of data. a. The inspection found that the audit trail feature for your GC instruments was not used until October 2013, even though your 2009 GC software validation included a satisfactory evaluation of the audit trail capability. b. There is no assurance that you maintain complete electronic raw data for the *(b)(4)* GC instruments, the Malvern particle size analyzer, and the ultraviolet (UV) spectrophotometer. Our inspection found that these instruments were connected to stand-alone computers that stored the data and that the data could be deleted. c. Prior to our inspection, your firm failed to have a backup system for the data generated by one of the *(b)(4)* Fourier transform infrared (IR) spectrometers, the polarimeter, the UV spectrophotometer, and the Malvern particle size analyzer.
Dr. Reddy's Laboratories	Not available	Not available	—	Data integrity. (Source: Health Canada) Regulatory partner.
IPCA Laboratories Ltd	Not available	Not available	—	Data integrity. (Source: Health Canada) Regulatory partner.
IPCA	Not available	Not available	—	Data integrity. (Source: Health Canada) Regulatory partner.

(*Continued*)

Table 2.1 (Continued) 2013–2016 Cases Relating to E-Records Integrity

Company Name	*Date*	*Type of Observation*	*Regulation*	*Note*
Polydrug Laboratories Pvt Ltd	Mar 2015	Statement of noncompliance with GMPs	Art. 111(7) of Directive 2001/83/EC as amended Art. 80(7) of Directive 2001/82/EC as amended	Deficient management of the computerized system. (Agency for Medicinal Products and Medical Devices of the Republic of Slovenia) A deficient GMP inspection report by the Slovenian Authority, caused a GMP noncompliance Report in EudraGMDP and the suspension of all CEPs of the company. The inspectors requested that the marketing authorization holders using APIs from Polydrug Laboratories to change their API supplier. Health Canada and the US FDA have used the GMP inspection report of the Slovenian Authority to decide on consequences for supplies to Canada and the United States. In June 2015, Health Canada issued a press release in which they requested Canadian importers to voluntarily quarantine drug products with APIs manufactured or tested by Polydrug Laboratories, in Ambarnath, Maharashtra, India, due to data integrity concerns. The US FDA has also issued an import alert. Products manufactured by Polydrug can no longer enter the US market due to serious GMP violations. It is very likely that the EU inspection was the initial trigger for actions taken by Canada and United States.
Hospira	Feb 2015	483	—	FDA 483 containing 14 observations mostly around responsibilities of the quality unit, e-records integrity (1), computer validation (1), and sterility.

Hospira (Injectables)	Mar 2015	WL	211.68(b) and 21CFR Part 211.194(a)	Your firm failed to exercise appropriate controls over computer or related systems to ensure that only authorized personnel make changes in master production and control records, and other records (21 CFR Part 211.68(b)). Your firm failed to ensure that laboratory records included complete data derived from all tests necessary to ensure compliance with established specifications and standards (21CFR Part 211.194(a)). In addition, violations (211.68(b) and 21CFR Part 211.194(a)), discuss similar documented violations in Hospira India, and state there is systemic violation at Hospira. It orders Hospira to implement specific global remediation action items.
Nosch Labs	April 2015	483	API	Nosch also lacked controls to ensure electronic records are equivalent to paper records and to prevent personnel from modifying or deleting information. The company did not return a request for comment by press time.
Yunnan Hande Bio-Tech. Co. Ltd	Apr 2015	WL	API	Failure to prevent unauthorized access or changes to data and to provide adequate controls to prevent omission of data in a laboratory IR spectrometer. It requests a "comprehensive" evaluation of the extent of the inaccuracy of the reported data. As part of your comprehensive evaluation, provide a detailed action plan to investigate the extent of the deficient documentation practices noted above.

(Continued)

Table 2.1 (Continued) 2013–2016 Cases Relating to E-Records Integrity

Company Name	*Date*	*Type of Observation*	*Regulation*	*Note*
VUAB Pharma	May 2015	WL	API	The second observation in the May 27, 2015 WL states that "Failure to prevent unauthorized access or changes to data and to provide adequate controls preventing data omissions." (In ICH Q7 GMP for API (10 Nov 2000) this observation is related to section 5.43) Your firm did not properly maintain a backup of HPLC chromatograms that form the basis of your product release decisions.
Megafine Pharma (Nashik)	May 2015	483	API	Manipulation of HPLC software "to obtain passing test results."
Minsheng Group Shaoxing Pharmaceutical Co. Ltd	May 2015	Statement of noncompliance with GMPs	Art. 111(7) of Directive 2001/83/EC	A major issue was found and related to the "no procedure in place for audit trail and there was no effective audit trail in place to determine any change or deletion of the chromatographic raw data." (French National Agency)
Zhejiang Hisun Pharma Company Ltd	Jun 2015	Not available	—	Data integrity. (Source: Health Canada) Regulatory partners.
Quest Life Science	Jun 2015	Notice of Concern (WHO)	Not available in the notice	The observation is related to the installation of Adobe Acrobat Editor in a QA station allowing the possibility of overwriting records with this software.

Wuxi Jida Pharmaceutical	Jun 2015	Statement of noncompliance with GMPs	Art. 111(7) of Directive 2001/83/EC as amended	Laboratory testing (deviation 28): Some deviations were found for the IR instrument, in particular that the IR software did not have controlled access via username and password and it was not forbidden to copy and rename files. (Italian Medicine Agency)
Parabolic Drugs Ltd	Jun 2015	Statement of noncompliance with GMPs	Art. 111(7) of Directive 2001/83/EC as amended	Falsification and security and integrity data. (Italian Medicine Agency)
Jinan Jinda Pharmaceutical	Jun 2015	Statement of noncompliance with GMPs	Art. 111(7) of Directive 2001/83/EC as amended	Breaches of data integrity in the context of HPLC analysis. (Italian Medicine Agency)
Jinan Jinda Pharmaceutical	—	Not available	Not available	Data integrity. (Source: Health Canada) Regulatory partners.
Mahendra Chemicals	Jul 2015	WL	API	The laboratory system lacked access controls to prevent the deletion or alteration of raw data and employees had uncontrolled access to operating systems and data acquisition software.
Mahendra Chemicals	—	Not available	Not available	Data integrity. (Source: Health Canada) Regulatory partners.
Agila Specialties Pvt Ltd Maylan	Aug 2015	WL	211.68(b)	Your firm failed to exercise appropriate controls over computer or related systems to ensure that only authorized personnel can change master production and control records, or other records (21 CFR Part 211.68(b)).

(Continued)

Table 2.1 (Continued) 2013–2016 Cases Relating to E-Records Integrity

Company Name	*Date*	*Type of Observation*	*Regulation*	*Note*
				Your Siemens computer-based BMS and NVPMS do not require passwords to access the network and servers. Your contractors' access is uncontrolled. Responsibilities for system administrators are undefined. This violation is recurrent (see above). On September 9, 2013, we cited your firm in WL 320-13-26 for failure to exercise appropriate controls over computer or related systems.
Svizara Labs Private Ltd	Sep 2015	Notice of Concern (WHO)	GMP or GCP	The company performed several analyses, e.g., with HPLC. However, there were no records and no data. These were found to be deleted for several test runs. Moreover, the company was not able to restore data that was archived or backed up for HPLC equipment.
Unimark Remedies Ltd	Sep 2015	WL	API	Failure to prevent unauthorized access or changes to data, and to provide adequate controls to prevent omission of data. (In ICH Q7 GMP for API [10 Nov 2000] this observation is related with section 5.43) Your laboratory systems lacked access controls to prevent raw data from being deleted or altered. For example:

				a. During the inspection, we noted that you had no unique usernames, passwords, or user access levels for analysts on multiple laboratory systems. All laboratory employees were granted full privileges to the computer systems. They could delete or alter chromatograms, methods, integration parameters, and data acquisition date and time stamps. You used data generated by these unprotected and uncontrolled systems to evaluate API quality. b. Multiple instruments had no audit trail functions to record data changes. We acknowledge your commitment to take corrective actions and preventive actions to ensure that your laboratory instruments and systems are fully compliant by January 15, 2015. In response to this letter, provide a copy of your system qualification to demonstrate that your electronic data systems prevent deletion and alteration of electronic data. Describe steps you will take (e.g., installing better systems or software) if your qualification efforts determine that the current system infrastructure does not ensure adequate data integrity. Explain the archival process your firm has implemented to address these issues and how you will evaluate the effectiveness of these corrections. Provide a detailed summary of the steps taken to train your personnel on the proper use of computerized systems.

(*Continued*)

Table 2.1 (Continued) 2013–2016 Cases Relating to E-Records Integrity

Company Name	*Date*	*Type of Observation*	*Regulation*	*Note*
				Failure to maintain *complete data derived from all testing and to ensure compliance with established specifications and standards.* Because you discarded necessary chromatographic information such as integration parameters and injection sequences from test records, you relied on incomplete records to evaluate the quality of your APIs and to determine whether your APIs conformed with established specifications and standards. For example: a. During the inspection, the investigator found no procedures for manual integration or review of electronic and printed analytical data for *(b)(4)* stability samples. Electronic integration parameters were not saved or recorded manually. When the next samples were analyzed, the previous parameters were overwritten during the subsequent analyses.
Iason Italia SRL	Oct 2015	Statement of noncompliance with GMPs	Art. 111(7) of Directive 2001/83/EC	Data integrity in the context of HPLC management, storage of materials, and documentation system. (Italian Medicines Agency)
Sandoz Private Ltd	Oct 2015	WL	211.68(b)	Your firm failed to exercise appropriate controls over computer or related systems to ensure that only authorized personnel make changes in master production and control records, or other records (21 CFR Part 211.68(b)).

				On August 25, 2014, we found there were no access restrictions to laboratory data generated by the *(b)(4)* instrument used to test and release raw materials and in-process drug products. Your laboratory computer systems lack necessary controls to prevent data tampering and to detect data that may have been compromised. We acknowledge that you are in the process of qualifying a new *(b)(4)* instrument. However, your response is still inadequate; you failed to evaluate the effects of potentially compromised data on release decisions that rely on data generated by this uncontrolled system. These examples are serious CGMP deficiencies and violations. They demonstrate that your quality system does not adequately ensure the accuracy and integrity of data generated and available at your facility. We strongly recommend that you hire a qualified third-party auditor/consultant with experience in detecting data integrity problems to help you come into compliance with CGMP regulations and statutory authorities.
Hubei Hongyuan Pharmaceutical Co., Ltd	Oct 2015	Statement of noncompliance with GMPs	Article 47 of Directive 2001/83/EC (API)	Two of 10 major deficiencies were related to data integrity, computer system validation, and change control. (Competent Authority of Czech Republic)

(*Continued*)

Table 2.1 (Continued) 2013–2016 Cases Relating to E-Records Integrity

Company Name	*Date*	*Type of Observation*	*Regulation*	*Note*
Dr. Reddy's Laboratories	Nov 2015	WL	API	Failure to prevent unauthorized access or changes to data, and to provide adequate controls to prevent omission of data, e.g., HPLC systems are configured so that no passwords are required to log in and no access controls to prevent alteration or deletion of data. Provide specific details of the steps you have taken to prevent unauthorized access to your electronic data systems and to ensure that data systems retain complete, accurate, reliable, and traceable results of analyses performed. Failure to prevent unauthorized access or changes to data. During the inspection, we found that QC laboratory analysts were authorized to release finished product in your firm's computerized SAP inventory management system. Release or rejection of finished product is a nondelegable responsibility of the quality unit, and cannot be shared with laboratory analysts or other personnel. However, your SAP system permitted QC laboratory analysts to release intermediates from one process to the next process, as well as to release finished product into the market without requiring quality unit oversight.
Sun Pharmaceuticals Industries Ltd	Nov 2015	WL	211.68(b)	Observation 6. "Your firm failed to establish appropriate controls over computers and related systems to ensure that changes in master production and control records or other records are instituted only by authorized personnel (21 CFR Part 211. 68(b)).

				You lacked audit trails or other sufficient controls to facilitate traceability of the individuals who access each of the programmable logic controller (PLC) levels or man-machine interface (MMI) equipment. You had no way to verify that individuals have not changed, adjusted, or modified equipment operation parameters. Access to production equipment used in parenteral manufacturing and solid (b)(4) dosage forms used a password shared by four or five individuals to gain access to each individual piece of equipment and access level. During our inspection, your Executive Production and QA manager confirmed that the password was shared. Neither your operators nor your supervisors had individual passwords. During our inspection, firm officials also confirmed that you had not established or documented a control program to describe the roles and responsibilities of production equipment system administrators. There was also no record documenting the individuals who have access to the production equipment or the manner in which individual personnel access production equipment."

(*Continued*)

Table 2.1 (Continued) 2013–2016 Cases Relating to E-Records Integrity

Company Name	*Date*	*Type of Observation*	*Regulation*	*Note*
Cadila Healthcare Ltd India (Zyfine)	Dec 2015	WL	API	Your firm failed to exercise sufficient controls over computerized systems to prevent unauthorized access or changes to data. Your firm failed to adequately control the use of computerized systems in the QC laboratory. Our inspection team found that the laboratory manager had the ability to delete data from the KF Tiamo software. During our limited review of your KF data, we found that one file had been deleted. However, because the audit trail function for the KF Tiamo software was not activated, and because eight different analysts share a single username and password, you were unable to demonstrate who performed each operation on this instrument system. You do not have a record of the acquisition of all data, nor do you have records of changes to or modifications of such data.
Wockhardt Ltd	Jan 2016	483		Multiple data files had been deleted from some machines.
Ipca Laboratories Ltd	Jan 2016	WL	211.68(b) and 211.194(a)	Failure to have computerized systems with sufficient controls to prevent unauthorized access or changes to data (Ratlam facility). Your firm failed to ensure that laboratory records include complete data derived from all tests necessary to ensure compliance with established specifications and standards. (21 CFR Part 211.194(a)) (Pithampur and Piparia Silvassa).

Farma Mediterrania, S.L	Jan 2016	Statement of Non-Compliance to GMPs	Art. 111(7) of Directive 2001/83/EC as amended Art. 80(7) of Directive 2001/82/EC as amended Art. 15 of Directive 2001/20/EC	Use in quality control a non-qualified chromatography equipment, with operating faults and an with an unvalidated computerized management system. As a result, the integrity, reliability, up-to-dateness, originality and authenticity of the data that are obtained cannot be guarantee. (Spanish Agency of Medicines and Medical Devices)
Rusa Pharma LTD	Jan 2016	Statement of Non-Compliance to GMPs	Art. 111(7) of Directive 2001/83/EC as amended Art. 80(7) of Directive 2001/82/EC as amended Art. 15 of Directive 2001/20/EC	No adequate evidence that the root causes of critical data integrity issues raised at the last inspection had been addressed. The control of electronic data and laboratory systems was not adequately robust and could not assure data traceability or security. (The competent authority of United Kingdom)
Cadila Healthcare Limited	Jan 2016	A Letter of Concern (WHO) GMP		Inaccuracies on environmental monitoring area. For the reason that these inaccuracies are related with a vaccine manufacturing facility, the environment issues are critical and generated a full investigation around the authentication of data for its traceability, accuracy and reliability. The action items associated with this investigation are discussed in this Letter of Concern.

(Continued)

Table 2.1 (Continued) 2013–2016 Cases Relating to E-Records Integrity

Company Name	*Date*	*Type of Observation*	*Regulation*	*Note*
Bend Research Inc.	Feb 2016	Statement of Non-Compliance to GMPs	Art. 111(7) of Directive 2001/83/EC as amended Art. 80(7) of Directive 2001/82/EC as amended Art. 15 of Directive 2001/20/EC	One major deficiency concerns data integrity. (The competent authority of Sweden)
Emcure Pharmaceuticals Ltd	Mar 2016	WL	211.194(a)	Your firm failed to ensure that laboratory records included complete data derived from all tests necessary to assure compliance with established specifications and standards (21 CFR 211.194(a)). (Spanish Agency of Medicines and Medical Devices)

Note: 2013–2016 cases e-records integrity, depicts the recent regulatory citations for e-records integrity at the time this book was sent to the publisher.

*US FDA, CPG 7356.002F, API Process Inspection, February 2006, requires the inspection of "quality and retention of raw data (e.g., chromatograms and spectra)." Laboratory Control records in US FDA Guidance for Industry Q7 GMP Guidance for API (August 2011) indicates that "laboratory control records should include complete data derived from all tests conducted to ensure compliance with established specifications and standards, including examinations and assays."

The deficiencies found in recent cases of poor e-records integrity include

- Insufficient controls on security
- Inconsistencies between e-records and paper-based records
- Ability of computer users to delete laboratory analysis data
- Disabling of software audit trail functions
- Lack of record-keeping for the acquisition, or modification, of laboratory data
- Shared systems login IDs
- No procedures in place for the backup and protection of data on stand-alone workstations
- Shared usernames and passwords for the Windows operating system
- Lack of computer locks to prevent unauthorized access to operating systems
- Unauthorized access to computer systems
- Unauthorized changes to data

Such e-records integrity issues, as uncovered by the regulatory agencies and competent authorities, have renewed industry dialogue on this topic.

The publication of the US FDA Code of Federal Regulations Title 21 Part 11, Electronic Records: Electronic Signatures and associated technologies has contributed to a better understanding by regulatory agencies, competent authorities, and the industry, and therefore has led to an increased focus on e-records integrity.

Additional Readings

Cosgrove, T., Data integrity, paper presented at the Third Annual ISPE-FDA CMP Conference, Baltimore, Maryland, 2–4 June 2014.

EudraGMDP, EMA: Noncompliance reports. http://eudragmdp.ema.europa.eu/inspections/gmpc/searchGMPNoncompliance.do.

FDA, U.S. and UK cite data integrity as compliance issue on the rise, *QMN Weekly Bulletin* 7, 33, 2015.

Health Canada, Inspection tracker: Drug manufacturing establishments, 2015, http://www.hc-sc.gc.ca/dhp-mps/pubs/compli-conform/tracker-suivi-eng.php.

US FDA, Inspections, compliance, enforcement, and criminal investigations, warning letters. http://www.fda.gov/ICECI/EnforcementActions/WarningLetters/default.htm

WHO (World Health Organization). Inspections, notices of concern. http://apps.who.int/prequal/assessment_inspect/info_inspection.htm#6.

Chapter 3

Electronic Records Life Cycle*

Introduction

E-records, as information objects, have a life cycle that begins "from initial data generation and recording, through processing (including transformation or migration), use, retention, archiving, and retrieval."†

The life cycle is needed to understand the controls necessary to properly manage e-records and ensure their integrity. Failure to address just one element of the data life cycle will weaken the effectiveness of the computer control systems‡ and the e-records integrity–related controls.

Figure 3.1 depicts a typical data life cycle.§ The typical stages associated with the e-records life cycle are: creation, access, use and reuse, migration, and physical deletion.

Note that the business requirements that underlie the e-records handling requirements drive the selection of appropriate supporting technologies. The technologies pose questions associated with ongoing internal and external secondary access to records, support the selection of appropriate technologies, and identify important system migration issues.

* López, O., Electronic records lifecycle, *Journal of GxP Compliance*, 19, 4, November 2015.

† MHRA, MHRA GMP data integrity definitions and guidance for industry, March 2015.

‡ Ibid.

§ ISPE/PDA, Good electronic records management (GERM), Figure 4.3, July 2002.

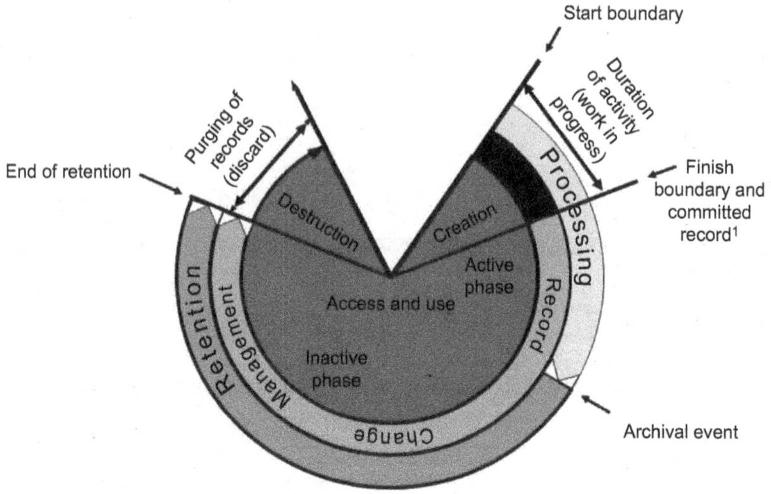

Figure 3.1 Typical data life cycle.

Creation

Initial e-records are generated during the Creation Stage as the result of activities. Some activities have defined boundaries. This means they have a start and an end point, during which information is recorded either by human action or by technology, such as process control and data acquisition, on a real-time basis.

There are two important elements during the Creation Stage. One, whether the raw e-records meets the requirements defined by business policy, governmental regulations, and by law. Two, that the raw e-record is correct, reliable, and accurately represents the particular activity recorded.

The "data" collected during the Creation Stage is considered to be "work in process" similar to draft documents.

An e-record becomes a CGMP record when the e-record is generated to satisfy a CGMP requirement. The e-record must save "the data at the time of performance to create a record in compliance with CGMP requirements."*

Access, Use, and Reuse

During the Access, Use, and Reuse Stage the records are stored and accessed for information on the particular activities they document. During the period of record-keeping, information must be authentic, trustworthy, and reliable

* US FDA, Guidance for industry: Data integrity and compliance with CGMP guidance for industry, (Draft) April 2016.

to inform the work of the principal stakeholders. During this period, it is important that the recorded information is stored in either processing (initial creation of records) or retention (storage of records) environments.

According to Medicines and Healthcare Products Regulatory Agency (MHRA) terminology, the data in the processing environment is raw data, whereas the data in the retention environment is known as a true copy.

Records retained in original processing environments are accessible by the tools and mechanisms used to create them. This means the raw data is easily modified. Although records are retained in their original processing environment, record authenticity, trustworthiness, and reliability are not solely a function of record access, but also access to tools and mechanisms associated with the creation of the original data. Should records require modification, it is imperative that compulsory change documentation procedures are in place to preserve an audit trail of changes throughout the period of time specified by the retention schedule.

This process also applies to record removal, should records be discarded before the period of time stipulated by the retention schedule. An audit trail should record the deletion event and the rationale for early disposal of records. Records are filed in record-keeping environments to preserve their integrity over the entire retention period. Within this environment, records may be reformatted for use with other software, different from that used to create the original data files. This approach maintains the integrity of the original files. However, retention environments can also be designed for use with the original processing tools to access stored records; in this case, it is essential that additional controls are used to secure the integrity of the original information.

Raw data that is transformed and placed in retention environments, separate from those used for original creation, should preserve the integrity of the source record and the protection mechanisms used to prevent informational loss and/or corruption. If records require modification in retention environments, it is essential that change documentation procedures are implemented to preserve an audit trail of change, or replacement, including the deletion of records.

Records that are transformed and placed in retention environments are referred to as data in MHRA terminology.

Once e-records have been transferred and placed in a retention environment, the e-records should never be directly modified. In the case of a modification in the retention environment, the same modification must first be performed to the record in the processing environment. The updated data set should then be uploaded to the retention environment using the same automated tool/interface used to load the records from the processing environment to the retention environment. If technical limitations require the e-record be modified in the retention environment, the change must be linked to the same alteration in the processing environment.

The primary purpose of e-records retention is to ensure authenticity, readability, and preservation of the data prepared by, and stored in, the computer system during the retention period stipulated by the retention schedule.*

Migration†

Data migration is the transporting of e-records from one system to another, or the transition of data from one state to another. It can occur either in the active or inactive phase of the e-records life cycle.

If system obsolescence forces a need to transfer e-records from one system to another, the process must be well documented and its integrity verified. If e-records are transferred to another data format or system, validation should include checks that data is not altered in value and/or meaning during data migration. Conversion of data to a different format is also considered to be data migration.

Migrated data should remain usable and retain its content and meaning. Risk assessment is a key instrument in data migration. The system owner should ensure system audit trails, electronic signatures, and metadata remain intact after migration. It is the system owner's responsibility to maintain the link between the readable audit trail, electronic signatures or metadata, and the audited data.

Transformation

Transformation of data can happen in two ways:

Over-rides: A program may be such that the sequence of program events or program edits can be over-ridden by the operator or automated. Any allowed over-rides must be under procedural control

* Ministry of Health, Labor and Welfare of Japan, Questions and answers (Q and A) regarding Guideline on management of computerized systems for marketing authorization holders and manufacturers of drugs and quasi-drugs, October 2010.

† OECD, The application of GLP principles to computerized systems, OECD Guidance Document (Draft), September 2014.

and, in case of operator over-ride, subject to audit trail. The over-ride procedural control should include error verification and correction verification. One area of concern in over-rides is the impact of over-rides at one computer related to operations at another computer in the system. The limits on information and command for distributed system should be clearly established by the regulated firm.

Integration: In typical data warehouses and business intelligence environments, the integration of e-records is performed. Each e-record to be integrated comes from difference sources. These rules, that are considered operational checks, are applied in order to prepare the data for loading into the end target (e.g., data mart). The transformation processing must be validated and changes must be controlled and tested. To maintain the e-records integrity in the integration of e-records, altering methods to reprocess will require a secured audit trail functionality, data, and access security.

See Appendix VIII for further information.

Physical Deletion

During the Physical Deletion Stage, company records that meet the approved retention time are tagged for deletion and removed in accordance with the approved procedures. The documentation that is purged typically includes content, metadata, audit trails, any pointers to the record, and links to related records. The associated records in the retention environment must also be simultaneously eliminated.

When a record is deleted prior to the date specified by the retention schedule, it is best practice to maintain an audit trail of the deletion until the end of the approved retention period.

Current good practice also includes, as part of a company's records handling program, a periodic review of approved retention periods of specific records in response to changing business, regulatory, or legal requirements. It is important, from a legal perspective, to remember that record handling programs include defined provisions to temporarily suspend the execution of a purge process (including backup tapes) if records are part of a legal discovery process during a pending litigation.

E-Records and Computer Systems Life Cycles

Table 3.1 compares the e-records and computer systems life cycles. In addition it shows how e-records are automatically created in a new computer system when data is migrated from a legacy, or other source, system.

All the repositories holding the e-records and associated records handling function are implemented as part of the software development.

Table 3.1 shows how e-records created before the retirement of a computer system can have a separate life expectancy. E-records that are not retired at the same time as the associated e-records managing system(s)

Table 3.1 E-Records and Computer Systems Life Cycles

	Computer Systems Life Cycle	*E-Records Life Cycle*
Definition	All phases in the life of the computer system from initial requirements until retirement including design, specification, programming, testing, installation, operation, and maintenance.	The E-records life cycle consists of all phases from initial generation and recording through processing (including transformation or migration), use, e-records retention, archive/retrieval, and physical deletion.
Requirements	√	Potential E-records migration requirements.
Design	√	E-records repository and security design.
Programming	√	Implementation of repository and security.
Testing	√	√
Installation	√	Potential E-records migration. (Creation)
Operation	√	√ (Creation, Access, Use, and Reuse)
Computer systems retirement	√	
E-records migration		√
E-records retirement		√

retire subsequently, upon completion of the e-records retention schedule. A preservation plan should be implemented that can include one of the following options.*

- Ensure that the new system will be able to retrieve the e-records from the retired computer system
- Maintain the previous application(s) that prepared the preserved electronic records.

Additional Readings

GAMP®/ISPE, Risk assessment for use of automated systems supporting manufacturing process: Risk to record, *Pharmaceutical Engineering*, Nov/Dec 2002.

ISPE/PDA, Good electronic records management (GERM), July 2002.

MHRA, MHRA GMP data integrity definitions and guidance for industry, March 2015.

Wyn, S., Data integrity throughout the computerized system lifecycle, paper presented at the Third Annual ISPE-FDA CMP Conference, Baltimore, Maryland, 2–4 June 2014.

* CEFIC, Computer validation guide, API Committee of CEFIC, January 2003.

Chapter 4

Electronic Records Related Definitions

Introduction

Centered on e-records integrity, the British Medicines and Healthcare Products Regulatory Agency (MHRA) is one of the first regulatory agencies to publish a broad data integrity guideline document.*

The Data Integrity Definitions and Guidance for Industry outlines data integrity governance and principles, defining elements to evaluate data (paper and e-records) integrity. The MHRA has interpreted the existing good manufacturing practices (GMP) requirements for e-records integrity contained in the European Medicines Agency (EMA) Annex 11† GMP guidelines.

One example of the MHRA guidance, enhancing the EU Annex 11, is the definition of raw data. The EU GMP Chapter 4‡ does not define the term *raw data,* but it is defined in the MHRA guidance document.

The MHRA guidance document also provides additional data-related terminology.

Using, as an example, a fully automated manufacturing system, this chapter discusses the data terminology introduced by the MHRA's Data Integrity Definitions and Guidance for Industry.

* MHRA, MHRA GMP data integrity definitions and guidance for industry, March 2015.

† EudraLex, Vol.4, *Good Manufacturing Practice, Medicinal Products for Human and Veterinary Use*—Annex 11: Computerized systems, European Commission, Brussels, June, pp. 1–4, 2011.

‡ EudraLex,Vol.4, *Good Manufacturing Practice, Medicinal Products for Human and Veterinary Use*, Chapter 4: Documentation, June 2011.

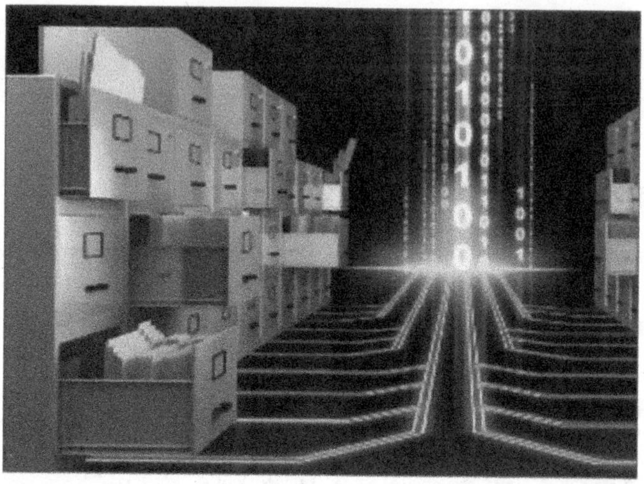

Beyond the scope of this chapter are the data integrity issues discussed in the MHRA guidelines. The data integrity–related issues and controls can be found elsewhere in this book.*

Data Terminology

The following are the terms introduced by MHRA in its Data Integrity Definitions and Guidance for Industry. These terms ensure a common understanding of usage in this book as well.

Term	*MHRA Definition*
Data	Information derived or obtained from raw data (e.g., a reported analytical result).
Original record	Data as the file or format in which it was originally generated, preserving the integrity (accuracy, completeness, content, and meaning) of the record, e.g., original paper record of manual observation or electronic raw data file from a computerized system.
Primary record	The record that takes primacy in cases where data that is collected and retained concurrently by more than one method fails to concur.

* Refer to Chapters 11 through 15 in this book.

Term	*MHRA Definition*
Raw data	Original records and documentation retained in the format in which they were originally generated (i.e., paper or electronic), or as a "true copy." Raw data must be contemporaneously and accurately recorded by permanent means. In the case of basic electronic equipment, which does not store electronic data, or provides only a printed data output (e.g., balance or pH meter), the printout constitutes the raw data.
True copy	An exact verified copy of an original record. Data may be static (e.g., a "fixed" record such as paper or pdf) or dynamic (e.g., an e-record that the user/reviewer can interact with).\

The following terms are included in this chapter as references. These terms can be compared with MHRA terminology.

Term	*Definition*
Certified copy	A copy of original information that has been verified, as indicated by a dated signature, as an exact copy having all of the same attributes and information as the original. *Source:* US FDA, Electronic Source Data in Clinical Investigations, September, 2013.
Certified copy	A copy of original information that has been verified as an exact (accurate and complete) copy having all of the same attributes, and information, as the original. The copy may be verified by dated signature or by a validated electronic process. *Source:* CDISC, (Clinical Data Interchange Standards Consortium) Clinical Research Glossary Version 8.0, December, 2009.
Critical data	Data with high risk to product quality or patient safety. *Source:* ISPE GAMP COP, Annex 11 Interpretation, July/August, 2011.
Electronic source data	Data initially recorded in electronic format. *Source:* US FDA CFR, Electronic Source Data in Clinical Investigations, September, 2013.
Raw data	All data on which quality decisions are based should be defined as raw data. It includes data that is used to generate other records. *Source:* EudraLex, Vol. 4, *Good Manufacturing Practice Medicinal Products for Human and Veterinary Use*, Chapter 4, June, 2011.

(*Continued*)

(*Continued*)

Term	*Definition*
Raw data	Any laboratory worksheets, records, memoranda, notes, or exact copies thereof, that are the result of original observations and activities of a non clinical laboratory study, and are necessary for the reconstruction and evaluation of the report of that study. In the event that exact transcripts of raw data have been prepared (e.g., tapes which have been transcribed verbatim, dated, and verified accurate by signature), the exact copy or exact transcript may be substituted for the original source as raw data. Raw data may include photographs, microfilm or microfiche copies, computer printouts, magnetic media, including dictated observations, and recorded data from automated instruments. *Source:* US FDA, Code of Federal Regulations, title 21, Vol. 1, part 58, subpart A, section 58.3(k), April, 2015.
Records	Records are made, manually and/or by recording instruments, during manufacture which demonstrate that all the steps required by the defined procedures and instructions were in fact taken and that the quantity and quality of the product was as expected. *Source:* EudraLex,Vol. 4, *Good Manufacturing Practice Medicinal Products for Human and Veterinary Use*, Chapter 1, June, 2011.
Records	Provide evidence of various actions taken to demonstrate compliance with instructions, for example, activities, events, investigations, and in the case of manufactured batches, a history of each batch of product, including its distribution. Records include the raw data, which are used to generate other records. For data regulated users should define which data are to be used as raw data. At least, all data, on which quality decisions are based, should be defined as raw data. *Source:* EudraLex,Vol. 4, *Good Manufacturing Practice Medicinal Products for Human and Veterinary Use*, Chapter 4, June, 2011.
Source data	All information in original records, and certified copies of original records of clinical findings, observations, or other activities in a clinical trial, necessary for the reconstruction and evaluation of the trial. Source data are contained in source documents (original records or certified copies). *Source:* EMA/INS/GCP/454280/2010 (GCP IWG), June, 2010.
Source data	All information in original records and certified copies of original records of clinical findings, observations, or other activities (in a clinical investigation) used for the reconstruction and evaluation of the trial. Source data are contained in source documents (original records or certified copies). *Source:* US FDA CFR, Electronic Source Data in Clinical Investigations, September, 2013.

Introduction to Automated Manufacturing System

Figure 4.1 depicts a total integrated manufacturing system, from plant floor all the way through the enterprise level.

In manufacturing systems, e-records integrity supports process reliability by making a regulated product of specified safety and quality. In nonclinical laboratory systems supporting GMP operations, both data capture and database management systems are used for product analysis studies. The integrity of e-records is an essential quality component in manufacturing.

In a plant floor environment, sensors, limit switches, and other control components, send information to diagnostic systems and control-based monitoring systems. These, in turn, send raw data to systems that manage maintenance, modeling, scheduling, tracking, and batching operations.

Cell controllers are used to control manufacturing process and data acquisition. In their most basic form, cell controller systems process inputs and direct outputs. Everything else is simply an activity, supporting inputs and outputs (I/Os).*

The primary concern of a cell controller is to perform precisely in the intended environment. Performing precisely in the intended environment is essential to ensure proper functioning of the process to manufacture quality product. The quality of the product is established by following the

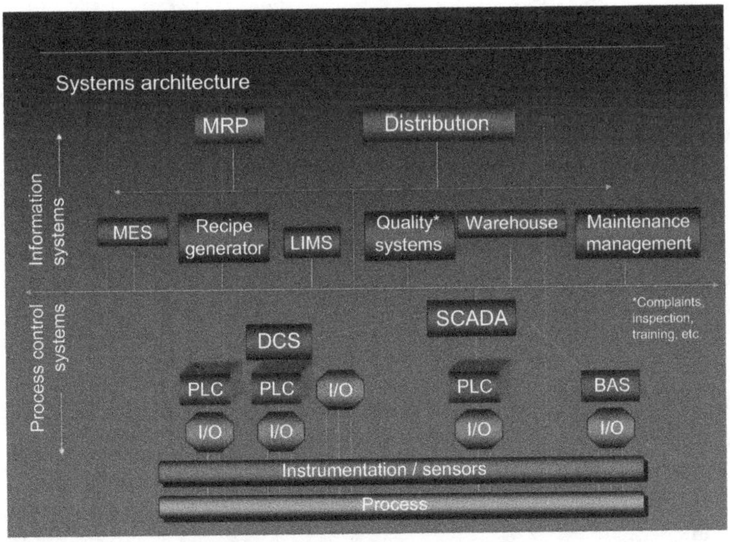

Figure 4.1 Total integrated manufacturing system.

* Snyder, D., Take advantage of control options, *A-B Journal*, March 1997.

determined sequence of operations and evaluating samples from the associated manufacturing batch by use of laboratory equipment and other type of verifications. The records of the history of each batch of product and/or associated utility are used to verify if the process was followed as established.

Cell controllers fall into a specific category, such as a distributed control system (DCS), a programmable logic controller (PLC), or supervisory control and data acquisition (SCADA). SCADA systems are typically used for collection.

SCADA systems are responsible for processing environment storage and handling manufacturing-related e-records, but they are not usually responsible for final storage.

In the context of this chapter the manufacturing execution system (MES) in Figure 4.1, is the other important element to consider.

MES tracks and documents the transformation of raw materials through finished goods. It works in real time to enable the control of multiple elements of the production process (e.g., inputs, personnel, machines, and support services). The server containing the MES application or accessed by the MES, may be used as the short retention environment.

In addition to the real-time controls provided by the MES, it creates the "as-built" record, capturing e-records, processes, and outcomes of the manufacturing process. This can be especially important in GMP-regulated activities,* where documentation, proof of processes, events, and actions are required.

MES is an intermediate step, between a manufacturing resource planning (MRP) system and a SCADA, or process control system, although historically, exact boundaries have fluctuated.

To understand the risk associated with the entire path that e-records follow, and where manipulations of those e-records can take place, it is important to describe the entire path. This description could start from the sensor in the field, and go as far as the MES "as-built" e-records and beyond.

The integration of all control and enterprise computer systems maximizes resources by identifying "common" solutions to manage the e-records. This integration is established by the ISA SP95, S88.01,† and S88.02‡ standards.

* In this book "GMP-regulated activities" is defined as the manufacturing-related activities established in the basic legislation compiled in Vol. 1 and Vol. 5 of *The Rules Governing Medicinal Products in the European Union*. http://ec.europa.eu/health/documents/eudralex/index_en.htm, and US FDA CFR, Title 21, Part 211, or any predicate rule applicable to medicinal products for the referenced country.

† International Society for Measurement and Control (ISA) Batch Control Standard (S88.01) defines a common set of models and terms for the design and operation of batch process control systems.

‡ S88.02 standard includes a section that defined the communication requirements between the functions of recipe procedure execution and equipment control.

How Are MHRA Definitions Applicable?

The automated enterprise and process control environments, explained before, illustrates the terminology introduced by the MHRA.

In this book, based on the MHRA definitions, "raw data" and "data," are considered to be e-records. When both are referred to (i.e., electronic raw data, and data) this book uses the term *e-records.*

Figure 4.2 depicts a simplified data flow diagram for a typical manufacturing system.

The SCADA system collects the raw data sent by the PLC, DCS, Building Automation System (BAS), and many other systems.

At the PLC level, the analog data is extracted from the PLC memory, transformed (digitized, validated, normalized, scaled, and so on), and sent to the SCADA. Similar sequencing is performed by the DCS and BAS. All data, on which quality decisions are based, should be defined as "raw data."* The regulated users define in the requirements specification which data are to be used as raw data.†

It is good practice to implement a quality control procedure to ensure that all raw data recorded at the SCADA level and during the course of manufacturing process is accurate and complete.

In the context of this example, the raw data saved in the SCADA is the earliest retainable record or "source data." The raw data saved in the SCADA is considered *original records* as well. As required by 21 CFR 211.180(d), original records must be retained "either as original records or true copies."

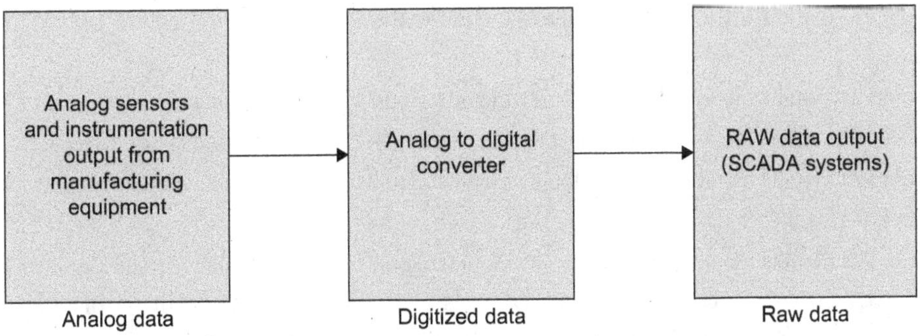

Figure 4.2 Simplified data flow diagram for a manufacturing system.

* EudraLex, Vol. 4, *Good Manufacturing Practice Medicinal Products for Human and Veterinary Use*, Chapter 4, June, 2011.

† EudraLex, Vol. 4, *Good Manufacturing Practice Medicinal Products for Human and Veterinary Use*, Chapter 4, June, 2011.

When raw data is modified in the SCADA environment, change related documentation must be enforced to preserve an audit trail of change, replacement history, or record removal. This is the fundamental concept to preserve the history of the raw data.

As part of this history, all deviations associated with the executed product recipe are documented and corrected. The raw data is reviewed. The data review process includes the review of the metadata and audit trail, as applicable. After the raw data review is successfully completed, the raw data is sent to the MES.

At the MES level, the raw data becomes data or information obtained from raw data. This raw data becomes part of the drug product batch documentation and control records. The product batch documentation incorporates other raw data of the associated batch, such as the in-process and laboratory control results.

In the context of the MES, the drug product batch documentation and control records are considered original records. This data set is generated combining raw data and/or data from diverse sources, and comprises unique information.

The functionality to receive the raw data from the different sources to populate the associated drug product batch documentation and control records residing in the MES, must be subjected to a very strict design, implementation, testing, and maintenance. The raw data load mapping is a critical functionality to write the correct raw data into the associated drug production record. In addition, this function cannot lose or corrupt raw data.

In case the load functionality modifies the format of the raw data, the validation must include verifications that data is not altered in value and/or meaning.

There must be a verification process to review and approve raw data, merged into the MES. In order to minimize the risk of incorrect and not secure entry and processing of the raw data into the MES, appropriate built-in checks must be included.

This verification process can be a visual or an automated process. In the case of an automated verification process, the referenced built-in checks must be validated, and during the Operational Phase, these built-in checks must be periodically verified.

Once raw data has been transferred to the MES, the data in the MES should never be directly modified. In the case of a modification in the raw data, the modification must be performed to the alike raw data set, and the updated raw data loaded to the MES using the same automated tool initially used to load data from the source to the MES. If technical limitations require the data to be modified in the MES, the change must have traceability to the same change in the source.

Finally, the raw data movements across repositories must be performed using qualified interfaces.

Raw data must always be archived and be sufficiently detailed to ensure it can be used to reconstruct any subsequent manipulation of data performed during or after the transformation, if any.

Primary Records

MHRA defines primary records as the data set that takes primacy in cases where there is an inconsistency between corresponding data sets.

Original records or true copies should be designated as "primary records." These two data sets contain (1) original record (raw data) and (2) exact verified copy of the raw data (true copy).

Note that a true copy of e-records must be accurate and complete, conveying all the information and revisions (e.g., metadata) as in the original e-records. The file format of the true e-records copy might differ from that of the original e-records.

Periodically, original records and true copies must be reconciled. In case of inconsistency between an original record and a true copy record, an investigation must be performed, the findings implemented, and any issue communicated across the organization.

As stated by the MHRA guideline, only one data set must be considered a primary record. The selected primary record is to be used for quality-related assessments.

Records Retention on Raw Data

Raw data, which supports information in the Marketing Authorization,* such as validation or stability, should be retained while the authorization remains in force. In some cases, up to 30 years of raw data must be retained. It may be considered acceptable to retire certain documentation

* EudraLex, Vol. 4, *Good Manufacturing Practice Medicinal Products for Human and Veterinary Use*, Chapter 4: Documentation, Section 4.12. June, 2011

where the data has been superseded by a full set of new data. In such cases, justification for this should be documented and should take into account the requirements for retention of batch documentation. The accompanying raw data should be retained for a period at least as long as the records for all batches whose release has been supported on the basis of that validation exercise.

For a medicinal product, the batch documentation shall be retained for at least one year after the expiry date of the batches to which it relates, or at least five years after the certification referred to in Article 51(3) of Directive 2001/83/EC, whichever is the longer period.

At least 2 years of data must be retrievable in a timely manner for the purposes of regulatory inspection.

In the case of the US FDA, the applicable pharmaceutical GMP regulations, 21 CFR 211.180(a), established that retention of data that is part of the drug product production and control records "shall be retained for at least one (1) year after the expiration date of the batch or, in the case of certain OTC drug products lacking expiration dating because they meet the criteria for exemption under 211.137, 3 years after distribution of the batch." As the results of the traceability requirement specified in 21 CFR 211.180(a), the raw data must be retained.

When computer systems are used instead of written documents, the manufacturer shall first validate the systems by showing that the e-records will be appropriately stored during the anticipated period. E-records stored by those systems shall be made readily available in legible form and shall be provided to the competent authorities at their request. The electronically stored e-records shall be protected against loss or damage, using methods such as duplication or backup and transfer to another storage system, and audit trails shall be maintained.

Summary

The MHRA Data Integrity Definitions and Guidance provides a wide data-related terminology use in support of this guidance.

The MHRA definitions are consistent with other regulatory agencies that use similar terminology, including the *Good Manufacturing Practice Medicinal Products for Human and Veterinary Use.*

In this chapter, these MHRA definitions are discussed based on a fully integrated enterprise and process control environments.

The concept of original records should consider if the data sets—the raw data and the certified copy—are the same. In the case of the MES example described in this chapter, it may not be prudent to designate the SCADA data set the original record. The content of each data set is different, even the SCADA data set is contained in the MES data set. But the MES data set contains additional data sets from other sources. It is not certain if, in the manufacturing environment, two data sets will be recorded concurrently, and the conflict about which data set turns out to be the original record will become an issue.

In any case, the GMP controls associated to preserve the integrity of GMP records do not change if these records in storage are data, original records, primary records, raw data, true copies, static data, and/or dynamic data.

These definitions create a better understanding of the electronic environment and outline how to recognize the risks associated with the entire path those e-records follow and where manipulations to those e-records can take place. This understanding is unmistakable in the paper domain.

Additional Readings

EudraLex, Good manufacturing practice, Annex 11: Computerized Systems, 2011.

ISPE/PDA, *Good Electronic Records Management (GERM)*, Figure 4.3, July 2002.

López, O., *EU Annex 11 Guide to Computer Validation Compliance for the Worldwide Health Agency GMP*, CRC Press, March 2015.

MHRA, MHRA GMP data integrity definitions and guidance for industry, March 2015.

Chapter 5

Electronic Records Handling: 21 CFR Part 211*

Introduction

The introduction of regulatory requirements to computer systems by the US Food and Drug Administration (US FDA) can be traced back to the first publication of the Good Manufacturing Process (GMP) regulations. These requirements are applicable to computer systems that have an effect on product quality, and to records known to be required by existing regulation. In 1963, the Code of Federal Regulations (CFR) Part 211.2(b) was incorporated as part of the first publication of the Current Good Manufacturing Practices (cGMP) regulations. It stressed the importance of backups and documentation, including the importance of keeping the hardcopy of master formulas, specifications, test records, master production and control records, and batch production records (i.e., batch production and control records) or calculations.

By 1976, the cGMP regulations combined Parts 211.2(b) and 211.68. The outcome of this combination was the updated 21 CFR Part 211.68 (Automatic, mechanical, and electronic equipment).

For all good practice disciplines regulated by competent authorities, it must be possible to reconstruct studies and reports from raw data, and

* López, O., Requirements for electronic records contained in 21 CFR 211, *Pharmaceutical Technology*, 36, 7, July 2008.

the electronic records may be needed to support any paper printouts.* Specifically, 21 CFR 211, 211.180(d) requires records to be retained "either as original records or true copies such as photocopies, microfilm, microfiche, or other accurate reproductions of the original records."

Speaking strictly about the integrity of the e-records retained by computer storage, the applicable requirements in 211.68† in 1976 were

- Computer systems e-record must be controlled including records retention, backup, and security.
- There must be procedural controls and technologies to ensure the accuracy and security of computer systems input/outputs (I/Os) data.
- Computer systems must have adequate controls to prevent unauthorized access, changes, inadvertent erasures, or loss of e-records.

The 2008 revision of the 211.68(b) maintains these requirements.

The revision of 2008 incorporates a new section in 211.68 that can be associated with a data integrity requirement, 211.68(c).

Based on these requirements, the relevant principles applicable to e-records in the 2008 cGMP are‡ access authorization, data I/Os, data storage, and backup and accuracy check.

Access Authorization Principles

- Computer systems should have sufficient controls to prevent unauthorized access or changes to e-records.§
- There should be controls to prevent omissions in e-records (e.g., the system turned off and data not captured). There should be a record of any data change made, a record of the previous entry, a record of who made the change and when the change was made.¶

* PI 011–3, *Good Practices for Computerised Systems in Regulated "GXP" Environments*, Pharmaceutical Inspection Co-operation Scheme (PIC/S), September 2007.

† US FDA 21 CFR 210 and 211, Federal Register, 41, 31, 6878–6891, February 13, 1976.

‡ US FDA 21 CFR 210 and 211, Federal Register, 73, 174, 51919–51933, September 8, 2008.

§ US FDA 21 CFR 211.68(b).

¶ US Federal Register, 43, 45013, September 29, 1978. US CGMP rev. comment paragraph 185.

Data Input/Output Principles

- Input to and output from the computer, or other records or data, must be checked for accuracy.*
- In the context of data integrity, computer systems must be validated to ensure accuracy, reliability, consistent intended performance, and the ability to discern invalid or altered records.†
- Where critical data is entered manually, there should be an additional check on the accuracy of the entry. This can be done by a second operator, or by the system itself.‡
- Computer systems exchanging data electronically with other systems should include appropriate built-in checks for the correct and secure entry and processing of data to minimize the risks.§,¶

Data Storage and Backup Principles

- A means of ensuring e-records protection should be established for all computer systems.**
- In addition to the security-related controls, regular backups of all files, e-records, and data entered into the computer should be made.††
- Measures must be taken to ensure that backup data is exact and complete, and that it is secure from alteration, inadvertent erasure, and loss.‡‡
- There must be written procedural controls describing periodic reviews, including e-records reviews. The objective of the e-records periodic review is to confirm that they have been accurately and reliably transferred.§§
- If system breakdowns or failures would result in the permanent loss of records, a back up system should be provided.

* Compliance Policy Guides associated to computer-related systems were issued by the FDA throughout the 1980s as guidelines or interpretations of the applicable CFRs.
† López, O., A guide to computer compliance guides, *Journal of cGMP Compliance*, January 1997.
‡ US Federal Register, 43, 45013, September 29, 1978. US CGMP rev. comment paragraph 186.
§ US FDA Compliance Policy Guides (CPG), Sec. 425.400 Computerized drug processing; input/output checking.
¶ US FDA 21 CFR 211.68(b).
** ICH Q7, GMPs Guide for Active Pharmaceutical Ingredients, 2007.
†† US FDA 21 CFR 211.68(b).
‡‡ US Federal Register, 43, 45013, September 29, 1978. US CGMP rev. comment paragraph 185.
§§ US FDA 21 CFR 211.68(b).

Accuracy Check

The control associated with 21 CFR Part 211.68(c) is similar to the accuracy checks associated with EU Annex 11 p6. It establishes that, for data entered manually, there should be an additional verification on the accuracy of the data entered. This verification can be done by a second person, or by a validated automated system.

21 CFR Part 211.68(c) states that

> (c) Such automated equipment used for performance of operations addressed by Sec. 211.101(c) or (d), 211.103, 211.182, or 211.188(b)(11) can satisfy the requirements included in those sections relating to the performance of an operation by one person and checking by another person if such equipment is used in conformity with this section, and one person checks that the equipment properly performed the operation.

Additional Readings

López, O., A historical view of 21 CFR 211.68, *Journal of GxP Compliance*, 15, 2 (Spring), 2011.

López, O., Requirements for electronic records contained in 21 CFR 211, *Pharmaceutical Technology*, 36, 7, July 2008.

US FDA, Code of Federal Regulations, Title 21, Food and Drugs, Parts 210 and 211, Final Rule; Amendments to the Current Good Manufacturing Practice Regulations for Finished Pharmaceuticals; Federal Register, 73, 174, 51919–51933, September 8, 2008.

Chapter 6

Electronic Records Handling: EMA Annex 11*

Introduction

E-records handling may include the classifying, storing, securing, and physical deletion (or in some cases, archival preservation) of records. The ISO 15489: 2001 standard defines records handling as "The field of management responsible for the efficient and systematic control of the creation, receipt, maintenance, use and disposition of records, including the processes for capturing and maintaining evidence of and information about business activities and transactions in the form of records."

The general principles of records handling apply to records in any format. Digital records (a.k.a. electronic records or e-records) raise specific issues. It is more difficult to ensure that the content, context and structure of records is preserved and protected when the records do not have a paper-based existence.

The European Medicines Agency's (EMA's) good manufacturing practice (GMP) requirements on data integrity for medicinal and veterinary products can be found in Article 9 item 2 Directive/2003/94/EC and 91/412/EEC, respectively. Undoubtedly, the area in which most Annex 11 recommendations are made is e-records and on how to manage e-records.

---

* López, O., Annex 11: Progress in EU Computer Systems Guidelines, *Pharmaceutical Technology Europe*, 23, 6, June 2011.

When electronic, photographic or other data processing systems are used instead of written documents, the manufacturer shall first validate the systems by showing that the data will be appropriately stored during the anticipated period of storage. Data stored by those systems shall be made readily available in legible form and shall be provided to the competent authorities at their request. The electronically stored data shall be protected, by methods such as duplication or backup and transfer on to another storage system, against loss or damage of data, and audit trails shall be maintained.

Directive/2003/94/EC/Article 9-2

The Annex 11 e-records handling guidelines can be categorized according to the e-record life-cycle concept. This categorization can be used to understand the discussion about the controls necessary to ensure the authenticity and reliability of records. Such a life cycle (Chapter 3) can be described as the creation, access, use, reuse, and physical deletion of records.

At the time of writing this book, EMA is developing guidance on data integrity for EU GMP.

Creation

4.8. If data are transferred to another data format or system, validation should include checks that data are not altered in value and/or meaning during this migration process.

The migration of e-records must be verified, there must be an additional check on the accuracy of the entry.

6. Accuracy checks: For critical data entered manually, there should be an additional check on the accuracy of the data. This check may be done by a second operator or by validated electronic means. The criticality and the potential consequences of erroneous or incorrectly entered data to a system should be covered by risk management.

Regulated users should define which data are to be used as raw data. As applicable, there should be special procedures for critical data entry, requiring a second check; for example, the data entry and check for a manufacturing formula, or the keying in of laboratory data and results from paper records. A second authorized person with a logged name and identification may verify data entry via the keyboard by entering the time and date. The inclusion and use of an audit trail (11 p9) to capture the diversity of the changes that could possibly impact the data may facilitate this check.

When automated equipment is used as described under US FDA 21 CFR 211.68(c), featuring direct data capture linked to other databases and intelligent peripherals, the verification by a second individual is not necessary. For example, firms may omit the second person component in weight check operations if scales are connected to a computer system that performs checks on component quality control release statuses and the proper identification of containers. The computer system must be validated—registering the raw materials identification, lot number, and expiry date—and integrated with the recorded accurate weight data.

Data integrity should be ensured by suitably implemented and risk-assessed controls. Accidental input of inappropriate data, data type, and/or out of range data should be prevented or should result in an error message. So-called boundary checks are encouraged.*

Access, Use, and Reuse

> *5. Data: Computerised systems exchanging data electronically with other systems should include appropriate built-in checks for the correct and secure entry and processing of data, in order to minimize the risks.*

Based on the complexity and reliability of computer systems, there must be procedural controls and technologies to ensure the accuracy and security of computer system inputs and outputs (I/Os) and e-records. The US FDA Compliance Policy Guide (CPG) 425.400 (formerly 7132a.07), "I/O Checking," establishes that computer I/Os should be tested for data accuracy as part of

* EMA, European Medicines Agency (EMA): GMP/GDP compliance—Questions and answers: Good manufacturing practice: Annex 11 Computerised Systems Question 2, http://www.ema.europa.eu/ema/index.jsp?curl=pages/regulation/q_and_a/q_and_a_detail_000027.jsp&mid=WC0b01ac05800296ca#section9

the computer system qualification and, after the qualification, as part of the computer system's ongoing performance evaluation procedure. The use of input edits may mitigate the need for extensive I/O checks.

The objective of the I/O checks is to develop a method to prevent inaccurate data inputs and outputs. I/Os should be monitored to ensure the process remains within the established parameters. When monitoring data on quality characteristics demonstrates negative tendencies, the cause should be investigated, corrective action taken, and revalidation considered.

Edits can also be used to make up information and give the erroneous impression that a process is under control.

These error overrides must be documented during design.

> *7.1. Data Storage: Data should be secured by both physical and electronic means against damage. Stored data should be checked for accessibility, readability and accuracy. Access to data should be ensured throughout the retention period.*

> *7.2. Data Storage: Regular backups of all relevant data should be done. Integrity and accuracy of backup data and the ability to restore the data should be checked during validation and monitored periodically.*

Computer system e-records must be controlled, covering record retention, backup, and security. Computer systems must also have adequate controls to prevent unauthorized access or changes to e-records, inadvertent erasures, or losses.

Regular training, in all of the relevant security/backup procedures, for the personnel providing security and performing backups is crucial. The validated backup procedure, including storage facilities and media, should ensure the integrity and availability of the e-records and the metadata of the e-records. The frequency with which backups are performed is dependent on the computer system functions and the risk assessment for the loss of e-records.

Procedures for regular testing, including a test plan, and for backup and disaster recovery should be in place. A log of backup testing, including the date of testing and the results, should be maintained and a record of the rectification of any errors should be kept. The physical security of the system should also be adequate to minimize the possibility of unauthorized access, willful or accidental damage by personnel, or the loss of e-records.

Before hardware and/or software are exchanged, a change control mechanism should be used to check that the e-records concerned can also be managed in the new configuration. If the impact assessment demonstrates that changes in the hardware and/or software mean that the stored e-records cannot be managed in the new configuration, one of the following procedures should be applied:

- The e-records in the format concerned should be converted into a format that can be printed in the new configuration.
- The components of the old hardware and/or software configuration required for printing should be retained. In this case it should be guaranteed that a suitable alternative system is available in case the retained system fails.
- The e-record is transferred to another medium.

The electronically stored e-records should be checked regularly for availability and integrity. Appropriate controls for electronic documents such as templates, forms, and master documents should be implemented. Appropriate controls should be in place to ensure the integrity of the record throughout the retention period.

Additional references associated with this principle can be found at: Article 9 Section 2, Commission Directives 2003/94/EC; PIC/S PI 011-3; EudraLex-Volume 4 Good manufacturing practice (GMP) Guidelines, Part I—Basic Requirements for Medicinal Products, Chapter 4—Documentation; and US FDA 21 CFR 211.68 and 21 CFR Part 11.10(c); 11.10(d); 11.10(e); 11.10(g); 11.10(h); 11.30.

> *9. Audit Trails: Consideration should be given, based on a risk assessment, to building into the system the creation of a record of all GMP-relevant changes and deletions (a system generated "audit trail"). For change or deletion of GMP-relevant data the reason should be documented. Audit trails need to be available and convertible to a generally intelligible form and regularly reviewed.*

Audit trails are control mechanisms generated by computer systems that allow all of the raw data entered and further processed by the system, to be traced back to the raw data. If the e-record needs to be changed, a second person should approve these changes along with the reasons given. The audit trail records should be reviewed regularly.

The date and time of the audit trail must be synchronized to a trusted date and time service.

One of the key controls for audit trails is the link of the e-record with the associated audit trail. Audit trails can be part of the record that has been modified or a stand-alone record linked to the modified record. Audit trails cannot be modified. The access rights for audit trail information must be limited to print and/or read only. The combination of authentication, digital certificates, encryption, and access control lists provides the technical mechanisms needed to control the access to audit trail files.

> *12.4. Management systems for data and for documents should be designed to record the identity of operators entering, changing, confirming or deleting data, including the date and time.*

Computer systems must have adequate controls to prevent unauthorized access or changes to e-records, as well as inadvertent erasures or losses. Procedures should ensure that

- Access rights for all operators are clearly defined and controlled, including physical and logical access.
- Basic rules exist and are documented to ensure that the security related to personal passwords or pass cards, and that the related system/e-record security requirements, are not reduced or negated.
- Correct authority and responsibilities are assigned to the correct organizational level.
- Identification code and password issuance is periodically checked, recalled, or revised.
- Loss management exists to electronically invalidate lost, stolen, or potentially compromised passwords. The system should be capable of enforcing regular changes to passwords.
- Procedures identify prohibited passwords.
- An audit log of breaches of password security should be kept and measures should be in place to address such breaches.
- The system should enforce access revocation after a specified number of unsuccessful login attempts.
- Validated recovery of original information and e-records, following backup, media transfer, transcription, archiving, or system failure.
- Attempted breaches of security safeguards should be recorded and investigated.

Some equipment, such as stand-alone computer systems and dedicated operator equipment interfaces and instruments, may lack logical (e.g., password.) capabilities. These should be listed, justified, and subjected to procedural controls.

> *17. Archiving: Data may be archived. This data should be checked for accessibility, readability and integrity. If relevant changes are to be made to the system (e.g. computer equipment or programs), then the ability to retrieve the data should be ensured and tested.*

The archived records need to be trustworthy and reliable as well as accessible, no matter where they are stored. The party having primary responsibility for record retention under the predicate regulations would be the party responsible for the adequacy of archiving these e-records.

Physical Deletion

The only activity not explicitly covered in the Annex 11 is the computer systems' and e-records' retirement. The retirement of computer systems and e-records is covered implicitly as part of Chapter 11, p10. Retirement is considered to be a change of the state of the computer, from active to inactive.

In the context of the computer system's retirement and the deletion of e-records:

- If the e-records are transferred to another e-records format or system, validation should include checks that the e-records are not altered in value and/or meaning during this migration process (11 p4.8).
- If the e-records are transferred to another system, the ability to retrieve the e-records should be ensured and tested (11 p7).

Controls Based on System Life Cycle

The following are a set of controls that should be in place to protect the e-records. These controls are compiled based on the Annex 11 computer system life cycle (SLC) phase* (Table 6.1).

* Life cycle: All phases in the life of the system from initial requirements until retirement including design, specification, programming, testing, installation, operation, and maintenance (EU Annex 11).

Table 6.1 Controls Based on SLC Phase

Computer SLC Phase	*Records Life Cycle*	*E-Records Controls*
General Phase—Requirements	Analysis	1. Identify the applicable critical records. Critical records are identified in the course of the risk analysis (11 p1). 2. Identify data and e-records integrity–related controls based on a risk assessment. Manage the controls to mitigate the risks through the SLC (11 p1). 3. If data are transferred to another data format, identify the new format. (11 p4.8 and 11 p8.1) and control requirements (11 p5). 4. Identify interfaces (11 p5) and the data to be entered manually (11 p6). 5. Based on the risk assessment, assess the need for audit trails (11 p12.4), and controls to prevent unauthorized access to the application and the operating systems (11 p7.1, 11 p12 and 21 CFR 11.10(g)). 6. The requirements documented must include the requirement(s) uncovered during the risk assessment. 7. Design the reports (11 p8.1), accuracy checks (11 p6), operational system checks (21 CFR Part 11.10(f)), authority checks (21 CFR Part 11.10(g)) and device checks (21 CFR Part 11.10(h)). 8. Timestamping controls. A timestamping service should be utilized. If the local clock is used, periodic coordination is expected between the service and the local computer clock. Limit access to the computer's local date and time function. The computer's local date and time function must not be accessed by users.

Project Phase—Specification, Design, Programming, Testing, Installation	Analysis	1. As part of the qualification of the application and associated controls, test the backup and restoration procedure(s) and verify the output of the backup (11 p7.2). Each backup set should be checked to ensure that it is error-free. 2. Verify audit trail capabilities, as applicable (11 p7.1). 3. Verify the accuracy of reports and audit trail reports (11 p8). 4. As applicable, and based on the operational sequencing, test the accuracy of the e-records (11 p7.1). 5. If e-records are transferred to another format, the qualification must include checks that the e-records' new formats are not altered during the migration process. (11 p4.8) 6. IT infrastructure must be qualified to ensure security and e-records integrity. (Principle b)
Operational and Maintenance Phases	Creation, Access, Use and Reuse, Archiving, Transfer, Archiving or Destruction	1. A means of ensuring e-records protection must be established for all computer systems (Health Canada GMP Guidelines for API (GUI-0104) Dec 2013, ICH Q7 Aug 2001, EMA Annex 11 p4.8, 11 p5, 11 p6, 11 p7, 11 p8.1, 11 p12). 2. Written procedures must be available for the operation and maintenance of computer systems.* Management of records, performance monitoring (11 p11), change control programs (11 p10) and e-records security (11 p12), calibration and maintenance (11 p10), personnel training (11 p2), emergency recovery (11 p16), management of incidents (11 p17), e-records entry (11 p6) and modifications (WHO 4.2), and periodic reevaluation (11 p11) are some of the procedures impacting e-records integrity.

(*Continued*)

Table 6.1 (Continued) Controls Based on SLC Phase

Computer SLC Phase	*Records Life Cycle*	*E-records Controls*
		3. The procedures and records pertaining to the security of the system and security of the e-records are very important and must be based on the IT policies of the regulated user and in conformance with the relevant regulatory requirements (11 p12.1). 4. There should be written procedures for the recovery of the system following a breakdown; these procedures should include documentation and record requirements to ensure the retrieval and maintenance of GxP information (11 p16). 5. E-records must be secured by both physical and electronic means against damage, including unauthorized access and changes to e-records (11 p12). As part of physical security, the security of devices used to store programs, such as tapes, disks, and magnetic strip cards must be considered. Access to these devices should be controlled. 6. Periodic (or continuous) reviews must be performed after the initial validation (11 p11). As part of a periodic review, verify the stored backups and archived e-records for accessibility, readability, and accuracy; verify the output of the backup; and the accuracy of the audit trail. As applicable, verify accurate and reliable e-records transfer (WHO 3.2). 7. Access to e-records should be ensured throughout the retention period (11 p7.1).

		8. The electronically stored e-records should be checked regularly for availability and integrity (11 p7.1). 9. Following changes to the system, change control should ensure the availability and integrity of the e-records on the backup copies by restoring the e-records on a trial basis (11 p10 and 11 p7.2). 10. E-record errors, complete loss of data, and loss of data integrity must be reported and investigated. Corrective action(s) must be taken in accordance with the investigation (11 p13). The GMP regulators expect any resulting recommendations to be implemented as soon as reasonably practical. 11. When applicable, there must be controls to prevent system failure and e-records not captured (11 p5). 12. For critical records entered or e-records amended (WHO 4.2) manually, there should be an additional check on the accuracy of the data and only entered by persons authorized to do so (11 p6). 13. Where an e-record is deleted prior to meeting its approved retention, an audit trail of the deletion is required until the end of the approved retention period (11 p7.1). 14. When outside agencies are used to provide a computer service, there should be a formal agreement including a clear statement of the responsibilities of that outside agency (11 p3.1).

(*Continued*)

Table 6.1 (Continued) Controls Based on SLC Phase

Computer SLC Phase	*Records Life Cycle*	*E-records Controls*
Retirement Phase	E-record Destruction	1. In the context of the computer system retirement, a. If the e-records are transferred to another e-record format or system, validation should include checks that e-records are not altered in value and/or meaning during this migration process (11 p4.8). b. If the e-records are transferred to another system the ability to retrieve the e-records should be ensured and tested (11 p7).

* O. López, Maintaining the validated state in computer systems, *Journal of GXP Compliance* 17, 2, August 2013 (http://www.ivt-network.com/article/maintaining-validated-state-computer-systems).

Additional Readings

EudraLex, EU Guidelines to Good Manufacturing Practice, Medicinal Products for Human and Veterinary Use, Annex 11: Computerized Systems, Volume 4, June 2011. http://ec.europa.eu/health/files/eudralex/vol-4/annex11_01-2011_en.pdf.

Heddell, G., Data integrity: An EU perspective, paper presented at the Third Annual ISPE-FDA CMP Conference, Baltimore, MD, 2–4 June 2014.

López, O., Annex 11 and electronic records integrity, in *EU Annex 11 Guide to Computer Validation Compliance for the Worldwide Health Agency GMP*, CRC Press, Boca Raton, FL, March 2015.

Chapter 7

Relevant Worldwide GMP Regulations and Guidelines

Introduction

In addition to the US FDA 21 CFR Part 211 and EU Annex 11, (Chapters 5 and 6 respectively), the following are relevant good manufacturing practice (GMP) regulations and guidelines containing references associated with the integrity of e-records.

> *Records shall be established and maintained to provide evidence of conformity to requirements and of the effective operation of the quality management system. Records shall remain legible, readily identifiable and retrievable. A documented procedure shall be established to define the controls needed for the identification, storage, protection, retrieval, retention time and disposition of records.*
>
> **ISO 13845**
> *Quality Management System, Section 4.2.4, Control of records*

Consistent with the globalization of the manufacturing of medicinal products for the healthcare industry, the reader may agree that the principles of e-records integrity are contained in all major worldwide regulations and guidelines. A comparison of key elements of recent guidelines and regulations covering e-records integrity can be found at http://www.computer-systems-validation.net/dataintegritycrosswalk.html.

API

Title: General Guidelines of Good Manufacturing Practices for Processors, Importers/Exporters of Medicines, ANMAT No. 2819/2004.
Regulation/Guideline: GMP
Organization: National Administration of Medicines, Food and Medical Technology
Country: Argentina
E-Records Integrity Items:
Documentation—Section 15.9

- If documentation is handled by electronic data processing methods, only authorized persons should be able to enter or modify the data in the computer and there must be a record of the changes and deletions that are made. Access should be restricted by keys or other mean and the entry of critical information must be verified independently.
- Batch records that are electronically stored should be protected by a backup, or by magnetic tapes, microfilms, printouts or other means.
- **Title:** Code of Good Manufacturing Practice for Human Blood and Blood Components, Human Tissues and Human Cellular Therapy Products, April 2013.

Regulation/Guideline: GMP
Organization: Therapeutic Goods Administration (TGA)
Country: Australia
E-Records Integrity Items:
Computers—Principle 1000

- Where a computerized system is implemented, there should be no adverse effects on product quality and safety, or the security and integrity of the data.

Computers—General 1008

- The following procedures and controls should be adopted for records retained by computer storage:
  - Records should be regularly and progressively backed up, and the backup should be retained at a location that is remote from the active file.
  - Data should be collected directly from equipment, and control signals between computers and equipment should be checked by verification circuits/software to confirm their accuracy and reliability.

- Interfaces between computers and equipment should be checked to ensure their accuracy and reliability.
- There should be documented contingency plans and recovery procedures in the event of a breakdown. The recovery procedures should be periodically checked for the return of the system to its previous state.
- The system should be able to provide accurate printed copies of the relevant data and information stored within. Printed matter produced by computer peripherals should be clearly legible and, in the case of printing onto forms, should be properly aligned onto the forms.

Computers—General 1009

- The system should include, where appropriate, built-in checks of the correct entry and processing of data.

Computers—General 1011

- Data should only be entered or amended by persons authorized to do so. Suitable methods of deterring unauthorized entry of data include the use of keys, pass cards, personal codes and the restriction of access to computer terminals. There should be a defined procedure for the issue, cancellation and alteration of the authorization to enter and amend data, including the changing of personal passwords. Consideration should be given to systems that allow for the recording of the attempts made by unauthorized persons to access them.

Computers—General 1012

- Critical data entered manually into a computer system should be checked for accuracy by a second person. The persons carrying out the data entry and verification should be identifiable.

Computers—General 1013

- The computer system should create an audit trail of any changes made to electronic data. The record should include the time of each change, the nature of the change, and the identity of the person involved.

Computers—General 1014

- Data should be secured by physical or electronic means against willful or accidental damage. Stored data should be checked for accessibility, durability and accuracy. If changes are proposed to the computer equipment or its programs these checks should be performed at a frequency appropriate to the storage medium being used.

Computers—General 1014

- Critical computer-dependent systems should have alternate systems available in their place in the event of a systems failure.

Title: Code of Good Manufacturing Practices for Medicinal Products
Regulation: GMP and Active Pharmaceutical Ingredients (APIs)
Organization: Therapeutic Goods Administration (TGA)
Country: Australia
Data Integrity Items: Refer to EU Annex 11 (Rev. Jan 1992)

On 29 July 2009, the Therapeutic Goods (Manufacturing Principles) Determination No. 1 of 2009 adopted the PIC/S Guide to Good Manufacturing Practice, 15 January 2009, PE 009-8, to be the code of GMP—except for its Annexes 4, 5 and 14, which are not adopted by Australia.

This updated code replaces the Australian Code of Good Manufacturing Practice for Medicinal Products (16 August 2002) as well as the Australian Code of Good Manufacturing Practice for Sunscreen Products (1994).

For both transitions, a one-year transition period was applied, ending on 1 July 2010. As of 1 July 2010, the 2002 code and the sunscreen code have both been revoked.

The 2009 code consists of two parts and fifteen annexes. Part I is applicable to the manufacturing of finished medicinal products, and Part II is applicable to the manufacturing of active pharmaceutical ingredients (APIs). Part II is identical to the ICH GMP Guide for APIs, which was already determined as a standard in the previous manufacturing principle.

The Annex-11 (Rev 0, January 1992) is applicable to the manufacturing of finished medicinal products, as well as to the manufacturing of APIs.

The 1992 Annex 11 data integrity-related items are the following:

6. The system should include, where appropriate, built-in checks of the correct entry and processing of data.
8. Data should only be entered or amended by persons authorized to do so. Suitable methods of deterring unauthorized entry of data include the use of keys, pass cards, personal codes and the restriction of access to computer terminals. There should be a defined procedure for the issue, cancellation, and alteration of authorization to enter and amend data, including the changing of personal passwords. Consideration should be given to systems allowing for recording of attempts to access by unauthorised persons.
9. When critical data are being entered manually (for example the weight and batch number of an ingredient during dispensing), there should be an additional check on the accuracy of the record which is made. This check may be done by a second operator or by validated electronic means.

10. The system should record the identity of operators entering or confirming critical data. Authority to amend entered data should be restricted to nominated persons. Any alteration to an entry of critical data should be authorized and recorded along with the reason for the change. Consideration should be given to building into the system the creation of a complete record of all entries and amendments (an "audit trail").
13. Data should be secured by physical or electronic means against willful or accidental damage, in accordance with item 4.9 of the guide. Stored data should be checked for accessibility, durability and accuracy. If changes are proposed to the computer equipment or its programs, these checks should be performed at a frequency appropriate to the storage medium being used.
14. Data should be protected by backing it up at regular intervals. Backup data should be stored as long as necessary, at a separate and secure location.

Title: Rules on Good Manufacturing Practice of Medicinal Products, Article 579 Item 2 in the Resolution of the Executive Board No. 17, April 2010
Regulation/Guideline: GMP
Organization: ANVISA
Country: Brazil
E-Records Integrity Items:
Title VII-Computerized Information Systems

Art. 577. The system should include, where applicable, verification of data entry and processing.

Art. 579. The entries and data modifications can only be performed by authorized persons.

§1 Measures should be taken that do not allow unauthorized persons to include, exclude or alter data in the system and can be used for system security; such as the use of passwords, personal codes, access profiles, keys or restricted access to the system.

§2 A procedure should be established for access management, defining how to issue, amend and cancel the passwords of persons who are no longer authorized to enter or change data in the system.

§3 Should be given preference to systems that allow registering attempting unauthorized access.

Art. 580. Where critical data is entered manually (example: the load and the lot number of a load input) there should be an additional verification ensuring the accuracy of the data entered.
The verification can be held by a second operator or electronically validated.

Art. 581. The system should record the identity of operators entering or confirming critical data. The authorization to change the data must be restricted.
§1 Any changes of critical data should be documented, describing the reason for the change.
§2 When data changes are made, the records of all of the entries, updates, users and dates should be kept.

Art. 583. In cases of quality audits must be possible to obtain printed copies of electronically stored data.

Art. 584. The data should be stored securely, by physical or electronic means against willful or accidental damage.
§1 The stored data should be checked for accessibility, durability and accuracy.
§2 If the proposed change in equipment or software, the checks must be carried out at a frequency appropriate to the storage medium in use.

Art. 585. The data should be protected by means of performing backup copies (backup) at regular intervals.
§1 The backup data must be stored for a set time and in separate and secure location.
§2 There should be procedures to ensure that the process of restoration and maintenance of backup data.
§3 Lost data should be treated as deviations.

Title: Good Manufacturing Practice for Active Pharmaceutical Ingredients, RDC Resolution #69, December 2014
Regulation/Guideline: API
Organization: ANVISA
Country: Brazil
E-Records Integrity Items:
Chapter VI—Documentation and Records

Art. 106 The data should be reliably recorded through a manual, electronic processing system or other means.

Paragraph 1. Standard/master formulas and written procedures for the system in use should be available, and the accuracy of the records should be checked.

Paragraph 2. If the data recording is done through electronic processing, it should be ensured that

I Only authorized people can modify the data stored on computers.

II There is a record of the changes made.

III Computer access is restricted by passwords or other means.

IV The entry of data that is considered to be critical is checked by a designated person other than the one who made the records, or else checked by the system itself.

V Electronic records of the batch data are protected by transferring copies onto magnetic tape, microfilm, paper or another medium.

Title: Good Manufacturing Practices (GMP) Guidelines for Active Pharmaceutical Ingredients (APIs), November 2013, GUI-0104.

Regulation/Guideline: API

Organization: Health Products and Food Branch Inspectorate

Country: Canada

E-Records Integrity Items:

15. Computerized systems should have sufficient controls to prevent unauthorized access or changes to data. There should be controls to prevent omissions in data (e.g. system turned off and data not captured). There should be a record of any changes made to data that includes the previous entry, who made the change, and when the change was made.
16. If computerized system breakdowns or failures would result in the permanent loss of records, a backup system should be provided. A means of ensuring data protection should be established for all computerized systems.

Title: Good Manufacturing Practice Guide for Active Pharmaceutical Ingredients, ICH Q7*

Regulation/Guideline: API

Organization: International Conference on Harmonization of Technical Requirements for Registration of Pharmaceuticals for Human Use

* Similar to ICHQ7, PE 009-10 Guide to GMP for Medicinal Products Part II, January 2013. This is the PIC/S guide applicable to API. Section 5.4 is related to computers. These computer-related sections in ICHQ7 and this API guide are equal.

Countries: Representatives from the following Regulatory Parties:

- European Union, the Regulatory Party is represented by the European Commission (EC) and the European Medicines Agency (EMA)
- Japan, the Regulatory Party is the Ministry of Health, Labor and Welfare (MHLW)
- USA, the Regulatory Party is the Food and Drug Administration (FDA)
- Canada, the Regulatory Party is the Health Products and Food Branch (HPFB)
- Switzerland, the Regulatory Party is the Swissmedic

As well as from the following Industry Parties:

- Europe, the European Federation of Pharmaceutical Industries and Associations (EFPIA)
- Japan, the Japan Pharmaceutical Manufacturers Association (JPMA)
- USA, the Pharmaceutical Research and Manufacturers of America (PhRMA)

E-Records Integrity Items:

Computerized Systems—Section 5.4

5.43 Computerized systems should have sufficient controls to prevent unauthorized access or changes to data. There should be controls to prevent omissions in data (e.g., in case a system turns off and the data is not captured). There should be a record of any change made, the previous entry, who made the change, and when the change was made to the data.

5.45 Where critical data is being entered manually, there should be an additional check on the accuracy of the entry. This can be done by a second operator or by the system itself.

REGULATORY GUIDANCE

A means of ensuring data protection should be established for all computerized systems.

Health Canada

GMP Guidelines for API (GUI-0104) Dec 2013 and ICH Q7 Aug 2001

5.48 If system breakdowns or failures would result in the permanent loss of records, a backup system should be provided. A means of ensuring data protection should be established for all computerized systems.

5.49 Data can be recorded by a second means in addition to the computer system.

Documentation and Records—Section 6.0

6.18 If electronic signatures are used on documents, they should be authenticated and secure.

Laboratory Control Records—Section 6.6

6.60 Laboratory control records should include complete data derived from all of the tests conducted to ensure compliance with established specifications and standards, including from examinations and assays.

Title: Guidance Computer Validation API, Rev 2, Jan 2003

Regulation/Guideline: API

Organization: Conseil Européen des Fédérations de l'Industrie Chimique (CEFIC)

Country: International. Three (3) European chemical industry groups: Corporate, Federation, Business (ABM). Refer to http://www.cefic.org/About-us/Our-Members/ for specific memberships. No Regulatory Party membership.

E-Records Integrity Items:

Compliance—Section 7.2

Critical compliance-related points to be considered include

- Access control/user management
- Data integrity including: prevention of deletion, poor transcription and omission
- Authorized/unauthorized changes to data and documents
- Audit trails
- Disaster recovery/backup and retrieval
- Training

Security—Section 7.4.12

There needs to be proper access control procedures on three levels:

1. Wide and/or local area network level
2. System, or application level
3. PC level

Items that need to be covered include the control of access, password policies and audit trails. At all three levels there should be continuously updated lists of approved users and their authorization levels.

Contingency planning—Section 7.4.15

In case of complete destruction of the hardware, software and data files, the knowledge and backups of the system should be available to build up a complete new system. It should be documented whether and how the process is continued in case of a disaster (unavailability of the system).

Audit trail—Section 7.4.20

Computer-generated and timestamped audit trails that independently record the date and time, entries and actions, that create, modify or delete electronic records. Record changes shall not obscure previously recorded information.

The audit trail should be searchable and be secured from any changes. It must be able to interrogate by dates, time, persons, type of change and reasons for change.

Periodic evaluation—Section 7.4.22

At predefined intervals (e.g., once a year) assessments should be made of the performance of the system by using the data from the change control and problem reporting documentation. A decision should be made and documented on the possible need for changes to and/or revalidation of the system. Decisions on periodic evaluation should be approved by at least the system owner and quality authority (QA).

Archiving—Section 7.4.23

All documentation generated in the operation, maintenance and change control procedures should be properly archived.

Data along with the necessary software to retrieve that data should be archived.

Retirement—Section 7.4.24

Refer to Chapter 6, Operation Activities.

GMP

Title: EudraLex, The Rules Governing Medicinal Products in the European Union Volume 4, Good Manufacturing Practice, Medicinal Products for Human and Veterinary Use, Chapter 4: Documentation, June 2011.

Regulation/Guideline: GMP and good clinical practices (GCP)

Organization: EMA

Country: EU (There are 28 Member States located in Europe: Austria, Belgium, Bulgaria, Croatia, Cyprus, Czech Republic, Denmark, Estonia, Finland, France, Germany, Greece, Hungary, Ireland, Italy, Latvia, Lithuania, Luxemburg, Malta, the Netherlands, Poland, Portugal, Romania, Slovakia, Slovenia, Spain, Sweden, and the United Kingdom.)

E-Records Integrity Items:

4.1 Appropriate controls should be in place to ensure the integrity of the record throughout the retention period.

4.10 Secure controls must be in place to ensure the integrity of the record throughout the retention period and validated where appropriate.

Title: EudraLex, The Rules Governing Medicinal Products in the European Union Volume 4, EU Guidelines for Good Manufacturing Practice for Medicinal Products for Human and Veterinary Use, Annex 15: Qualification and Validation, March 2015.

Regulation/Guideline: GMP and GCP

Organization: EMA

Country: EU

E-Records Integrity Items:

1.8 Appropriate checks should be incorporated into qualification and validation work to ensure the integrity of all of the data obtained.

Title: EudraLex, The Rules Governing Medicinal Products in the European Union Volume 4, EU Guidelines for Good Manufacturing Practice for Medicinal Products for Human and Veterinary Use, Part 1 Chapter 3: Premises and Equipment, August 2014.

Regulation/Guideline: GMP

Organization: EMA

Country: EU

E-Records Integrity Items:

3.41 Measuring, weighing, recording and control-related equipment should be calibrated and checked at defined intervals by appropriate methods. Adequate records of these tests should be maintained.

Title: Good Manufacturing Practices (GMP) Guidelines, 2009 Edition, Version 2, GUI 0001

Regulation/Guideline: GMPs

Organization: Health Products and Food Branch Inspectorate

Country: Canada

E-Records Integrity Items: Refer to EU Annex 11 (Rev. Jan 1992)

5.3 Equipment used during the critical steps of fabrication, packaging/labeling, and testing—which includes computerized systems—is subject to installation and operational qualification. Equipment qualification is documented. Further guidance is provided in Health Canada's document, entitled Validation Guidelines for Pharmaceutical Dosage Forms (GUI-0029) and PIC/S Annex 11: Computerized Systems.

Refer to the Australian's Code of Good Manufacturing Practices for Medicinal Products, GMP and API, for analysis.

Title: GMP Annex 2 Computerized Systems, December 2015.
Regulation/Guideline: GMP
Organization: China Food & Drug Administration (CFDA)
Country: China
E-Records Integrity Items:

3. As part of product quality risk management, the degree of validation and data integrity control should depend on documented risk assessment results.
9. Systems must be validated to ensure that no change to the value and meaning of data occurs, despite the format or migration of data.
14. System entering and using are performed only be authorized personnel. There should be means to avoid unauthorized personnel trying to enter system.

    A procedure should be created for authorization, cancel authorization, authorization changing of system entering and using. Meantime, system should record unauthorized access. A documented procedure, related record note and physical isolation means should be performed to ensure that only authorized personnel can operate system, when defects of system makes not to achieve personnel access control.
15. For critical data entered manually, there should be an additional check on the accuracy of the data. This check may be done by a second operator or by validated electronic means. If necessary, a double check function should be set for a computerized system to ensure the accuracy of data entering and handling.
16. Computerized systems should record the ID of personnel who enter or check critical data. Only authorized personnel can modify data input. Each change to the input data should be approved and the reason should be recorded. According to risk assessment, that should be considered that an integrated audit trail system is created in computerized system to record data entering and modification, and system using and modification.

18. When electronic data and paper data exist in a site, and the policy about which form as primary data, electronic or paper data, should be documented.
19. When an electronic record is considered to be primary data, the following requirements should be met:
    - The electronic data could be printed to clear file for audit trail.
    - Data should be secured by both physical and electronic means against intentional or accidental damage. Storage data access and integrity checking should be performed, while daily maintenance and system changed (for example, computerized device or program).
    - A procedure should be created for data backup and recovery, and regular backups of data should be made to ensure that it will be reviewed. All backups of data should be set in an individual and safe place. The duration of the retention period should follow the requirements for documentation and records in this guideline.
24. (VI Data Integrity: It is data accuracy and reliability to describe all stored data is in objectively truth state.

Title: TS066: Good Practice Guidelines for Elements of the Quality System, November 2013.
Regulation/Guideline: GMP
Organization: European Committee on Blood Transfusion (CD-P-TS) of the Council of Europe
Country: EU
E-Records Integrity Items:

4.2 Data processing systems.

4.2.1 When computerized systems are used, software, hardware and backup procedures must be checked regularly to ensure reliability, be validated before use, and be maintained in a validated state. Hardware and software must be protected against unauthorized use or unauthorized changes. The backup procedure must prevent loss of or damage to data at expected and unexpected downtimes or function failures (Directive/2005/62/EC/Annex 4.5).

4.2.4 There must be a hierarchy of permitted user access to enter, amend, read or print data. Methods of preventing unauthorized entry must be in place, such as personal identity codes or passwords that are changed on a regular basis.

4.2.5 All necessary measures must be taken to ensure the protection of data. These measures must ensure that safeguards against unauthorized data additions, deletions or modifications, and against the transfer of information, are in place in order to resolve data discrepancies and to prevent unauthorized disclosure of such information.

Title: Guideline on Management of Computerized Systems for Marketing Authorization Holders and Manufacturers of Drugs and Quasi-Drugs, October 2010.
Regulation/Guideline: GMP
Organization: Ministry of Health, Labor and Welfare of Japan
Country: Japan
E-Records Integrity Items:

The actual Japanese requirements on computer systems in the area of GMP and good quality practice (GQP) are laid down in the "Guideline on Management of Computerized Systems for Marketing Authorization Holders and Manufacturers of Drugs and Quasi-Drugs."

4.2 Documentation of User Requirement Specifications
 (4) Data
 1) Lists of input and output information
 2) Retention methods

4.5 Documentation of Design Specification
 4.5.2 Software Design Specifications
 (1) Details of input/output information
 (2) Files and data structure
 (3) Details of data processing
 (5) Details of interfaces

6. Activities in Operations Management
 (4) Information security management
 1) Controlling access privileges for persons in charge of the input, modification and deletion of data, and the prevention of unauthorized accesses.
 2) Control of identification components.
 3) Limited access to the hardware installation areas.

Title: Guidance on Good Practices for Computerized Systems in Regulated "GXP" Environments (PI 011-3), September 2007.
Regulation/Guideline: GMP

Organization: PIC/S*

Country: 39 regulatory agencies, within 37 countries, are members of the PIC/S (Pharmaceutical inspection cooperation scheme, http://www.picscheme.org/pics.php).

E-Records Integrity Items:

4.5 The inspector will consider the potential risks, from the automated system to product/material quality or data integrity, as identified and documented by the regulated user, in order to assess the fitness for purpose of the particular system(s).

4.12 In addition to the validation considerations, the inspector will also be concerned with assessing the basic operational controls, quality system and security features for these systems, as indicated in the PIC/S GMP Annex 11.†

8.4 It is important to acknowledge that the scope and level of documentation and records needed to formalize and satisfy basic project management requirements for critical systems will be dependent upon

- The complexity of the system and variables relating to quality and performance.
- The need to ensure data integrity.
- The level of risk associated with its operation.
- The GxP impact areas involved.

14.3 Validation scope should include GxP compliance criteria, ranked for product/process quality and data integrity risk criticality, should the system fail or malfunction.

16.5 The validation exercise for an ongoing evaluation of legacy systems should involve the inclusion of the systems under all of the documentation, records and procedural requirements associated with the current system; for example, change control, audit trail(s), (where appropriate), data and system security, additional development or modification of software under QMS, 29 maintenance of data integrity, system backup requirements, operator (user) training and an ongoing evaluation of the system operations.

---

* PIC/S organization develops and promotes guidance documents for regulatory inspectors. These guides are very valuable for the industry too because they represent the inspectors perspective by regulatory inspection. These guides could be considered as a kind of "common denominator" in order to enable Mutual Recognition Agreements (MRA) between the regulatory Agencies of the country members.

† EMA Annex 11, Rev 0, January 1992.

17.3 Common IT infrastructural features may need to be controlled centrally by IT systems and security management.

19.1 The security of the system and security of the data are very important and the procedures and records pertaining to these aspects should be based on the IT policies of the regulated user and in conformance with the relevant regulatory requirements. The use of a computerized system does not reduce the requirements that would be expected for a manual system of data control and security. The system owner will be responsible for managing access to their system, and for important systems, the controls will be implemented through an information security management system (ISMS).

19.2 It is very important for the regulated user to maintain the procedures and records related to accessing the system(s). There should be clearly defined responsibilities for system security management, suitable for both small and complex systems, including

- The implementation of the security strategy and delegation.
- The management and assignment of privileges.
- Levels of access for users.
- Levels of access for infrastructure (firewall, backup, etc.).

19.5 The validated backup procedure including storage facilities and media should ensure data integrity.

19.7 The physical security of the system should also be adequate to minimize the possibility of unauthorized access, willful or accidental damage by personnel or loss of data.

20.1 Where applicable, the audit trail for the data integrity may need to include functions such as authorized users, creations, links, embedded comments, deletions, modifications/corrections, authorizations, privileges, time and date, inter alia.

21.13 Additional security arrangements and controls will be needed for GxP computerized systems, which electronically generate regulatory records, allow for external access, or enable key decisions and actions to be undertaken through electronic interfaces.

23.14 If satisfied with the validation evidence, inspectors should then study the system when it is being used and call for printouts of reports from the system and archives as relevant. All points in Annex 11 (6, 8–19)* may be relevant to this part of the assessment. Look for correlation

* EMA Annex 11, Rev 0, January 1992.

with validation work, evidence of change control, configuration management, accuracy and reliability. Security, access controls and data integrity will be relevant to many of the systems particularly EDP.

Title: PIC/S GMP Guide for Blood Establishments, PE 005-3, September 2007.
Regulation/Guideline: GMP
Organization: PIC/S
Country: 39 regulatory agencies, within 37 countries, are members of the PIC/S (Pharmaceutical Inspection Cooperation Scheme, http://www.picscheme.org/pics.php).
E-Records Integrity Items:
Computers

9.8 The hardware and software of the computers should be checked regularly to ensure reliability. The software (program) should be validated before use.

9.9 Computer hardware and software should be protected against use by unauthorized persons. The users of computers should be trained and should be authorized only to handle the data required for the task(s) that they perform.

9.10 There should be documented procedures for backup protection against the loss of records in the event of planned and unplanned function failures.

9.12 Changes to computerized systems (hardware, software or communication) should be validated, applicable documentation revised (if appropriate) and personnel trained before the change is introduced into routine use. Only authorized persons should make changes to software.

Title: Data Integrity and Compliance with CGMP – Guidance for Industry (Draft)

Regulation/Guideline: 21 CFR Parts 210, 211 and 212.

Organization: US FDA

Country: United States
E-Records Integrity Items:
Following the guidance in CPG 7132a.11*, this guidance confirms the applicability of the regulations to computer hardware and software. In the absent of explicit regulations addressing computer systems, the CPG

* FDA, CPG 7132a.11, "Computerized Drug Processing, CGMP Applicability to Hardware and Software," 9/4/87.

provides the connection between the regulations and the computer systems to meet the agency's expectations.

In a Q&A format, the data integrity guidance establishes a correlation between e-records and the CGMP. The corresponding reference points in parts 21 CFR 211 and 212 are listed in detail in the data integrity guidance document. As an example:

211.68 (requiring that "backup data are exact and complete," and "secure from alteration, inadvertent erasures, or loss")

212.110(b) (requiring that data be "stored to prevent deterioration or loss")

211.100 and 211.160 (requiring that certain activities be "documented at the time of performance" and that laboratory controls be "scientifically sound")

211.180 (requiring that records be retained as "original records," "true copies," or other "accurate reproductions of the original records")

211.188, 211.194, and 212.60(g) (requiring "complete information," "complete data derived from all tests," "complete record of all data," and "complete records of all tests performed").

Title: 21 CFR Part 11 Electronic Records; Electronic Signatures

Regulation/Guideline: Any predicate rule in which the e-records are under the scope of this regulation. Refer to the US FDA Guidance on Part 11, Section III.B.2.

Organization: US FDA

Country: United States

E-Records Integrity Items:

Subpart B—Electronic Records

11.10 Controls for closed systems.

Persons who use closed systems* to create, modify, maintain, or transmit electronic records shall employ procedures and controls designed to ensure the authenticity, integrity, and, when appropriate, the confidentiality of electronic records, and to ensure that the signer cannot readily repudiate that the signed record is not genuine. Such procedures and controls shall include the following:

(a) The validation of systems to ensure the accuracy, reliability and consistency of the intended performance, and the ability to discern invalid or altered records.

---

* Note from the author: Because the US FDA Guidance on Part 11 (Guidance for Industry Part 11, Electronic Records; Electronic Signatures—Scope and Application, August 2003) does not address the open/closed topic, the author of this book believe that the open/closed distinction will be important for FDA in the future. It is not a "critical" subject.

(b) The ability to generate accurate and complete copies of records in both human readable and electronic forms, suitable for inspection, review, and copying by the agency. Persons should contact the agency if there are any questions regarding the ability of the agency to perform such review and copying of the electronic records.
(c) Protection of records to enable their accurate and ready retrieval throughout the records retention period.
(d) Limiting system access to authorized individuals.
(e) Use of secure, computer-generated, time-stamped audit trails to independently record the date and time of operator entries and actions that create, modify, or delete electronic records. Record changes shall not obscure previously recorded information. Such audit trail documentation shall be retained for as long as it is required, and shall be available for agency review and copying.
(f) Use of operational system checks to enforce permitted sequencing of steps and events, as appropriate.
(g) Use of authority checks to ensure that only authorized individuals can use the system, electronically sign a record, access the operation or computer system input or output device, alter a record, or perform the operation at hand.
(h) Use of device (e.g., terminal) checks to determine, as appropriate, the validity of the source of data input or operational instruction.
(i) Determination that persons who develop, maintain, or use electronic record/electronic signature systems have the education, training, and experience to perform their assigned tasks.
(j) The establishment of, and adherence to, written policies that hold individuals accountable and responsible for actions initiated under their electronic signatures, in order to deter record and signature falsification.
(k) Use of appropriate controls over systems documentation including
  (1) Adequate controls over the distribution of, access to, and use of documentation for system operation and maintenance.
  (2) Revision and change control procedures to maintain an audit trail that documents time-sequenced development and modification of systems documentation.

Title: Guidelines on Good Data and Records Management Practices (Draft), September 2015.
Regulation/Guideline: GMP
Organization: World Health Organization (WHO)
Country: All countries that are members of the United Nations may become members of WHO by accepting its constitution. There are a total of 194 Member States. (http://www.who.int/countries/en/).
E-Records Integrity Items:

The WHO released in September 2015 is a draft guidance* document that tries to associate gaps between the principles of good data and record management and actual practices. The scope of this guideline consists of predicate rules.

This guidance goes further than the typical data integrity issues covered by the MHRA guideline.

According to the guidance, organizations need to first establish an organizational structure that includes written policies and procedures documenting processes to prevent and detect situations that may have an impact on data integrity.

Senior management has the final accountability to guarantee that an effective quality system is in place in which employees are stimulated to communicate e-record failures and inaccuracies.

Quality units should also report on metrics related to data integrity, to help identify opportunities for improvement. These include tracking and trending invalid and aberrant data, as well as a regular review of audit trails and routine inspections.

WHO recommends monitoring contract organizations, as well as tracking and trending associated quality metrics for those sites.

Finally, management needs to ensure that all personnel are trained in data integrity polices and agree to abide by them.

Title: Guidelines on good manufacturing practices for blood establishments, WHO Technical Report Series, No. 961, Annex 4, 2011.
Regulation/Guideline: GMP
Organization: World Health Organization (WHO)

* GMP News, New WHO draft on "Good Data and Record Management," 2015, http://www.gmp-compliance.org/enews_05073_New-WHO-Draft-on-%22Good-Data-and-Record-Management%22.html.

Country: All countries that are Members of the United Nations may become members of WHO by accepting its constitution. There are a total of 194 Member States. (http://www.who.int/countries/en/).

E-Records Integrity Items:

6.3 Computerized systems

Hardware and software should be protected against unauthorized use or changes.

A backup procedure should be in place to prevent the loss of records in cases of expected or unexpected downtime or function failures. The archival and retrieval processes should be validated to ensure the accuracy of the stored and retrieved data.

Once in routine operation, critical computer systems should be maintained.

The manual entry of critical data, such as with laboratory test results, should require independent verification and release by a second person. When a computerized system is used, an audit trail should be guaranteed.

Title: Specifications for Pharmaceutical Preparations (Technical Report Series 961), 2011.

Regulation/Guideline: GMP

Organization: WHO

Country: All countries that are members of the United Nations may become members of WHO by accepting its constitution, a total of 194 Member States (http://www.who.int/countries/en/).

E-Records Integrity Items:

15.9 Data (and records for storage) may be recorded by electronic data processing systems or by photographic or other reliable means. Master formulae and detailed standard operating procedures (SOPs) relating to the system in use should be available and the accuracy of the records should be checked. If documentation is handled by electronic data-processing methods, only authorized persons should be able to enter or modify data in the computer, and there should be a record of the changes and deletions made. Access should be restricted by passwords or other means and the entry of critical data should be independently checked. Batch records stored electronically should be protected by back-up transfer on magnetic tape, microfilm, paper print-outs or other means. It is particularly important that, during the period of retention, the data is readily available.

Title: Supplementary Guidelines in Good Manufacturing Practice: Validation. Validation of Computerized Systems, WHO Technical Report Series, No. 937, Annex 4, Appendix 5, 2006.

Regulation/Guideline: GMP

Organization: World Health Organization (WHO)

Country: All countries that are members of the United Nations may become members of WHO by accepting its Constitution, a total of 194 Member States (http://www.who.int/countries/en/).

E-Records Integrity Items:

2.1 There should be a control document or system specification. The control document should state the objectives of a proposed computer system, the data to be entered and stored, the flow of data, how it interacts with other systems and procedures, the information to be produced, the limits of any variable and the operating program and test program.

3.3 The following general GMP requirements are applicable to computer systems.

- Checks: Data should be checked periodically to confirm that they have been accurately and reliably transferred.

4.2 Data should be entered or amended only by persons authorized to do so. Suitable security systems should be in place to prevent unauthorized entry or manipulation of data. The activity of entering data, changing or amending incorrect entries and creating backups should all be done in accordance with written, approved standard operating procedures (SOPs).

4.3 The security procedures should be in writing. Security should also extend to devices used to store programs, such as tapes, disks and magnetic strip cards. Access to these devices should be controlled.

4.4 Traceability is of particular importance and it should be possible to identify the persons who made entries/changes, released material, or performed other critical steps in manufacturing or control.

4.5 The entry of critical data into a computer by an authorized person (e.g., entry of a master processing formula) requires an independent verification and the release for use by a second authorized person.

5.1 Regular backups of all files and data should be made and stored in a secure location to prevent intentional or accidental damage.

7.2.2 Records are considered as software*: the focus is placed on accuracy, security, access, the retention of records, reviewal, double checks, documentation and the accuracy of reproduction.

Additional Reading

Schmitt, S., Data integrity: FDA and Global Regulatory Guidance, *JVT*, 20, 3 October 2014.

* This statement is similar to the original intention of the US FDA Compliance Policy Guide (CPG) Computerized Drug Processing; CGMP Applicability to Hardware and Software (Sec. 425.100). The equivalence of software and records in this CPG has been superseded by the approach taken in the Guidance on Part 11 Scope and Application.

Chapter 8

Trustworthy Computer Systems*

Previous articles[†,‡] discussed the issues of good manufacturing practice (GMP) controls to preserve the integrity of critical e-records and how to assess the effectiveness of these controls. However, to ensure the integrity of e-records, it is essential that the system handling these e-records must be, at the same time, trustworthy.

This chapter describes the concept of trustworthy computer systems in a GMP-regulated activity[§] and the regulatory requirements and key guidelines associated with the trustworthiness of computer systems within the scope of the referenced competent authority. Examples of such computer systems performing GMP-regulated activity are those that

- Make decisions on the market release of drugs and create and retain market distribution records
- Create and retain manufacturing orders and manufacturing records

* López, O., Trustworthy computer systems, *Journal of GxP Compliance* 19, 2, July 2015.

† López, O., EU annex 11 and the integrity of erecs, *Journal of GxP Compliance* 18, 2, May 2014.

‡ López, O., A computer data integrity compliance model, *Pharmaceutical Engineering*, March/April 2015.

§ In this chapter, "GMP regulated activities" is defined as the manufacturing-related activities established in the basic legislation compiled in Volume 1 and Volume 5 of the publication "The rules governing medicinal products in the European Union," http://ec.europa.eu/health/documents/eudralex/index_en.htm, US FDA 21 CFR Part 211, "Current Good Manufacturing Practice In Manufacturing, Processing, Packing or Holding of Drugs; General and Current Good Manufacturing Practice For Finished Pharmaceuticals" or any predicate rule applicable to medicinal products for the referenced country.

- Control/manage manufacturing processes and retain relevant data
- Manage storage, inventory, and so on, of raw materials and products (including intermediates)
- Control/manage laboratory instruments used for quality control (QC) tests and systems to retain QC test results and relevant data
- Control/manage equipment and facilities, including heating, ventilation, and air conditioning (HVAC), water supply systems, and so on, which may have a significant impact on the quality of products, and systems to retain relevant data
- Create, approve, and retain documents (standard operating procedures [SOPs], quality standard codes, product standard codes, and so on).

This chapter covers the key requirements of trustworthy computer systems and provides guidelines from worldwide competent authorities and related organizations (e.g., Pharmaceutical Inspection Convention [PIC] and the Pharmaceutical Inspection Co-operation Scheme [PIC/S]).

For the purpose of this chapter, the terms and definitions given in 9000-3 and ISO 12207 are applicable. In the event of a conflict in terms and definitions, the terms and definitions specified in ISO 9000-3 apply.

Introduction to Trustworthy Computer Systems

The latest e-records integrity issues from regulated users* uncovered by competent authorities have revived the dialog among those in the industry on the GMP controls around e-records. There has been a better understanding of the topic by the competent authorities and the regulated users after the US Food and Drug Administration (FDA) 21 CFR Part 11, Electronic Records: Electronic Signatures† became effective in 1997.

Nevertheless, to ensure the integrity of the e-records, it is essential to ensure that the computer systems are trustworthy. Trustworthy computer systems are the first line of defense to protect the critical e-records managed by these systems.

Trustworthy computer systems consist of computer infrastructure, applications, and procedures that

* Computer System Validation, Data Integrity Deviations, 2016, http://www.computer-systems-validation.net/dataintegritydeviations.html.

† 62 FR 13464, Mar. 20, 1997.

- Are reasonably suited to performing their intended functions
- Provide a reasonably reliable level of availability, reliability, and correct operation
- Are reasonably secure from intrusion and misuse
- Adhere to generally accepted security principles

The driver of the computer systems validation process is to ensure an acceptable degree of evidence (documented, raw data), confidence (dependability and thorough, rigorous achievement of predetermined specifications), intended use, accuracy, consistency, and reliability,* or that the computer system is a trustworthy system.

In the context of e-records integrity, the objectives of a trustworthy computer system are to ensure

- Consistency of data, in particular, preventing unauthorized creation, alteration, or destruction of data (integrity)
- That legitimate users are not improperly denied access to information and resources (availability)
- That resources are used only by authorized persons in authorized ways (legitimate use)

Computer Systems Suited to Performing Their Intended Functions

This is one condition that links the intended use† of a computer system and the functionality of the computer system provided by the developer. A trustworthy computer system conforms to GMP controls and to the efficacy of the computer system to perform the prescribed operation.

Related to GMP controls, computer systems executing GMP-regulated activities should‡ follow the quality management system requirements of the

* WHO, Technical Report Series No. 937, Annex 4. Appendix 5, Validation of computerized systems, 2006.

† Intended use: Use of a product, process, or service in accordance with the specifications, instructions, and information provided by the regulated user.

‡ Should: Used to express a nonmandatory provision. Statements that use "should" are best practices, recommended activities, or options to perform activities to be considered in order to achieve quality projects results. Other methods may be used if it can be demonstrated that they are equivalent.

International Organization for Standardization (ISO) 9001 (e.g., ISO 9000-3), or an equivalent acceptable development methodology* (e.g., ISO 12207, ISO 12119). As an example, the origins of good automated manufacturing practices (GAMP) embraced ISO 9000-3.

The intended use of a computer system is established during the requirements analysis and settles in the requirements specification.

The requirements specification describes the required functions of the computer system, and it is based on a documented risk and a GMP impact assessment. This specification must be managed† and the requirements contained traceable throughout the computer system life cycle (SLC) (EMEA Annex 11-4.4). The requirements specification is based on inputs from many sources, including computer system users, quality assurance, applicable regulations, information technology, infrastructure architecture, potential data migration, engineering, and safety. Based on this specification, the system is developed or configured following the applicable best compliance practices transcribed as procedural controls.

The precise execution of an approved comprehensive quality management system enables both the regulated user and the competent authority to have a high level of confidence in the integrity of both the processes executed within the controlling computer system(s) and those processes controlled by and/or linked to the computer system(s), within the prescribed operating environment(s).

The evidence to demonstrate the conformance of the computer systems with the established process requirements and applicable regulatory requirements of computer systems performing GMP-regulated activities is accomplished via the computer validation‡ process.

> *Software quality is the fitness for use of the software product.*
>
> **Schulmeyer and McManus**

---

* Software life cycle process that contains the activities of requirements analysis, design, coding, integration, testing, installation and support for acceptance of software products (ISO 9000-3).

† López, O., Requirements management, *Journal of Validation Technology*, May 2011.

‡ Computer validation: Formal assessment and reporting of quality and performance measures for all the life-cycle stages of software and system development, its implementation, qualification and acceptance, operation, modification, re-qualification, maintenance, and retirement. (PI 011-3. *Good Practices for Computerised Systems in Regulated "GXP" Environments*, Pharmaceutical Inspection Co-operation Scheme (PIC/S), September 2007.)

The definition of computer systems validation by PIC/S makes reference to the "formal assessment and reporting of a computer systems validation." This reference can be interpreted as requiring controlled documented methodology and records based on best compliance practices. The controlled documented methodology and records ensure that the regulated user has generated documented evidence (electronic and/or paper based) that gives a high level of assurance that both the computer system and the computerized system will consistently perform as intended, designed, implemented, verified, tested, and maintained.*,†

The relevant requirements and/or guidelines about this topic are as follows.

ISO 9000-3

Section 7.3.6.1 states that validation of software is aimed at providing reasonable confidence that it will meet its operational requirements.

US FDA

The FDA considers software validation to be the confirmation by examination and provision of objective evidence that software specifications conform to user needs and intended use, and that the particular requirements implemented through software can be fulfilled consistently.

The computer validation process takes place within the environment of an established SLC. The SLC contains software engineering tasks and documentation necessary to support the software validation effort. In addition, the SLC contains specific verification and testing tasks that are commensurable to the risk associated to the computer system.

---

* PI 011-3. *Good Practices for Computerised Systems in Regulated "GXP" Environments*, Pharmaceutical Inspection Co-operation Scheme (PIC/S), September 2007.

† Cappucci, W.; Chris Clark, C.; Goossens, T.; Wyn, S., ISPE GAMP CoP Annex 11 interpretation, *Pharmaceutical Engineering*, July/August 2011.

European Medicines Agency (EMA) Annex 11, Therapeutic Goods Administration (TGA),* and China's SFDA†

According to the interpretation of the GAMP Community of Practice (CoP) Task Team,‡ the second principle in the EMA Annex 11, "The application should be validated; IT infrastructure should be qualified," reflects the GAMP 5 definition of computer system validation as achieving and maintaining compliance with applicable GxP§ regulations and fitness for intended use.

PIC/S PI-011-3, Association of Southeast Asian Nations (ASEAN),¶ and Canadian HPFBI**

Some of the specifics of PIC/S PI-011-3 intended for inspectors may need some modification to account for the updated EMA Annex 11, but overall it remains a good resource.

Consistent with the US Food and Drug Administration (FDA) expectations on software validations, PIC/S considers that computer validation is the formal assessment and reporting of quality and performance measures for all the SLC stages of software and system development as well as its implementation, qualification and acceptance, operation, modification, re-qualification, maintenance, and retirement.

---

* On 29 July 2009, the Therapeutic Goods Administration (Manufacturing Principles) Determination No. 1 of 2009 adopted the PIC/S Guide to Good Manufacturing Practice—15 January 2009, PE 009-8, to be the Code of GMP, except for its Annexes 4, 5, and 14, which are not adopted by Australia. Annex 11, Computerized systems, was one of the PIC/S Guide to Good Manufacturing Practice annexes adopted. TGA is Australia's regulatory authority for therapeutic goods.

† The China State Food and Drug Administration (SFDA) released in December 2015 GMP Annex 2 Computerized System. Actually, this document is based on the 1992 EMA GMP Annex 11.

‡ Cappucci, W.; Chris Clark, C.; Goossens, T.; Wyn, S., ISPE GAMP CoP Annex 11 interpretation, *Pharmaceutical Engineering*, July/August 2011.

§ GxP: The underlying international life science requirements such as those set forth in the US FD&C Act, US PHS Act, FDA regulations, EU Directives, Japanese MHL.W regulations, Australia TGA, or other applicable national legislation or regulations under which a company operates (GAMP Good Practice Guide, IT Infrastructure Control and Compliance, ISPE 2005).

¶ Based on the ASEAN Mutual Recognition Agreement recognition of GMP inspections, it will follow PIC/S GMPs.

**In the Health Products and Food Branch Inspectorate (HPFBI) GMP Guidelines (2009 Edition, Rev 2), Health Canada establishes that guidance to validate computer systems performing GMP regulated activities is provided in PIC/S PI-011-3.

International Conference on Harmonization of Technical Requirements for Registration of Pharmaceuticals for Human Use (ICH)

The ICH Q7A GMP Guidance for API (Chapter 5) calls for the suitability of the computer system to be demonstrated during an "appropriate installation and operational qualifications."

World Health Organization (WHO)

The Technical Report Series (No. 937, Annex 4, Appendix 5, "Validation of computerized systems") establishes that the purpose of validation of a computer system is to ensure an acceptable degree of evidence (documented, raw data), confidence (dependability and thorough, rigorous achievement of predetermined specifications), intended use, accuracy, consistency, and reliability.

Japanese MHLW

The Japanese Ministry of Health, Labor and Welfare (MHLW) published the Guideline on Management of Computerized Systems for Marketing Authorization Holders and Manufacturers of Drugs and Quasi-Drugs in October 2011. The purpose of this guideline is to specify the activities during the development of computerized systems, validation items to verify such systems, and the activities to be observed during the operations of such systems, with the purpose of ensuring that such systems perform as intended.

Brazil ANVISA

Article 572 of the Brazilian Agência Nacional de Vigilância Sanitária (ANVISA) rules on GMP of medicinal products establishes that the extent of validation depends on a number of factors, including the intended use of the system, the type of validation to perform (prospective, concurrent, and retrospective), and inserting new elements.

Provide a Reasonably Reliable* Level of Availability, Reliability, and Correct Operation

The best application will not meet the user's need if it is unavailable. In the technical sense, availability is the measure of the percentage of time that an

* Reliable: Consistently good performance.

application is available for use. The typical end user expects an application to be available 24/7/365; anything else is deemed unacceptable. But uptime is not the only indicator of availability. Offutt* suggests that "using features available on only one platform" makes the application unavailable to those with a different platform. The user invariably will go elsewhere.

Maturity, fault tolerance, and recoverability are related to reliability or the amount of time that the computer system is available for use.

In the event of a system failure, there should be a general procedure to remedy and restore the hardware or software from any situation to a correctly functioning and basic condition and to reconstruct the relevant data reliably† (EMA Annex 11-16).

The procedure to remedy and restore system errors should consider the following:

- Conduct error analysis
- Commission and carry out repairs
- Implement additional organizational measures (work around)
- Test software components
- Check stored data
- Reconstruct data
- System release for reuse
- Documentation instructions

All performance requirements, including reliability and recovery, that the software must meet must be specified in the requirements specification.

Testing of the recovery-related requirements include challenging the ability of the system to recover from programming errors, data errors, and hardware failures. If the recovery is automatic, reinitialization, checkpoints mechanism data recovery, and restart should be evaluated.

Incidents related to computer systems that could affect the reliability of records should be recorded and investigated.

GAMP5 Appendix M4 (Section 3.1.14) provides guidance on reliability and error recovery.

---

* Offutt, J., Quality attributes of web software applications, *IEEE Software*, March/April 2002, pp. 25–32.

† APV, *Guideline Computerized Systems based on Annex 11 of the EU-GMP Guideline*, April 1996.

The correct operation consists of those attributes of the computer system that provide full implementation of the required functions. The application-dependent algorithms consisting of manufacturing procedures, control, instructions, specifications, and precautions to be followed within such automated systems are embodied in the computer program(s) that drive the computer. They include those instructions to enforce process sequencing with significant impact on drug product quality.

The lack of operational checks to enforce event sequencing is significant if an operator's ability to deviate from the prescribed order of computer system operation steps results in an adulterated or misbranded product and/or data integrity.*

The relevant requirements and/or guidelines about this topic are as follows.

ISO 9000-3

The operational environment requirements (Section 7.2.1.1) may include, but not be limited to, the following characteristics: functionality, reliability, usability, efficiency, maintainability, and portability.

US FDA

The *General Principles of Software Validation*† establishes reliability as a quality factor to be addressed during quality planning and is clearly established in the requirements specification.

21 CFR 11.10(a) requires computer systems to be reliable and perform the correct operation.

EMA and TGA

Annex 11-11 stipulates that, during periodic reviews, the reliability of a computer system must be evaluated.

* López, O., Operational checks, in *21 CFR Part 11: Complete Guide to International Computer Validation Compliance for the Pharmaceutical Industry*, Eds. (Interpharm/CRC, Boca Raton, FL, 1st edn, 2004).

† US FDA, *General Principles of Software Validation; Final Guidance for Industry and FDA Staff*, CDRH and CBER, January 2002.

PIC/S PI-011-3, ASEAN, and Canadian HPFBI

Understanding that the majority of the software used in the health-care industry is developed by suppliers, the PIC/S guideline stresses the quality of the software engineering processes followed during the development of the software product by the supplier.

To have confidence in the reliability of the products, the regulated user should evaluate the quality methodology of the supplier for the design, construction, supply, and maintenance of the software. Refer to GAMP 5 Appendix M2, Supplier Assessment.

After acquiring a system, software product, or service, the regulated user needs to execute the activities, defined in the applicable procedural controls, to demonstrate the correct operation of the components associated with the computer system and the integration of the components.

ICH

There is no explicit statement related to the availability and reliability of the computer systems. Implicit requirements linked with the correct operation of the computer systems can be found in the requirements associated with validations of the computer systems.

WHO

Refer to the previous note related to the WHO in which reliability and correct operation are referenced.

China SFDA

As in the ICH, there is no explicit statement related to the availability and reliability of the computer systems. Implicit requirements associated with the correct operation of the computer systems can be found in Article 6:

> Computerized system validation, including application validation and infrastructure qualification, the scope and extent should depend on scientific based risk assessment. Risk assessment should adequately consider the scope and purpose of use a computerized system. Verification should be run throughout the life cycle of a computerized system.

Brazil ANVISA

As in the ICH and China SFDA, there is no explicit statement related to the availability and reliability of the computer systems in the ANVISA's Rules on Good Manufacturing Practice of Medicinal Products in the Resolution of the Executive Board No. 17 (Title VII-Computerized Information).

Implicit requirements associated with the correct operation of the computer systems can be found in Articles 577 and 578:

> The system should include, where applicable, verification of data entry and processing.
>
> Before starting to use a computerized system, one must test and verify the ability of the system to store the desired data, ensuring the technological infrastructure necessary to its full operation.

Secure from Intrusion and Misuse

To avoid intrusions into computer systems, physical and/or logical controls must be established enabling access to authorized persons only.* For those users allowed to access a computer system, the precise access level to the applications and resources must be assigned based on an authorization level. Documentation regarding the creation, change, and cancellation of access authorizations and the level of authorization must be maintained at all times.†

To minimize intrusion risks to computer systems, computers input and output (I/O) must be monitored for the correct and secure entry and processing of data. One illustration of an I/O monitoring is an intrusion detection system. This is a device or software application that monitors network or system activities for malicious activities or policy violations. These systems produce reports that can be used to strengthen the security controls.

The misuse of computer systems by users can be remediated by the system owner implementing a training program of the intended use of the related applications and all computer resources.

---

* Section C.02.005 Item 15 in the Computer Systems GMP Guidelines for API in Canada's GUI-0104, December 2013.

† Article 579 Item 2 in the Resolution of the Executive Board No. 17, Brazilian GMPs, April 2010.

All intrusion and misuse incidents should be reported and assessed. The root cause of an intrusion and misuse should be identified and should be the basis of corrective and preventive actions.

The relevant requirements and/or guidelines about this topic are as follows.

ISO 9000-3

During the review of the requirements, risks associated with security issues are to be assessed (Section 7.2.2.2). Management of the security controls is performed during the system development life cycle. ISO 9000-3 recommends writing a plan specifically to manage the implementation of the security controls. During the operational phase, the security controls are maintained and their effectiveness evaluated as applicable.

US FDA

Overall, 21 CFR Part 211.68 symbolizes the US FDA security-related requirements. Computer systems must have adequate controls to prevent unauthorized access or changes to data, inadvertent erasures, or loss.

211 CFR Part 11, 11.10(d) requires that access to e-records on a computer system be granted only to authorized individuals.

EMA, TGA, and China SFDA

According to EMA Annex 11-12, physical and/or logical controls to restrict access to computer systems and data storage areas should be in place and based on a risk assessment. The users' authorization levels and the changes to such levels must be controlled and documented.

Similar to the 2003 US FDA 21 CFR Part 11 Guideline, high-risk computer systems handling critical e-records should implement audit trail functionality.

PIC/S PI-011-3, ASEAN, and Canadian HPFBI

PI-011-3 provides a complete section, Section 19, covering the security of computer systems.

Summarizing this section, the security of the system and data is very important, and the procedures and records pertaining to these aspects should be based on the policies of the regulated user and in conformance with the relevant regulatory requirements. It is very important for the regulated user to maintain the procedures and records related to accessing the system(s). There should be clearly defined responsibilities for system security management, suitable for both small and complex systems, including:

- Implementation of the security strategy and delegation
- Management and assignment of privileges
- Levels of access for users
- Levels of access for infrastructure

ICH

Section 5.43 calls for sufficient controls by the computer system to prevent unauthorized access or changes to data. There should be controls to prevent omissions in data (e.g., system turned off and data not captured). There should be a record of any data change made, the previous entry, who made the change, and when the change was made.

ICH Q7, Section 6.6, requires a complete record of all raw data generated during each test using laboratory equipment. The information to be collected by testing includes graphs, charts, and spectra from laboratory instrumentation. A second person must verify this information for accuracy, completeness, and compliance with established standards.

WHO

The Technical Report Series (No. 937, Annex 4, Appendix 5) establishes that the security procedures should be in writing. Security should also extend to devices used to store programs, such as tapes, disks, and magnetic strip cards. Access to these devices should be controlled.

Brazil ANVISA

Article 579 establishes that the entries and data modifications can be performed only by authorized persons.

- Measures should be taken that do not allow unauthorized persons to include, exclude, or alter data in the system and can be used for security measures, such as the use of passwords, personal code, access profiles, keys, or restricted access to the system.

- A procedure should be established for access management, defining how to issue, amend, and cancel the passwords of persons who are no longer authorized to enter or change data in the system.
- Preference should be given to systems that allow registering attempted unauthorized access.

Adhere to Generally Accepted Security Principles

Each predicate rule (e.g., 21 Code of Federal Regulations [CFR] Part 211.68(b)) or guideline (e.g., Guidance for Industry Computerized Systems Used in Clinical Investigations) requires/outlines appropriate security-related controls over applications, infrastructure, and infrastructure components, to ensure that only authorized personnel have a hierarchy of permitted access to enter, amend, read, or print out e-records and the information stored within. These controls must be addressed adequately during the development, validation, operation, and maintenance of any computer system.

The following are essential practices relevant to the security of applications.* The applications can be networked or stand-alone. If the application is networked, supplementary practices are contained in the next section.

1. All applications must have a qualified authentication mechanism to control access (EMA Annex 11-Principle #2).
2. Software "virus checking" must take place periodically to protect of the applications and data.
3. Procedural controls must be established to specify the manner in which application security is administered (ICH Q7 Section 5.44).
4. The process for setting up access to applications must be defined and executed by the appropriate application-specific security administration personnel. The technical preparation, education, and training for personnel performing administration tasks, and associated documented evidence, are a key regulatory requirement (EMA Annex 11-2).
5. The management of the user application accounts is a key procedural control. This procedural control includes requesting the addition, modification, and removal of application access privileges (EMA Annex

* O. López, *Computer Technologies Security. Part 1: Key Points in the Contained Domain*, Sue Horwood Publishing, Pulborough, 2002.

11-12.3). The request is approved by the appropriate manager, carefully documented, and submitted to the application security administration for execution of the request.

6. There must be a procedure to grant temporary application-specific access for personnel (21 CFR Part 11.10(d)).
7. In the event that a user leaves the company, there must be a process to notify the appropriate security administration *as soon as* the employee departs (EMA Annex 11-12.3).
8. A procedure must exist that defines the escalation process and actions to be taken on discovery of unauthorized access (EMA Annex 11-13).
9. A documented record of security administration activities must be retained.
10. Procedures must exist to control remote modem access to applications via the applicable infrastructure.*
11. In cases where data or instructions are only available from specific input devices (e.g., instruments, terminals), the system should be checked for, and the operator should verify, the use of the correct device (EMA Annex 11-5).
12. When an individual has been authorized to use the system, time-stamped audit trails (EMA Annex 11-9) must record write-to-file operations and changes, and independently record the date and time of the application-specific operator's actions or entries.
13. Time-stamped audit trails (EMA Annex 11-9) must be used to keep track of modifications by the database administrator to the application-related e-records.
14. The use of operational checks is recommended to enforce sequencing (21 CFR Part 11.10(f)).
15. Authority checks (21 CFR Part 11.10(g)) must be used, when applicable, to determine if the operator can use the system, operate a device, or perform the operation at hand.
16. The e-records must not be altered, browsed, queried, or reported via external software applications that do not enter to the data repository area through the protective technological controls (US FDA,† EMA Annex 11-7.1 and Annex 11-17, and TGA.‡

* PI 011-3. *Good Practices for Computerised Systems in Regulated "GXP" Environments*, Section 21.8, Pharmaceutical Inspection Co-operation Scheme (PIC/S), September 2007.

† US FDA, *Guidance for Industry Computerized Systems Used in Clinical Investigations*, May 2010.

‡ TGA, *CGMP Human Blood Tissues*, Section 1011, April 2013.

17. Unauthorized modification to the system clock must be prevented (21 CFR Part 11.10(d)). One possible technological control around this item is the use of a digital time-stamping service or an infrastructure that supports time stamping from a trusted time service (e.g., coordinated universal time).

An example of item 17 is a recent Statement of Noncompliance with GMPs issued on December 2014* following an inspection by the Italian Medicines Agency in accordance with Art. 111(7) of Directive 2001/83/EC as amended. One of the concerns was that the "analysts routinely use the terminal administrator privileges to set the controlling time and date settings back to overwrite previously collected failing and/or undesirable sample results. This practice is performed until passing and/or desirable results are achieved."

The relevant requirements and/or guidelines discussed in this chapter under the "Secure from Intrusion and Misuse" are also applicable in this section.

Trustworthy Computer Systems Infrastructure

The following items are the key practices that are applicable for the security of the networked environments (local area networks or wide area networks).

1. Network resources have a qualified authentication mechanism for controlling access (EMA Annex 11-12.1). Table 8.1 shows the authentication requirements and the methods of implementation. These authentication requirements and methods of implementation are relevant to applications security as well.

   Access control decision functions are defined using access-right lists, such as access control lists (ACLs), which allow the allocation of use, read, write, execute, delete, or create privileges. Access controls enable a system to be designed in such a way that a supervisor, for example, will be able to access information on a group of employees, without everyone else on the network having access to this information.

* http://eudragmdp.ema.europa.eu/inspections/gmpc/searchGMPNonCompliance.do?ctrl=searchGMPNCResultControlList&action=Drilldown&param=26750.

Table 8.1 Authentication

Requirement	*Implementation*
The following features must be implemented: • Automatic logoff. • Unique user identification. • In addition, at least one of the other listed implementation features must be a procedure that corroborates that an entity is who it claims to be.	• Automatic logoff • Biometrics • Password • PIN • Telephone callback • Token • Unique user identification

The access controls are an element of the authority check requirements.

2. The process for setting up user access to a network is the responsibility of the appropriate network security administration personnel. The technical preparation, education, and training for personnel performing administration tasks are fundamental (EMA Annex 11-2). The determination of what is required and the provision of documented evidence of the technical preparation, and the education and training of personnel is a key regulatory requirement (21 CFR Part 11.10(i)).
3. Procedural controls, which specify the manner in which network security is administered, must be established and documented. Network users must be trained in the policies, practices, and procedures concerning network security.
4. The management of network user accounts is a key procedural control. This process includes the request for the addition, modification, and removal of access privileges (EMA Annex 11-12.3). The request must be approved by the appropriate manager, documented, and submitted to the network security administration for implementation.
5. There must be a procedure for granting controlled temporary network access for personnel (21 CFR Part 11.10(d)).
6. In the event that a user leaves the company, there must be a process for notifying the appropriate security administration as soon as the employee departs (EMA Annex 11-12.3).
7. Provisions must be made for the regular monitoring of access to the network. There must be an escalation procedure for defining the actions to be taken if unauthorized access to the network is discovered (EMA Annex 11-13).

8. A documented record of security administration activities must be retained.
9. Procedures must be established to control remote access to the network. Systems that have connections to telephone communications through modems should have strict access controls and restrictions. Access restrictions on these systems should be designed to prevent unauthorized access or change. One possible method for controlling remote access is telephone call back.
10. Remote access to applications must be performed through the protective technological controls.
11. Time-stamped audit trails (21 CFR Part 11.10(c) and € and EMA Annex 11-9) to record changes must be used to record all write-to-file operations, and to independently record the date and time of any network system administrator actions or data entries/changes.
12. Unauthorized modification of the system clock must be prevented (21 CFR Part 11.10(d)).

Computer System Procedures

Refer to Chapter 11.

Summary

To ensure the integrity of e-records, it is essential that the system handling these e-records must be, at the same time, trustworthy.

Trustworthy computer systems consist of computer infrastructure, applications, and procedures that

- Are reasonably suited to performing their intended functions
- Provide a reasonable level of availability, reliability, and correct operation
- Are reasonably secure from intrusion and misuse
- Adhere to generally accepted security principles

No matter the selected model (traditional or cloud), the requirements for trustworthy and compliant computer systems performing regulated activities are the same.

Finally, consistent with the globalization of the health-care industry, the preceding principles are contained in all key regulations and guidelines.

Additional Readings

López, O., A computer data integrity compliance model, *Pharmaceutical Engineering* 35, 2, March/April 2015.

López, O., Computer systems alidation, in *Encyclopedia of Pharmaceutical Science and Technology*, 4th Edition, Taylor and Francis: New York, August 2013, pp. 615–619.

López, O., *Computer Technologies Security Part I: Key Points in the Contained Domain*, Sue Horwood Publishing, Pulborough, England.

López, O., EU Annex 11 and the integrity of erecs, *Journal of GxP Compliance* 18, 2, May 2014.

López, O., *EU Annex 11 Guide to Computer Validation Compliance for the Worldwide Health Agency GMP*, CRC Press, Boca Roton, FL, March 2015.

Chapter 9

MHRA Guidance

Introduction

The Heads of Medicines Agencies (HMA) and the European Medicines Agency (EMA) had determined in early 2015 "the need to ensure the integrity of the data on which regulatory decisions about medicines are based. Concerns about data integrity may arise for many reasons, for example, poor training, inadequate implementation or occasionally due to suspicions of falsification. The integrity of the data in the studies used to support market authorization is fundamental to trust and confidence in the products themselves."*

The HMS and EMA "will ensure that all suspicions of problems with data integrity are thoroughly investigated working closely with other international partners where these data may have been generated or used."†

As part of the strategy by the HMA and EMA, the Medicines and Healthcare Products Regulatory Agency (MHRA, United Kingdom [UK] Medicines and Medical Devices Regulatory Agency) is setting emphasis on the integrity of the critical data during inspections at regulated manufacturing sites. In addition, the MHRA is stressing self-inspections programs to address the effectiveness of the current good manufacturing practice (cGMP) controls to ensure data integrity and traceability.‡

* HMA and EMA, EU medicines agencies network strategy to 2020 (Draft), March 2015.

† HMA and EMA, EU medicines agencies network strategy to 2020 (Draft), March 2015.

‡ MHRA, MHRA expectation regarding self-inspection and data integrity, September 2014.

Prior to any inspection, entities that fall under the pre-inspection compliance are required to include the following data integrity measures for inspection purposes:

- Confirmation that a data integrity/data governance policy is in place (Chapter 10).
- Confirmation that computer system owners/personnel with administrative-level permissions are available during the GMP inspection.
- Information on the computer systems that are used for storage, control, and processing is available.

A list of all principal computer systems and stand-alone systems, including qualification dates, is required during the inspection.

In preparation for these inspections, the MHRA introduced the Data Integrity Definitions and Guidance.* This guidance document outlines a data integrity governance system and supplementary principles for defining quality and data integrity into processes and systems. The guidance provides notes and examples about the definitions and the controls associated with e-records integrity.

The Data Integrity Definition and Guidance supplements the EMA Annex 11† GMP guidelines to the UK pharmaceutical industry on how to implement cGMP data integrity controls. It is an excellent reference for other regulated users and inspectors that ensures a common understanding of terms and concepts.

At the time of writing this book, a cross-MHRA inspectorate group is writing a consolidated guidance document that will apply across all GxPs. According to the MHRA, there is a need to consider data integrity across the board.

Based on the National Institutes of Standards and Technology (NIST) definition of data integrity, this chapter discusses the technical and procedural controls–related guidance provided by the MHRA on e-records integrity and the relationship with those relevant elements in EMA Annex 11. Organizational controls are out of the scope of this chapter.

---

* MHRA, MHRA GMP data integrity definitions and guidance for industry, March 2015.

† EC, Volume 4: EU guidelines to good manufacturing practice: Medicinal products for human and veterinary use—Annex 11: Computerized systems, European Commission, Brussels, June, pp. 1–4, 2011.

Data Governance

The MHRA guidance provides critical points to consider when implementing Annex 11 elements related to e-records integrity.* The approach is based on the typical Annex 11 system life cycle (SLC) phases: project, operations, and retirement.

The MHRA guidance document endorses a strong data governance approach. The majority of the lack of e-records integrity cases have to do with bad practices, poor organizational controls, and/or with lack of the technical controls that open possibilities for e-records manipulations. These deficiencies are corrected by applying good e-records integrity practices (GEIP) within all the components in the regulated user's organization.

The e-records governance is met by

- Training all computer systems users about e-records integrity
- Making senior management accountable to totally support the controls associated with e-records integrity
- Addressing e-records ownership and the responsibilities associated with this role (EMA Annex 11 definition: System Owner)

A robust data governance approach will ensure that data is complete, consistent, and accurate, irrespective of the format in which the data is generated, used, or retained.†

The MHRA requires cGMP-regulated users to complete a cGMP Pre Inspection Compliance Report‡ before an inspection, unless it is a triggered inspection, which is given only short notice. One area covered in this compliance report is data integrity. In this data integrity section, the questionnaire includes if the regulated user has a policy on data integrity governance.

Figure 9.1 suggests an approach of the integration of the GEIP with the typical EMA Annex 11 SLC. This approach is combined with the subject of this chapter.

* López, O., EU Annex 11 and the integrity of erecs, *Journal of GxP Compliance*, 18, 2, May 2014.

† Churchward, D., Good Manufacturing Practice (GMP) data integrity: A new look at an old topic, Part 2 of 3, July 2015.

‡ MHRA, Comply with good manufacturing practice (GMP) and good distribution practice (GDP), and prepare for an inspection, December 2014.

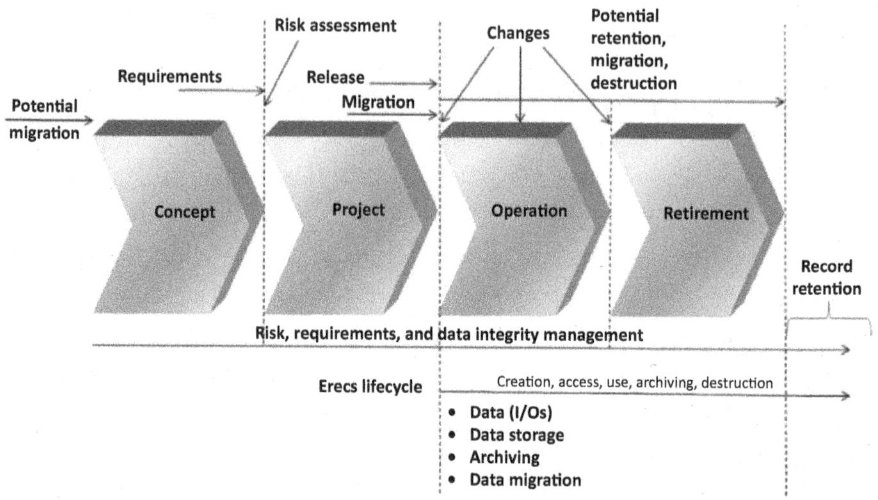

Figure 9.1 Data integrity management.

Computer Systems Validation

An element in e-records governance is the computer validation process. This process provides the initial assurance of the successful implementation of the e-records integrity controls. These controls are to be maintained throughout the operation, maintenance, and retirement of the computer system.

Computer systems validation is the formal assessment and reporting of quality and performance measures for all the life-cycle stages of software and system development, its implementation, qualification and acceptance, operation, modification, re-qualification, maintenance, and retirement. This should enable both the regulated user and competent authority to have a high level of confidence in the integrity of both the processes executed within the controlling computer system(s) and in those processes controlled by and/or linked to the computer system(s), within the prescribed operating environment(s).*

The MHRA guideline established validation of computer systems based on the EMA Annex 11 guidelines.

* PI 011-3, Good practices for computerised systems in regulated "GXP" environments, Pharmaceutical Inspection Co-operation Scheme (PIC/S), September 2007.

Requirements

Business requirements* are gathered as part of the feasibility study at the beginning of the automated project, including the data integrity–related requirements. These data integrity–related requirements are traced to the regulated company data governance (11, p. 4.4).

The following data integrity requirements are critical.

- Identify the critical data.†
- Based on a risk assessment, identify the e-records integrity–related controls. The identified risk must be managed through the SLC (11, p. 1).
- If data is transferred to another data format, the new format must be established‡ (11, p. 4.8 and 11, p. 8.1).
- Identify interfaces (11, p. 5) and the data to be entered manually (11, p. 6).
- Based on risk assessment, assess the need of audit trails (12.4) and controls to prevent unauthorized access to the application and the operating systems (11, p. 7.1; 11, p. 12; and 21 CFR 11.10(g)) by restricting access via passwords or other means.
- Record the access attempts.
- A reliable time source must be used to update server's time. This reliable time must be used for the generation of time stamps.
- Design the applicable reports (11, p. 8.1), operational system checks (21 CFR Part 11.10(f)), authority checks (21 CFR Part 11.10(g)), and device checks (21 CFR Part 11.10(h)).

The appropriate methods to prevent unauthorized manipulation of data include the use of

- Keys
- Passwords
- Personal codes
- Restricted access to computer terminals

---

* Business requirements are the critical activities of an enterprise that must be performed to meet the organizational objective(s) while remaining solution independent.

† Critical data: Data with high risk to product quality or patient safety. (ISPE GAMP COP Annex 11—Interpretation, July/August 2011.)

‡ Establish is defined in this book as meaning to define, document, and implement.

Of special interest are the system administrator access and the access to the e-records retained by computer storage (11, p. 7.1). According to the Data Integrity Definitions and Guidance document, the MHRA expects that each system administrator should have unique access to the computer system. Every employee with administrative privileges is logged into the computer system with his or her distinct password, to ensure that there is traceability of actions performed in the computer and the respective user, including an audit trail.

During the implementation of a new system in which a legacy system is replaced, the Requirements Stage must consider the data migration from the legacy system to the new system. It will be required to

- Consider storage and infrastructure requirements
- Map source and destination fields
- Specify the mandatory fields for data
- Extract and load requirements
- Specify the data inputs (e.g., format, decimal places, units, ranges, limits, defaults, and the conversion requirements)
- Determine what constitutes an error and how errors must be handled
- Verify requirements to ensure that the source data is the same as the data in the destination

As the reader can evaluate from the above requirements, this is a project by itself.

The business requirements are transformed to user requirements or capabilities needed by a user to solve or achieve an objective. Finally, the user requirements are translated to functional requirements or requirements that specify the behavior or functions of the computer system (11, p. 4.4).

Risk Assessment

A mature data governance system adopts a "quality risk management" approach across all areas of the quality system* (11, p. 4.5). The critical data integrity risk will vary depending on the degree to which data generated by

* Churchward, D., Good Manufacturing Practice (GMP) data integrity: A new look at an old topic, Part 2 of 3, July 2015.

the computer system can be configured, and therefore potentially manipulated* (11, p. 12.2).

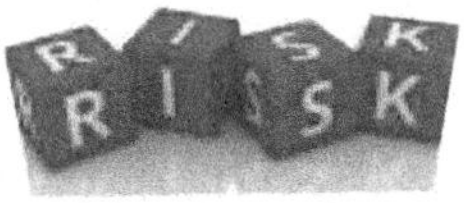

Based on the foregoing statements, an evaluation of risks is performed to uncover potential data manipulations in an unauthorized manner and, via a root analysis, finding the mitigation(s) to the potential unauthorized manipulation of the data. These analyses may lead to architecture and design trade-offs during system development.

The MHRA guidance suggests mitigations to address the risk of data manipulations in an unauthorized manner.

- Access controls to ensure that only authorized individuals can access and use the system based on their job role (11, p. 12.1 and p. 12.2). The access controls are applicable to database servers or any server containing GMP-related data.
- The regulated entity must have documentation about users and access level (11, p. 12.3).
- In cases where technological or design constraints do not allow unique access to the computer application and/or database server(s), a paper-based method must provide access traceability.
- The access to system administrators should be minimal, unique per administrator, and traceable. The preferred traceability method for actions performed by a system administrator is audit trails (11, p. 9). It is not specified if the audit trails must be recorded electronically.
- Separation of roles must be enforced on data maintenance.
- Data maintenance must be controlled (11, p. 12.4) and an approval method must be implemented (11, p. 10).

Another area to consider is the risk associated with data migration from existing system(s) over to a new system. The risk of data migration may be mitigated by verifying "that data are not altered in value and/or meaning during this migration process" (11, p. 4.8).

* Churchward, D., Good Manufacturing Practice (GMP) data integrity: A new look at an old topic, Part 1 of 3, June 2015.

Annex 20* summarizes an approach to a quality risk management pertinent to computer systems and computer-controlled equipment.

- Determine the GMP criticality of the system, impact on patient safety, product quality, or data integrity; identify the critical performance parameters; determine the extent of validation.
- Develop requirement specification considering the basis of the criticality; perform a detailed risk assessment to determine critical functions.
- Select the design of computer hardware and software (e.g., modular, structured, fault tolerance); implement appropriate controls via design as much as possible.
- Perform code review, as applicable.
- Determine the extent of testing and test methods of the controls implemented during the design.
- Evaluate the reliability of electronic records and signatures, as applicable.
- The risks uncovered during this activity must be managed through the SLC (11, p. 1).

The risk management process supports the assessment against the computer requirements and within its operational environment. Decisions regarding risks identified must be made prior to starting the design of the computer system.

According to the MHRA guidance, "the effort and resource assigned to data governance should be commensurate with the risk to product quality."

In addition, the MHRA communicated to the regulated user that he or she must carry out a routine effectiveness review of his or her governance systems to ensure data integrity and traceability are maintained. The effectiveness review can be performed during the periodic review.

The requirements document must include requirement(s) related to the mitigation of the uncovered risks.

* EudraLex, *The Rule Governing Medicinal Products in the European Union*, Volume 4, *EU Guidelines for Good Manufacturing Practices for Medicinal Products for Human and Veterinary Use*, Annex 20, Quality Risk Management, February 2008.

Data Migration and Computer Systems Release to Operations

As part of the Project Phase, the application is delineated, documented, and implemented.

The following is addressed by the MHRA guideline:

- As part of qualifying the application and associated controls, test the backup and restoration procedure(s) and verify the output of the backup (11, p. 7.2). Each backup set should be checked to ensure that it is error-free, including the metadata and all configuration-related files.
- The ability to retrieve the e-records and audit trails should be ensured and tested (11, p. 7.1).
- Verify the accuracy of reports and audit trail reports (11, p. 8).
- As applicable and based on the operational sequencing, test the accuracy of the e-records (11, p. 7.1).
- Information technology (IT) infrastructure must be qualified to ensure security and electronic records integrity (11, Principle b).

At the same time, if e-records are transferred to a new environment, changing the format of the e-records, the qualification must include test cases and the associated verifications that the electronic records' new format does not alter the content of the records and associated metadata during the migration process (11, p. 4.8). The migrated records and application(s) are integrated, and testing is executed to demonstrate such integration.

As part of the implementation, one of many data integrity–related requirements addressed in the MHRA guideline is the recording of transactions contemporaneously by computer systems. These are typical transactions in which the user agrees, completes by performing certain predefined actions, or acknowledges a deviation. These actions must not be combined into a single computer system transaction with other operations.

The preceding guideline can be traced to section 4.8 in volume 4, chapter 4 (Documentation) from the EudraLex, the rules governing medicinal products in the European Union.

> Records should be made or completed at the time each action is taken and in such a way that all significant activities concerning the manufacture of medicinal products are traceable.

Recording data contemporaneously is a key factor related to data reliability.*

Operations

During this stage, e-records are generated, recorded, transformed, access, used, logically deleted, migrated, and retired. This is when the integrity of the e-records can be compromised. All the technical controls designed and implemented are used to preserve the integrity of the e-records. Applicable to the Operational Stage, Chapter 3 describes the life cycle of the e-records.

During the Operational Stage, the procedural controls must be enforced:

- Only authorized people can modify the e-records stored on data servers or any other media.
- There are records of changes made.
- Entry of data considered critical is checked by a designated person other than the one who made the records or checked by the system itself.
- A procedural control is available for cancellation, changes to the level of approval, and for entering or editing data, including changing of personal password.

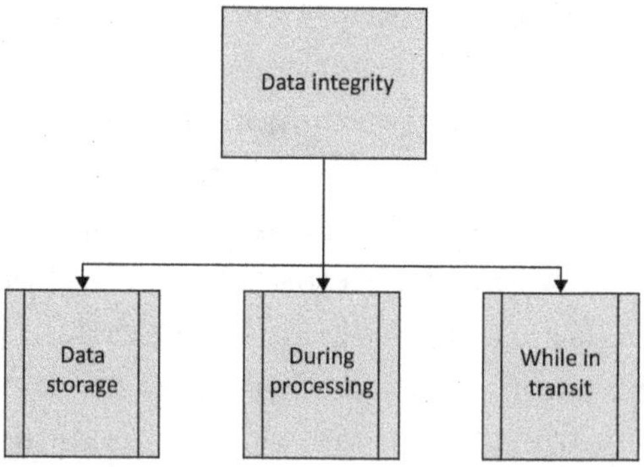

To keep the focus on the data integrity technical controls during the Operational Stage, the data integrity controls can be categorized in three spaces: data storage, data during processing, and data while in transit.

* Data reliability is a state when data is sufficiently complete and error free to be convincing for their purpose and context. In addition to being reliable, data must also meet other tests for evidence.

Chapters 13 through 15 describe the records integrity controls associated with these three categories.

Computer System Retirement: E-Records Migration

The activities to migrate e-records as part of a computer system retirement are no different from the migration of e-records as part of the transfer of e-records to a new computer system, discussed previously.

E-records must be preserved as part of the planning to retire the computer system generating e-records.*

The e-records preservation plan must include one of the following options:

- Make sure that a new system will be able to retrieve e-records from previous systems.
- Preserve previous applications (not contemplated, the system is to be retired).
- Archive hard copies (when allowed).
- Complete system documentation and validation dossier.

If archiving hard copies, computer records reproduced in paper copies is the selected method to migrate the e-records, the paper copies must be certified as true copies of the original e-records, and the paper copies are to be signed and dated as verified true copies. All electronic metadata must also be part of the fixed record. The verified hard copy must then be stored with other paper-based records.

After executing the e-records preservation plan, ensure that the quality assurance (QA) unit of the regulated user performs an audit on the preserved records. The audit will verify the traceability between planning and implementation, and will assess the successful execution of the preservation plan.

E-records migration must ensure the protection of e-records from deliberate or inadvertent alteration or loss.

Refer to Chapter 8, "E-Records Migration."

* CEFIC, Computer validation guide, API Committee of CEFIC, December 2002.

E-Records Archiving

Refer to Chapter 13, "E-Records Archiving and E-Records Storage."

The MHRA guidance document recommends that archive e-records should be locked such that they cannot be altered or deleted without detection and an audit trail.

The archive arrangements must be designed to permit recovery and readability of the e-records and metadata throughout the required retention period.

E-Records Destruction

Refer to Chapter 3, "Destruction."

Additional Reading

MHRA, MHRA GMP data integrity definitions and guidance for industry, March 2015.

Chapter 10

Electronic Records Governance

Introduction

Governance is a collection of written procedures that are directed by a strong management commitment with the power to implement and enforce the procedures. It ensures that strategy, policies, and procedures are actually implemented, and that required processes are followed correctly. Governance includes defining roles and responsibilities, measuring and reporting, and taking actions to resolve any issues identified.* E-records governance refers to an organizational structure that includes written policies and procedures documenting processes to prevent and detect situations that may have an impact on e-records integrity.

> *The FDA relies on accurate information to ensure drug quality, and data integrity problems break trust.*
>
> **Brooke Higgins**
>
> *Senior policy advisor for CDER's Office of Compliance, and Office of Manufacturing Quality*

* *ITIL Service Design*, 2011.

The following are e-records management essentials.

- Availability is the ensurance of consistent access to the information by authorized people.
- Usability is a quality attribute that assesses how easy user interfaces are to use.
- E-records integrity is the property that the e-records have not been altered in an unauthorized manner. The focus is on security, access, retention of records, review, double checks, documentation, and accuracy of reproduction.
- E-records security refers to protective digital privacy measures that are applied to preclude unauthorized access to computers, databases, and websites. E-records security also protects e-records from getting corrupted.

These e-records management essentials are related to trustworthy computer systems (Chapter 8). To ensure the integrity of e-records, it is necessary that the computer system handling these e-records must be, at the same time, trustworthy.

The Medicines and Healthcare Products Regulatory Agency (MHRA) stresses e-records governance in its good manufacturing practice (GMP) Data Integrity Definitions and Guidance for Industry (Chapter 9). A strong e-records governance approach ensures that e-records are "complete, consistent and accurate."*

According to the MHRA, the scope of e-records integrity governance should include

- Relevant policies
- Training in the importance of e-records integrity
- Procedures
- Computer system access controls

Note that implementing technology by itself will not solve e-records integrity issues. In a Notice of Concern by the World Health Organization (WHO) in September 2015† associated with e-records deleted on laboratory

* Churchward, D., Good manufacturing practice (GMP) data integrity: A new look at an old topic, Part 1 of 3, MHRA Inspectorate Blog, June 2015.

† WHO, Notice of concern to Svizera Labs, September 2015.

equipment, it was stated that "new equipment and usage of a server, on its own, is not deemed sufficient to ensure the absence of data integrity issues and to prevent the manipulation of analytical data." The implementation of effective behavioral, procedural, and technical steps based on a clear understanding of risk will ensure that the system will encourage the right behaviors, improve compliance, and provide greater assurance of product quality.*

Based on the MHRA guidance, this chapter discusses e-records governance. It highlights the e-records integrity elements in the governance.

The governance system to be implemented must adopt a "quality risk management" approach across all areas impacted by the e-records integrity.†

E-records governance should address e-records ownership throughout the life cycle and consider the design, operation, and monitoring of processes/systems to comply with the principles of e-records integrity including control over intentional and unintentional changes to the information.

The goal of defining, documenting, and implementing e-records governance is achieved by following a systematic process that includes implementing policy, strategy, plan, procedures, and guidelines. The implementation of these documents will involve a staff to plan, perform training, and enforce the governance-related documents.

E-Records Integrity Strategy

The e-records integrity strategy is a high-level plan of actions designed to bring about compliance e-records integrity in the regulated entity, including mobilizing resources to execute the actions.

The e-records integrity strategy emerges as the regulated entity adapts to the current regulatory agencies or competent authorities' concerns.

The e-records integrity strategy should have three parts: (1) a diagnosis that defines or explains the nature of the e-records integrity; (2) a guiding policy for dealing with the e-records integrity strategy; and (3) clear actions designed to carry out the guiding policy.

The senior leadership of the regulated entity is generally tasked with determining strategy.

---

* Churchward, D., Good manufacturing practice (GMP) data integrity: A new look at an old topic, Part 3 of 3, MHRA Inspectorate Blog, August 2015.

† MHRA, MHRA GMP data integrity definitions and guidance for industry, March 2015.

E-Records Integrity Policy

The e-records integrity policy is derived from the regulated entity strategy.

The e-records policy communicates the philosophy and expectations of the senior management to attain e-records integrity states in all levels of the regulated entity and defines the general principles that are required within a regulated entity.

This e-records integrity policy is intended to establish responsibilities and expectations as well. All GMP-regulated activities and associated procedures and guidelines must be consistent with the e-records integrity policy.

It is anticipated that the e-records integrity expectations of senior management will be incorporated into the e-records life cycle (Chapter 3).

The e-records integrity policy, procedural controls, and guidelines should be interlinked so that regulated users know where and how the e-records governance is implemented in detail.

E-Records Integrity Plan

Consistent with the e-records integrity strategy and policy, the e-records integrity plan is a document that tailors the specific activities, schedule, costs, and responsibilities necessary to monitor the implementation and remediation to bring e-records into compliance.

The e-records integrity plan will require continued interactions between quality assurance (QA), operations, and other parts of the regulated entity.

The plan should include

- Organizational structure of the e-records integrity program
- Schedule and time line
- Individuals responsible
- Resource availability
- Definition of the e-records integrity quality attributes
- How to measure each attribute
- Quality standards
- E-records integrity requirements
- Risk assessment and management
- Establishment of an inspection program
- Deliverables
- Overall acceptance criteria

- How to correct causes of nonconformance
- Process improvement

This document states which person is responsible for implementing the activities described in the plan and outlines the framework to follow to accomplish e-records integrity.

As part of the plan, an assessment must be designed and implemented to uncover all compliance gaps. The planning to remediate the uncovered gaps can be part of the e-records integrity plan or it can be part of a remediation plan by itself. If the second alternative is implemented, the remediation plan must be connected with the e-records integrity plan. This will enable consistency between both plans.

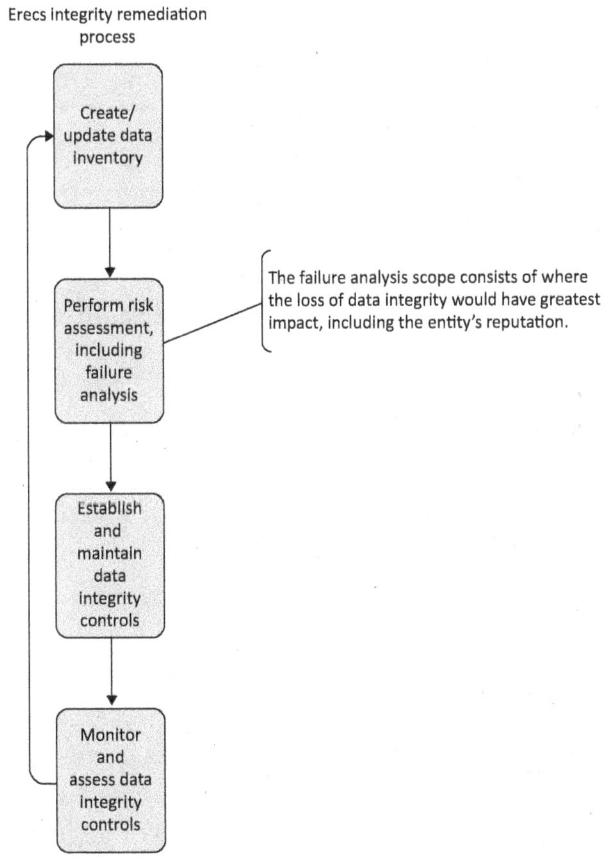

The plan containing the remediation activities should identify any existing technological/procedural controls that may need to be remediated or new technological/procedural controls that need to be implemented to ensure that any compliance gaps are corrected in a consistent and uniform manner.

Using the evaluation reports, the remediation activities, available resources, and project schedule, the business cost of the remediation approach can be estimated. This will enable the business to make a decision regarding the remediation or replacement of the current system based on the cost- effectiveness of the system and its operational feasibility.

The plan must contain activities that place emphasis on achieving consistent, high-quality, and sustainable compliance solutions.

Refer to Chapter 19 on "Remediation Project."

E-Records Integrity Procedural Controls

Refer to Chapter 11.

E-Records Integrity Guidelines

Guidelines may be written to help when implementing the procedures associated with e-records integrity. It is imperative to recognize that guidelines contain recommendations or acceptable methods for complying, but other methods may be used if it can be demonstrated that they are equivalently associated with a procedure. This is probably the reason why guidelines should not be referenced in procedural controls.

The applicability of e-records integrity guideline(s) for a particular project must be evaluated based on the intended use of the implementation. E-records integrity guidelines can be developed for each e-records integrity procedural control contained in Chapter 11.

Organization

Many groups establish and support the e-records integrity program. However, it is the responsibility of senior management to provide adequate resources to support the execution of the e-records integrity program.

In addition, senior management has the ultimate responsibility to ensure that an effective quality system is in place in which employees are encouraged to communicate e-records failures and mistakes.

In order to manage the execution and supervision of e-records integrity activities, it is necessary to establish an organizational structure. This structure will provide planning, audits, evaluations, remediation, training, reporting, and ongoing support.

As part of the organization, one critical item to consider is the segregation of duties. The segregation of duties ensures that the assignment of authority is appropriately divided between individuals to protect systems, program libraries, and e-record files from unauthorized access and modifications.*

E-Records Repository Inventory

An e-record repository inventory containing all critical e-records should be collected and maintained. The inventory should feature a description of the content of the repository, repository steward,† type of e-record (raw data, data, or true copy), key dependencies, interfaces, applications that update and/or read the repository, server names holding each e-records, security settings, location of design documentation, and other significant information. This inventory can become the e-records portfolio and the starting point of the e-records integrity gaps analysis.

Training

It is imperative that everyone related to a computer system is alert to the need for security concerns. Management should make sure that users are alert to the significance of e-records security, the procedures and system features that are accessible to provide suitable security, and the concerns of security gaps.

The e-records governance system should include training the staff in the importance of e-records integrity principles and the creation of a working environment that encourages an open reporting culture for errors, omissions, and aberrant results.

Personnel operating, maintaining, and programming computer systems must have suitable training and understanding of the e-records integrity issues and how their roles affect these issues.

Personnel will be required to train all regulated users in a regulated entity in all procedural controls associated with the implementation of the

---

* ISPE/PDA, *Good Practice and Compliance for Electronic Records and Signatures. Part 1 Good Electronic Records Management (GERM)*, July 2002.

† Repository steward: 1. Accountable for the business data and the repository content. 2. Responsible for ensuring that the repository remains validated. 3. Responsible for the periodic reconciliation between original records and true copies.

e-records integrity governance. Training activities associated with this task include

- Development of syllabuses.
- Managing training and training records.
- Coordination between governance training programs and the change management process. Any modification to the procedures associated with the governance is translated to training requirements, development, and training session(s).
- Maintenance of training materials.

The training program includes training internal auditors to understand what to look for to detect e-records integrity deficiencies. This training can also be performed via computer. The cost will relate to the computer resources and maintenance of the training records.

Enforcement

It is required that e-records integrity–related records and security profiles be routinely audited by designated competent person(s). The objective of these audits or self-inspection activities is to monitor the implementation and compliance with current good manufacturing practice (cGMP) principles, company policies, and procedures. In case of deviations from the applicable requirements, necessary corrective measures will be proposed.*

In particular, the GMP Data Integrity Definitions and Guidance for Industry stresses that QA should "review a sample of relevant audit trails, raw data and metadata as part of self inspection to ensure on going compliance with the data governance policy/procedures."

Similar reviews must be performed with the applicable service providers (e.g., cloud computing) by the regulated entity as part of their service providers program.

Until an acceptable level of understanding and conformance of the e-records integrity program is reached, the regulated entity should look for

* EudraLex, The rules governing medicinal products in the European union, Volume 4 *EU Good Manufacturing Practice (GMP) Medicinal Products for Human and Veterinary Use*, Chapter 9: Self Inspections, 2001.

external support to ensure absolutely unbiased, third-party investigations and/or to enhance the internal investigation program.

Additional Readings

MHRA, MHRA GMP data integrity definitions and guidance for industry, March 2015.

ISPE GAMP COP, Considerations for a corporate data integrity program, March 2016.

Chapter 11

Procedural Controls for Handling E-Records

Introduction

When using a computer system to perform good manufacturing practice (GMP)-regulated operations, the owner of the system should ensure that the computer system and the associated e-records conforms to the established requirements for intended use, availability, reliability, correct operation, and adherence to security principles. Refer to Chapter 8.

In addition to the foregoing, as part of GMP controls, it is also necessary to have procedural controls for the development, operation, maintenance, and retirement applicable to computer systems and associated e records in manufacturing environments.

The procedural controls should cover system setup, installation, deployment and use, validation and functionality testing, e-records collection and handling, system maintenance, system security measures, security settings, security user's profiles, change control, e-record backup, recovery, contingency planning, and decommissioning.

The responsibilities of the owner and other parties E with respect to the use of the computer system should be clear and documented. Users should be trained in the use of the computer system and managing e-records.

All procedural controls are to be associated with the intended use, associated requirements, and, specially, addressing the source of possible failures. Training of the users should be associated with the procedural controls developed, paying attention to the manual-related controls and addressing as well the source of the failures found during the failure analysis.

The documentation associated with the computer system must address manual and technical e-records integrity controls. The software supporting team must address these controls and take them into account during the neglect stage of the system.

E-Records Integrity Procedural Controls

The e-records integrity procedural controls should clearly define the management and accountability after the user to the applicable e-records.

Related to accountability to the e-records, a procedure should address e-records ownership throughout the life cycle and consider the operation, monitoring, and retirement processes to comply with the principles of e-records integrity. One key aspect to address is who will be accountable for the active records management after the retirement of the computer systems handling those e-records.

The number and type of procedural controls needed vary with each computer system, but it is important that all procedures be written, suitable, clear, accurate, and approved by designated individuals.

The following e-records management essentials are related to trustworthy computer systems (Chapter 8). Procedural control must be in place to ensure these features.

- Availability is an ensurance of consistent access to the e-records by authorized people.
- Usability refers to e-records being located, retrieved, and presented during their retention.
- E-records integrity is the property that the e-records have not been altered in an unauthorized manner.
- E-records security refers to protective digital privacy measures that are applied to preclude unauthorized access to computers, databases, and websites. E-records security also protects e-records from corruption.

Other e-records quality attributes, such as reliability* and authenticity,† are established via validation and monitoring processes. After establishing the

* Reliability: Record must be complete and accurate.

† Authenticity: Record must be proven to be what its purpose is to be.

authenticity and reliability of the e-records, the consistent implementation of the e-records integrity controls maintains this quality attribute over the e-records life cycle.

Procedures for the operation of a computer system should also describe a secondary raw data recording method in case the main recording method fails. The raw data subsequently entered into the computer should be clearly identified as such, and should be retained as the original e-records. Manual backup procedures serve to minimize the risk of any data loss and ensure that these alternative e-records are retained.

E-records management procedures must cover:

- E-records creation
  - It is the outcome of a validated/qualified practice (qualified equipment, validated process, or validated method).
  - If e-records is transferred via interfaces, the authenticity and integrity of the received data must be ensured (validation, monitoring).
  - Manual interaction during e-records creation requires additional controls, including an additional check on the accuracy of the e-records. This additional check can be done by a second operator or by a validated electronic means.
  - Manual recording of critical values from display requires a secondary verification of the values entered before the e-records are committed.
- E-records modification
  - Ensure that the systems are designed to permit e-records changes in such a way that the e-records changes are documented and that there is no physical deletion of entered e-records (e.g., maintain an audit trail, data trail, edit trail) and associated metadata (e.g., data that describe the context, content, and structure of the e-records).
  - Maintain a list of the users who are authorized to make e-records changes.
- E-records review
  - Verification of e-records.
  - Traceability to raw e-records.
  - Changes to critical data are traceable (analysis results, method parameters).
  - What manual activities have been performed by whom and when?
  - If unprocessed raw e-records are not printed, the review must also include an electronic system to check for any user manipulation of e-records.

- E-records security: User access
  - The other key issue about security of e-records is the segregation of duties (analysis, review, admin tasks).
    - Operational safeguards must be used to prevent unauthorized use of passwords and/or identification codes, and to detect and report any attempt to misuse such codes. Operational safeguards include that all the procedural controls and policies are established to provide security for passwords and identification.
    - The operational safeguards also include the procedures for issuing passwords, verifying identities, constructing passwords, determining the frequency of password changes, training employees, auditing for effectiveness, and monitoring the entire process of these safeguards.
    - In addition, there must be policies that cover the use of various identifiers and physical access to systems.
    - The analyst and reviewer must not have administrator rights.
    - There should be different personalized accounts for analysis and administration with additional mitigating controls (e.g., review of user access log) if the recommended solution is not possible for organizational reasons—controls needs to be defined in a procedure.

The objective of all operational safeguards is to ensure the monitoring and detection throughout the operation of the computer system and associated infrastructure to preserve the reliability of the computer system. Refer to Chapter 8.

- E-records availability
  - Procedures should be in place to ensure that essential information remains complete and retrievable throughout the specified retention period.
    - Back up and restore.
    - Disaster recovery.
    - Archival.
  - Restore and recovery procedures need to be tested to ensure e-records integrity is not compromised by technical controls.
  - Restore and recovery procedures must require an appropriate authorization mechanism to prevent misuse.

E-records management procedures need to consider different computer systems:

- Computer system, fully electronic e-records handling
  - Maintain all relevant raw e-records as e-records.
  - Paper printouts are copies of e-records (11 p 8.1) and may be used for further regulated activities if following a defined procedure.
- Hybrid systems (highest risk due to incompatible media management)
  - Create and maintain raw data partly as e-records and partly as paper records (e.g., approval on paper).
  - Require procedural or technical links between e-records and paper records.
    - Validate printout (e.g., qualified procedure or verification by a second operator on the accuracy of the printout)
    - Link and synchronization of printout and e-records
- E-records not to be deleted in system (need for the existence of a version control and/or audit trail)
- Written procedure to keep changes to e-records and paper records synchronized
- Pass through system
  - Raw e-records passed through to paper or compliant computer system.
  - E-records integrity to be ensured by creating an implemented automated control (preferred) or procedural controls until printout/pass through to next system.
  - The controls depend on system complexity and risk.

Other Related Procedural Controls*: Operational Activities

Routine use of computer systems during the operational life requires procedural controls describing how to perform operational activities. These operational procedural controls must be in place and approved by the appropriate individuals. The execution of these procedural controls should be monitored by the regulated user to verify accurate implementation and adherence.

* López, O., Maintaining the validated state in computer systems, *Journal of GxP Compliance*, 17, 2, August 2013.

These procedural controls should be reviewed on a periodic basis as in line with the local retention policy. In addition, it is vital that the system owners ensure that the relevant users are trained accordingly.

Key operational procedural controls are

Archiving

In the context of the regulated user, archives consist of e-records that have been selected for permanent or long-term preservation on the grounds of their evidentiary value.

As applicable, all computer system baselines should be archived in an environmentally controlled facility, which is suitable for the material being archived, and which is both secure and, where possible, protected from environmental hazards. An e-record of all archived materials should be maintained.

Refer to Chapter 13.

Backups

This control provides the ability to protect the e-records from system failure and the ability to recover the e-records. For these reasons, e-records must be regularly and progressively backed up, and a copy of the backup retained at a remote and secure location.

These back-ups must be "a true copy of the original data that is maintained securely throughout the record retention period. This backup file should contain the data (which include the metadata) and should be in the original format or in a format compatible with the original format".

The procedural control establishing the backup process must be in place to ensure the integrity of backups (secure storage location, adequately separated from the primary storage location, and error-free). This backup may be part of a more general disaster recovery plan.

Following changes to the system and/or backup utility, change control should ensure the availability and integrity of the backup files and stored e-records by comparing backup e-records and the original files backed up on a trial basis.

The integrity and accuracy of backup data and the ability to restore the data should be checked during validation and monitored periodically. Refer to "Checks" elsewhere in this chapter.

The frequency of backups depends on e-records criticality, the amount of stored data, and the frequency of data generation.

Business Continuity

In the event of a computer-related breakdown, the business continuity procedural control is the appropriate procedure to follow for preserving a computer system's trustworthiness.

Business continuity procedural control, including disaster recovery procedural control, ensures minimal disruption in the event of accidental or deliberate damage to the e-records. It is necessary to ensure that the integrity of the e-records is not compromised during the return to normal operation. At the lowest level, this may mean the accidental deletion of a single file, in which case procedural controls should be in place for restoring the most recently backed-up copy. At the other extreme, a disaster such as a fire could result in the loss of the entire system.

The business continuity procedural control is contemplated as part of the documented contingency planning. For critical computer-dependent systems, the contingency plan should consider alternate systems accessible in the event of a systems failure.

The procedural control employed should be tested regularly and all relevant personnel should be made aware of its existence and trained to use it. A copy of the procedural controls should be maintained off-site.

Refer to NIST, "*Contingency Planning Guide for Federal Information Systems*," Special Publication 800-34, May 2010.

*E-Records Quality Control**

The aim of e-records-related quality control procedures is to minimize the effects of missing and inaccurate data. The e-records editing process should be part of the standard operating procedures documentation that describes the process for confirmation and correction of e-records. The standard operating procedure for e-records editing should guarantee that any queries about data validation are brought rapidly to the attention of the data entry manager and quality control.

An audit trail should be available to trace the nature of any changes to data, the dates of changes, and the person responsible for the changes.

Data collection and entry should be performed continuously. It should be checked either by double-entry (preferable) or by proofreading for the primary variables and on a random basis for other parameters.

* Department of Health, 2006. Guidelines for good practice in the conduct of clinical trials with human participants in South Africa. Department of Health: Pretoria, South Africa.

Checks should be manual as well as automated. In the latter case, it should be combined with data entry (e.g., immediate automatic checks or batch checking) to speed up feedback on data requiring clarification.

E-records Storage

For the purpose of e-records' short- or long-term retention, when investigating after an incident and/or business continuity, it is necessary to guarantee the availability of all files and stored e-records to reconstruct all GMP-relevant documentation.

The procedures providing for future access to the e-records should be established. These procedures should address the stability of the storage media and the availability of the necessary hardware and software to provide for future use of the e-records.

Specifically to e-records storages, there must be procedures to establish and maintain e-records security and logical arrangements of e-records.

Related with the retention times of the e-records, it must be referenced the applicable predicate rule when establishing retention times.

Infrastructure Maintenance*

The procedural controls applicable for the preventive maintenance and repair of the infrastructure provide a mechanism for anticipating problems and, as a consequence, possible loss of e-records.

In addition to the typical infrastructure elements such as system-level software, servers, wide area network, local area manager, and the associated components, the infrastructure includes uninterruptable power supplies (UPSs) and other emergency power generators.

Modern infrastructure hardware usually requires minimum maintenance because electronic circuit boards, for example, are usually easily replaced and cleaning may be limited to dust removal. Diagnostic software is usually available from the supplier to check the performance of the computer system and to isolate defective integrated circuits. Maintenance procedural controls should be included in the organization's procedural control. The availability of spare parts and access to qualified service personnel are important for the smooth operation of the maintenance program.

Refer to Chapter 13.

---

* López, O., *Computer Infrastructure Qualification for FDA Regulated Industries*, PDA and DHI Publishing, 2006.

Problem Reporting

The malfunction or failure of a computer system's components, incorrect documentation, or improper operation that makes the proper use of the system impossible for an undetermined period characterizes some of the incidents that can affect the correct operation of a computer system. These system incidents may become nonconformances.

To remedy the problem quickly, a procedural control must be established for the users of the system to record any computer system failures. This enables the reporting and registration of any problem encountered by the users of the system.

Problem Management

Reported problems can be filtered according to whether their cause lies with the user or with the system itself, and fed back into the appropriate part of the supplier's organization. To remedy a problem quickly, a procedural control must be established if the system fails or breaks down. Any failures, the results of the analysis of the failure, and, as applicable, any remedial actions taken must be documented.

Those problems that require a remedial action involving changes to any baseline are then managed through a change control process.

Retirement

The retirement of computer systems performing regulated operations is a critical process. The purpose of the Retirement Period is to replace or eliminate the current computer system and, if applicable, ensure the availability of the e-records that have been generated by it for conversion, migration, or retirement.

In case of system retirement, the following steps should be taken*:

- Set up an e-records preservation plan that could include one of the following options:
  - Make sure that a new system will be able to retrieve e-records from previous systems
  - Preserve previous applications
  - Archive hard copies (when allowed)

---

* CEFIC, *Computer Validation Guide*, API Committee of CEFIC, January 2003.

- Completion of system documentation and validation dossier
- Execution of the e-records preservation plan
- Quality assurance (QA) audit on the preservation of documentation.

Restore

A procedural control for regular testing of restoring backup data, to verify the proper integrity and accuracy of e-records, must also be in place.

Risk Management

The basis for all these processes enabling e-records integrity is the initial risk assessment as part of the risk management. Refer to Risk Management in Chapter 12.

An excellent source on security-related management of risks can be found in *An Introduction to Computer Security: The NIST Handbook*, chapter 7, Computer Security Risk Management (Special Publication 800-12).

Security

Regulated entities must be able to control the access to the regulated user's that are permitted to access e-records and in what circumstances. E-records to protect include specifications, process parameters, or manufacturing methods.*

Computer systems security includes the authentication of users and access controls. Security is a key component for maintaining the trustworthiness of a computer system and its associated e-records. Security is an ongoing element to consider and is subject to improvement.

In particular, after a system has been released for use, it should be constantly monitored to uncover any security gap and violations.

As an example, a good laboratory practice (GLP)-related warning letter (WL) to Colorado Histo-Prep on March 2014, highlights the statement, "You failed to monitor access and record changes (via an audit trail) of electronic statistical data and statistical analyses. Thus, the quality and integrity of your data and analyses cannot be ensured." The predicate rule associated with this WL is 21 CFR Part 58.81(b)(10).

---

* US FDA, Guidance for industry: Data integrity and compliance with CGMP guidance for industry, (Draft) April 2016.

Any security violation must be followed up, analyzed, the root causes found, and proper action taken to avoid a recurrence.

Training

All staff maintaining, operating, and using computer systems performing regulated operations must have documented evidence of training in the area related to the scope of the work. For users, the training will concentrate on the correct use of the computer system, how to report any failure or deviations from the normal operating condition, and security.

Staff training should focus on the importance of e-records integrity principles and the creation of a working environment that encourages an open reporting culture for errors, omissions, and aberrant results.

There should be documented training on the importance of security including the need to protect and not share passwords as well as enforcement of security systems and processes.

Other Related Procedural Controls*: Maintenance Activities

The validated status of computer systems performing regulated operations is subject to threat from changes in its operating environment, which may be either known or unknown.

Procedural controls must be established for the following.

Verification and Revalidation

There should be written procedural controls for performance monitoring, change control, applications, infrastructure and e-records security, calibration and maintenance, personnel training, business continuity, and periodic reevaluation.†

After a suitable period of running a new system, it should be independently reviewed and compared with the system specification and functional specification. The periodic verification must include e-record checks and audit trails.

* López, O., Maintaining the validated state in computer systems, *Journal of GxP Compliance*, 17, 2, August 2013.

† WHO, Technical Report Series No. 937, Annex 4. Appendix 5, Validation of computerized systems, Section 1.6, 2006.

Computer systems used to control, monitor, or record functions that may be critical to the safety of a product should be checked for accuracy at intervals of sufficient frequency to provide ensurance that the system is under control. If part of a computer system that controls a function critical to the safety of the product is found not to be accurate, then the safety of the product back to the last known date that the equipment was accurate must be determined.

Change Control

Change control procedural control should ensure e-records integrity. Infrastructure and application changes must provide for sustained access to and retention of the raw data without e-records integrity risks.

Ensurance that changes to computer software (system and applications), infrastructure hardware, configuration files, e-records, and process equipment are verified and documented and made only by authorized personnel.

Modifications and adjustments to computer systems shall only be made in accordance with a defined procedural control that includes provisions for checking, approving, and implementing the modification and/or adjustment.

The correct implementation of a change management ensures the integrity of the e-records to be modified including any data that describe the context, content, and structure of the data. This is particularly important when making changes to computer systems, such as software upgrades or migration of e-records.

Checks

Software, hardware, e-records, and backups must be verified periodically to ensure reliability. The backup procedure must guarantee e-records integrity. Each backup set should be checked to ensure that it is error-free.

The critical hardware and interfaces between computers and equipment should be checked periodically or continuously to ensure accuracy and reliability. The periodic input/output (I/O) verification is clearly established in the US FDA Compliance Policy Guides (CPG), Sec. 425.400 Computerized Drug Processing; Input/Output Checking.

In addition to the periodic verifications such as I/O checking, the majority of the worldwide computer regulations and guidelines concur that a periodic review is necessary "to confirm that they remain in validation state and are compliant with the GMP" (11, p. 11). During the periodic review, the e-records that were transferred to another format or system (11, p. 4.8) must be verified to ensure that the stored e-records are accessible, readable, and accurate.

Specifically related to e-records:

- E-records should be verified after being transferred to another data format or system.
- Periodically stored e-records should be verified for accessibility, readability, and accuracy.
- If data is exchanged electronically, there should be verifications for the receiving system for the correct processing.
- Critical data* entered manually by an authorized person into the computer system requires input validation. Refer to Chapter 5 under "Accuracy Check," and Chapter 6 under "Creation."

Additional Readings

European Compliance Academy (ECA), Which SOPs are required by GMP? August 2014, http://www.gmp-compliance.org/enews_4431_Which-SOPs-are-required-by-GMP_8382,9074,Z-QAMPP_n.html.

McDowall, R.D., What is data integrity training, *Spectroscopy* 30, 11, 34–41, November 2015.

* Critical Data—data with high risk to product quality or patient safety. (ISPE GAMP COP Annex 11—Interpretation, July/August 2011).

Chapter 12

Electronic Record Controls: Supporting Processes*

The following controls maintain the e-records integrity as part of the life cycle of the system.

Business Continuity

Based on risk, business continuity ensures the continuousness of the operation in the event of a system breakdown. Business continuity refers to the prepared measures that will secure business operations in case of system failure or trouble. The procedural control employed to restore the system must be adequately documented and tested regularly. All relevant personnel should be made aware of its existence and trained to use it. A copy of the procedure should be maintained off-site.

At the lowest level, business continuity applies to the accidental deletion or corruption of a file, in which case a procedure should be in place for restoring the most recently backed-up copy. At the other extreme, a disaster such as the complete destruction of the hardware, software, and e-records files and, until recovering from the disaster, transitioning back to a paper-based system.

* López, O., A computer data integrity compliance model, *Pharmaceutical Engineering* 35, 2, March/April 2015.

Incident Management

The faults, incorrect documentation, e-records errors, improper operation, or interface errors of computer system components illustrate some of the incidents that can affect the correct operation of a computer system. These incidents are also known as *nonconformances*.*

Effective monitoring of the operation of a computer system involves users or operators trained in the associated operational procedure. This facilitates their ability to recognize unexpected responses and outputs, react to the incident properly, and fully document such incidents to aid in the evaluation and debugging process.

Manage by corrective and preventive actions (CAPA), the initial assessment of the incident includes root cause analysis.†

Periodic Reviews

Periodic (or continuous) reviews must be performed after the initial validation of the computer system. The periodic review‡ procedure should describe the process to verify stored, backed up, and archived e-records and associated metadata for accessibility, readability, accuracy, and all controls at all levels.

If an error or omission is identified during the periodic review, the action to be taken must be described in the procedure. This procedure should enable e-records corrections or clarifications to be made in a current good manufacturing practice (cGMP) compliant manner, providing visibility of the original record and audit trailed traceability of the correction.§

In addition, during the periodic review, the output of the backup and accuracy of the audit trail should be verified. As applicable, the periodic review must verify accurate and reliable e-records transfer from backups.

---

* Non conformance A departure from minimum requirements specified in a contract, specification, drawing, or other approved product description or service.

† EudraLex, The rules governing medicinal products in the European Union, Volume 4, EU guidelines for good manufacturing practice for medicinal products for human and veterinary use, Chapter 1, *Pharmaceutical Quality System*, Section 1.4A (xiv), January 2013.

‡ "*What does periodic mean? What period of times is expected as a minimum, for example?* Periodic in this case means regularly and recurrently. No minimum period of time is defined. It must be substantiated that the period of time is adequate in order to control the process risk." Mangel, A., Q&A on Annex 11, *GMP Journal*, 8, April/May 2012.

§ MHRA, MHRA GMP data integrity definitions and guidance for industry, March 2015.

The periodic review should also cover a review of the access restrictions of those with specific access rights to computer systems. The access restrictions must remain current and appropriate.

Personnel

Access to the computer systems and associated repositories must be restricted to authorized users only. The level of access must be based on the user's assigned task(s).

Data must only be entered or amended by regulated users who are authorized to do so. The segregation of duties between data entries, reviewers, and system administrators is very critical. Reviewers and system administrators must not have access to enter and/or amend data to the data storage areas. If the application software security service does not allow the implementation of configurable segregation of duties, it will be required to establish these controls in a procedure.

There must be records documenting the individuals who have any access to the computer systems handling critical e-records. This includes users, reviewers, system administrators, analysts, programmers, and so on.

Requirements Document*

This specification must include both structural and functional analyses. These evaluations take into account the required e-records integrity controls.

Based on the intended use of the system, the associated requirements, and the failure analysis, the appropriate e-records integrity controls pertinent to the application and the infrastructure supporting the application are selected.

The requirements document is the basis for the final quality of the system to be implemented and the source of all the implementation and maintenance activities.

Like all requirements associated with a computer system, the e-records integrity requirements must be traceable through the life cycle.

* López, O., Requirements management, *Journal of Validation Technology* 78–86, May 2011.

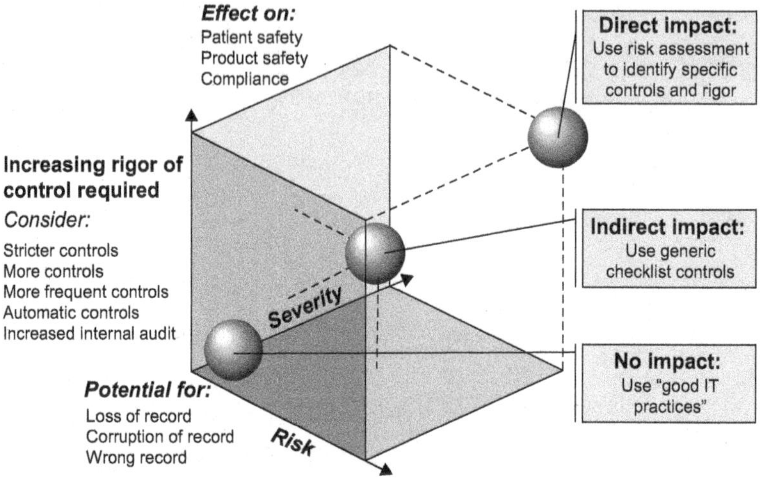

Figure 12.1 Controls based on risk and impact. (From Perez, A.D., New GAMP Good Practice Guide for Electronic Record and Signature Compliance, paper presented at the FDA Part 11 Public Meeting, June 2004.)

Risk Management*,†

Risk management is integral to the e-records management process. Risk management is about identifying what the risks to compliance are and having an understanding of the impact of the risk.

The initial risk assessment associated with e-records integrity determines the necessary controls that must be taken into account based on the environment and the utilization context of those e-records. Controls should be appropriate to ensure the security, integrity, and confidentiality of records (Figure 12.1).‡

The controls based on the risk assessment can be determined by the type of impact of the e-records on patient safety, product safety, and compliance. Procedures, processes, and systems managing these records are to be developed to achieve the integrity of the e-records.

* NIST, *An Introduction to Computer Security: The NIST Handbook*, Chapter 7, Computer Security Risk Management (Special Publication 800-12).

† Graham, L., Compliance matters, Good laboratory practice, Blog MHRA Inspectorate, September 2015.

‡ ISPE GAMP Forum, Risk assessment for use of automated systems supporting manufacturing processes: Part 2—Risk to records, *Pharmaceutical Engineering* 23, 6, November/December 2003.

Table 12.1 Controls Based on the Impact of E-Records on Patient Safety, Product Safety, and Compliance

Control	*No Impact*	*Indirect Impact*	*Direct Impact*
Access control	Controlled access	• Authorization process • Access management • Password management • Documentation	• Rigorous authorization control • Strict and proactive access management • User profiles • Unique accounts • Stringent PW management • Physical security • Full documentation
Backup and restore	• Checking of outcome • Multiple copies (redundancy)	• Checking of outcome • Multiple copies (redundancy) • Formal periodic testing • Documentation	• Checking of outcome • Multiple copies (redundancy) • Formal periodic testing • Full documentation • Remote storage locations • Automated processes

Table 12.1 is an example of controls based on the impact of the e-records on patient safety, product safety, and compliance. Risk mitigation strategies need the understanding of many factors, including*:

- The degree to which data can be configured
- Understanding system complexity
- User access permissions and system configuration
- Transaction windows
- Understanding data structure
  - Dynamic versus static data
  - Access, security, and hosting of data
  - File structure
- Validation for intended purpose versus functional verification
- Audit trails and metadata

* Churchward, D., GMP compliance and data integrity, paper presented at the PDA/PIC's Quality and Regulations Conference, Brussels, Belgium, June 2015.

The selected mitigation strategy(ies) will determine the associated controls. The integration of the system life cycle (SLC) and the risk management must exist to effectively implement and maintain the e-records integrity controls.

As part of the assessment of the risks associated with the possible issue about e-records integrity, a failure analysis is performed to find out where the loss of e-records integrity would have the greatest impact, including the regulated entity reputation.

It is important that the risks are reviewed periodically and, if appropriate, the mitigation systems revised. The effectiveness of a risk management process is dependent on the quality of information fed into the risk assessment process, which in turn is reliant on the robustness of the quality system in place.

Failure to manage e-records integrity risk can have the following impacts:

- Authorization, completeness, and accuracy of transactions may be incorrect as they are entered, processed, summarized, and reported.
- There may be inadequate management controls concerning the integrity of processed e-records or databases, which ultimately may impact the quality of a product.

Security

REGULATORY EXPECTATION

The electronically stored data shall be protected, by methods such as duplication or backup and transfer on to another storage system, against loss or damage of data, and audit trails shall be maintained.

Chapter II, Article 9(2), the Commission Directive 2003/94/EC

Since maintaining data integrity is a primary objective of the GMP principles, it is important that everyone associated with a computer system is aware of the necessity for security considerations. The regulated entity must ensure that personnel are aware of the importance of data security, the procedures, and system features that are available to provide appropriate security and the consequences of security gaps. Such system features could include routine surveillance of system access, the implementation of file verification routines, and exception and/or trend reporting.

As a function related to security, e-records integrity service maintains information exactly as it was inputted and is auditable to affirm its reliability.

Security controls must be established for all computer systems as a means of ensuring e-records protection. Computer security is the principal enabler to create the integrity of e-records.

A number of unrelated regulated entities have had problems linked to the proper control of computer systems to prevent unauthorized changes in e-records. Usually, these regulated entity sites alter or delete critical e-records.

The system owner* is the person responsible for providing suitable records protection controls over the application, infrastructure (e.g., network, database server), and database components. These record protection controls ensure that only authorized personnel can make changes to any component of the computer system and the security of the e-records residing on the system.

Security must be instituted at several levels. Procedural controls must govern the physical access to computer systems (*physical security*). As part of the physical security, security of devices used to store programs also must be considered, such as tapes, disks, and magnetic strip cards. Refer to Chapter 13, related to physical security.

Access to individual computer system platforms is controlled by network-specific security procedures (*network security and database server*). Access to these devices should be controlled (*logical security*).

Unnecessary networked services should be disabled and secured. Database software, like most operating systems and complex applications, provides a number of services that allow remote system management, distributed processing, and other network-related functions. In many cases, those services are enabled by default and are often "protected" by using either no password or a vendor-supplied default password.

As with applications and operating systems, database servers can also have vulnerabilities that lead to unauthorized e-records access, loss of e-records integrity, or total system compromise. To minimize the impact of

* System owner: The person responsible for the availability and maintenance of a computerized system, and for the security of the data residing on that system (EU Annex 11).

vulnerabilities, eliminate known security vulnerabilities by keeping the database servers up-to-date with security patches released by vendors.

Without the ability to selectively grant access to a database and its data, arbitrary users can add and delete information at will. Even if access controls are enforced by web applications, e-records contained within the database are still at risk if a malicious user circumvents the web application and accesses the database directly. If possible, use database access controls that can restrict what users, groups of users, or applications can access or change the database.

E-records security includes the integrity, reliability, and availability of these records. During validation of a database or inclusive system, consideration should be given to*

- Implementing procedures and mechanisms to ensure data security (e.g., user access to the e-records and user permissions to perform activities in the database) and keeping the meaning and logical arrangement of data
- Load-testing, taking into account future growth of the database and tools to monitor the saturation of the database
- Precautions for necessary migration of data (11, p.17) at the end of the life cycle of the system

Procedures and technical controls should be put in place to prevent the altering, browsing, querying, or reporting of e-records via external software applications that do not enter through the protective system software.

Finally, application-level security and associated authority checks control access to the computer system applications (*applications security*).

A defined procedure(s), at all levels, should be established for the issue, cancellation, and alteration of authorization to enter and amend, including changing of personal passwords.

Where a record is deleted prior to meeting its approved retention, an audit trail of the deletion is required until the end of the approved retention period.

Recording activities of unauthorized attempts to access the computer system and/or e-records storage devices also should be considered.

---

* European Medicines Agency (EMA): GMP/GDP compliance, *Questions and answers: Good manufacturing practice: Annex 11 Computerised Systems Question 4*, http://www.ema.europa.eu/ema/index.jsp?curl=pages/regulation/q_and_a/q_and_a_detail_000027.jsp&mid=WC0b01ac05800296ca#section9.

In those cases in which is critical the use of an explicit terminal as the source of data inputs or operational instructions entered by the user terminal, verification may be implemented.

An example of a potential security issue is the elevated access level by the database administrator. The database administrator could alter e-records in the database table without any traceability of the modification(s) to these e-records.

The database system administrator can modify, without traceability, any field in signed records including the signature field, time stamp, and reason for the signature. It should be ensured that electronic signatures applied to e-records are valid over the storage period of the e-records and documents. The updated signature will make the complete e-record invalid and the signature will not be permanently linked to the signed record.

There are three possibilities to fix the preceding example:

- Implement procedural control to maintain the segregation of duties,* including not allowing record changes by the system administrator. In addition, for all modification to the records, each record must be submitted for electronic reapproval.
- Implement database software that provides audit trail capabilities at all access levels, including the database administrator. Establish procedural controls to maintain the segregation of duties, including not allowing record changes by the system administrator.
- Incorporate digital technologies (e.g., hashing†) into the database software. A minor change in the e-record will result in a change in the output of the hashing. An automated service verifies the original hashing and the calculated hashing, reporting any change to the hashing and invalidating the record and associated signature if applicable.

Use all of the capabilities provided in the database to restrict the database administrator's access to any features beyond account management (and possibly configuration controls), your procedures, and training materials.

During the validation of a database system, considerations should be given to implementing procedures and mechanisms to ensure data security

* Segregation of duties: A process that divides roles and responsibilities so that a single individual cannot subvert a critical process.

† López, O., Technologies supporting security requirements in 21 CFR Part 11: Part I, *Pharmaceutical Technology*, Feb 2002.

and the segregation of duties. The implementation of these procedures and mechanisms must be verified and/or tested.

Upon placing the e-records in retention environments, the same level of e-records security that was controlled throughout their earlier life cycle still needs to be maintained.

The Federal Information Processing Standards Publication (FIPS PUB) 199, Standards for Security Categorization of Federal Information and Information Systems, is a security categorization standard for information and information systems. It is another method to perform a risk assessment.

Suppliers and Service Providers

Refer to Chapters 16 and 17.

Timestamping Controls*

Time stamping is recognized as a valuable service that supports nonrepudiation of transactions. It adds integrity and trust to messages and records sent by means of a network. Accordingly, unauthorized modifications to the system clock and time drift† between servers must be prevented. The certificate server and client clocks must remain synchronized as closely as possible. Kerberos‡ recommended maximum tolerance settings for computer clock synchronization to be 5 minutes. Kerberos uses time stamps to determine the validity of entities' authentication requests and to help prevent replay attacks.

The system date and time are included as part of the audit trails and electronic signatures. The digital timestamping service (DTS) issues a secure time stamp that includes the time, a hash of the digital information being time stamped, and a time certification, which can be used for digital signatures. A message digest is produced from the record and sent to the DTS. The DTS sends back the time stamp, as well as the date and time that the

* López, O., Overview of technologies supporting security requirements in 21 CFR Part 11: Part II, *Pharmaceutical Technology*, March 2002.

† Time drift is when two or more servers do not have identical times. The discrepancy can vary from seconds to minutes and can become extensive if left unchecked.

‡ Kerberos (http://www.isi.edu/gost/info/Kerberos/) is an industry-standard authentication system. suitable for distributed computing by means of a public network.

time stamp was received, with a secure signature. The signature proves that the document existed on the stated date. The document contents remain unknown to the DTS—only the digest is known. The DTS must use lengthy keys because the time stamp may be required for many years.

DTS and digital certificates provide the mechanism to authenticate the source (device checks) of the time stamp in audit trails and electronic signatures. Access-right lists and digital certificates can be used to control access to the DTS.

In addition to the DTS, other supporting time controls include an infrastructure that supports time stamping from a trusted time such as the coordinated universal time at http://www.datum.com/tt. This technology, which in some cases is compliant with X.509 (Public Key Infrastructure Certificate and Certificate Revocation List [CRL] Profile), is linked with a time-calibration service. Applications or computer logs may require timestamping services on the server.

In addition to the utilization of a timestamping service, attention must be paid to the periodic coordination between the service and the local computer clock, and to limit the access of the computer date and time local function. The local computer date and time function must not be accessed by users.

Additional Readings

Cooper, L. and Moore, T., Complying with FDA's 21 CFR Part 11 regulation: A secure time management primer, Larstan Business Reports, 2002.

ISO/IEC 18014 Information Technology - Security Techniques - Time-stamping Services. https://en.wikipedia.org/wiki/Timestamp.

ITIL Service Design, *Appendix M: Risk Assessment and Management*, 2011 Edition.

NIST, *An Introduction to Computer Security: The NIST Handbook*, Special Publication 800-12, 59–70, 1995.

Chapter 13

Electronic Records Controls: Records Retained by Computer Storage*

Introduction

When e-records are retained in computer storage, the security-related procedures describe the access controls to the e-records that are retained throughout the retention period.†

The risk assessment for data servers, or any infrastructure that retains e-records, identifies potential hazards and vulnerabilities. In the context of e-records that are retained by computer storage (e.g., e-records in data servers), such hazards may result in threats to the integrity of the e-records, including modification and/or accidental destruction of the e-records without having proper authorization from the e-records owner(s).

The procedure addressing the security of e-records in storage should also address the stability of the storage media and the availability of the necessary hardware and software to provide future access to and use of the e-records.

* López, O., A computer data integrity compliance model, *Pharmaceutical Engineering* 35, 2, March/April 2015.

† EudraLex, *The Rules Governing Medicinal Products in the European Union Volume 4, Good Manufacturing Practice, Medicinal Products for Human and Veterinary Use*, Chapter 4: Documentation, June 2011.

The procedural controls associated with the e-records' storage comprises e-records archiving, migration, and storage.

Where e-records retention is contracted to a third party, particular attention should be paid to the ownership and retrieval of e-records held under this arrangement. The physical location in which the e-records are held, including the impact of any laws applicable to that geographic location, should also be considered.

The requirements for the storage of e-records and electronic documents do not differ from that of paper documents. It should be ensured that the electronic signatures applied to e-records are valid for the entire storage period for those documents,* or until the e-records are modified.

Physical security is a key element to the e-records in computer storage as well.

E-Records Archiving

In the context of e-records that are no longer active, these e-records are archived. This is considered to be a long-term retention environment.

E-records archiving is the process of moving e-records that are no longer actively used to a separate records storage device for long-term retention, often disabling the e-records from any further changes. The retention period of these e-records had not been finalized.

The controls addressed in "E-Records Storage," described in this chapter, are also applicable to archived records.

The archiving process is an activity that may involve a modification of format, media, and/or physical storage. It must be performed in a controlled manner in accordance with a procedural control.

There are multiple types of archiving disposition:

- Extract/Migrate: The migration of digital information from one hardware/software configuration to another, or from one generation of computer technology to a later one, offers one method of dealing with technological obsolescence. Data is extracted from the current system and moved to another location or the entire instance is migrated elsewhere.

---

* European Medicines Agency (EMA)—GMP/GDP compliance—Questions and answers: Good manufacturing practice: Annex 11 Computerised Systems, Question 8, http://www.ema.europa.eu/ema/index.jsp?curl=pages/regulation/q_and_a/q_and_a_detail_000027.jsp&mid=WC0b01ac05800296ca#section9.

- Host: These are single-instance database systems that are not typically managed by the site and are hosted elsewhere.
- Archive: Will contain the following types:
  - Report: In this case, the official record is considered to be in hard copy currently, or the most effective end state will be a hard copy.
  - Physical to Virtual (P2V) (Encapsulate): In order to be able to access the e-record effectively, in some cases it is necessary to have both the application and the database in a virtual environment. Encapsulation is a technique for grouping together a digital object and anything else necessary to provide access to that object. In this case, software will be used to encapsulate the data and application and the product will be housed in a server designated for this purpose.
  - Technology emulation creates an environment that behaves in a hardware-like manner. It potentially offers substantial benefits in preserving the functionality and integrity of digital objects.
  - Keeping every version of software and hardware: The requirement for keeping every version of software and hardware, operating systems, and manuals, as well as the retention of personnel with the relevant technology skills. This option makes the preservation of obsolete technologies to access the archived e-records unfeasible.

If the e-records in storage are transferred to another format, media, or system, the archiving process must include verification that the e-records are not altered in value and/or meaning during this migration process. The metadata must also be transferred and verified. Refer to "Data Migration" in this chapter.

The computer system holding the archived records must implement all security-related functions to restrict access to authorized persons only. Periodically, archived records need to be verified for accessibility, readability, integrity, and the state of security control.

If changes are implemented to the computer infrastructure and/or application, then it is required to ensure and test the ability of the application to access the e-records.

E-records may be retained on archived media for a very long period of time. The procedure addressing the e-records in storage should also address the stability of the storage media itself.*

---

* Brown, A., Selecting storage media for long-term preservation, The National Archives, DPGN-02, August 2008, https://www.nationalarchives.gov.uk/documents/selecting-storage-media.pdf.

After completing the specified record retention requirements, the records can be physically deleted.

Each country has their particularity about each of the best practices discussed in this book. One example of such particularity is the clinical e-records archiving guidelines established in South Africa. In South Africa, e-records must be reproduced as hard copies, which should be signed and dated as verified accurate copies of the original data. The verified hard copies should then be stored with other paper-based records. This requirement in South Africa is established to overcome the possibility of a loss or inability to read the information due to technological redundancy.*

E-Records Migration

E-records migration is the process of transferring e-records between storage types, formats, or computer systems. It is a key consideration for any system implementation, upgrade, or consolidation.

E-records migration is usually performed programmatically to achieve an automated migration, freeing up human resources from tedious tasks. E-records migration occurs for a variety of reasons, including server or storage equipment replacements or upgrades, the retirement of computer systems, website consolidation, server maintenance, and data center relocation.†

Before any e-record can be migrated from one system to another, it is important to identify differences between systems and how they might affect how reliably the migrated e-record can preserve and present information.

Changes in factors that affect how reliably an e-record can preserve and present information might not always be readily apparent. Examples of such changes include, but are not limited to, the following:

- Moving from one type of record storage media to a different one
- Installing a new version of an application or operating system software program
- Moving from one electronic file format to another

* Department of Health, Guidelines for good practice in the conduct of clinical trials with human participants in South Africa, Section 6.7 Department of Health, Pretoria, 2006.

† Janssen, C., Data migration, http://www.techopedia.com/definition/1180/data-migration (retrieved 12 August 2013).

Verification must be performed after concluding the migration process to ensure that information in the original e-records has not been altered in, or deleted from, the electronic copy of the e-records. The verification should include corroboration that the e-records are not altered in value, meaning, structure, context and links (e.g., audit trails, metadata), and/or meaning during this migration process.

Accessibility and readability verifications of the migrated e-records are also applicable after the migration of e-records.

In addition to these verifications, migration testing should be performed long before migration is complete. Testing must be performed throughout the migration process to catch errors and problems while they're still fixable. As soon as the migration process is complete, a team of data small and medium-sized enterprises (SMEs) must perform a more comprehensive set of tests to assess and accept the new system before the users start using the migrated data set.

The migrated set of e-records must be assessed to ensure a high level of quality once the new repository becomes available to current and future users. The e-records quality assessment process should involve the removal of duplicate content and all files that are not relevant to current or future business processes, and, if applicable, the creation of a master data file.

When system-level software is used to make an identical copy of an e-record, the system-level software typically has a built-in error-checking mechanism to help ensure that the copy is, in fact, a true copy.

The migration process must be well documented.

E-Records Storage

E-records storage is a device that records (stores) or retrieves (reads) information (e-records) from any medium, including the medium itself. This is considered to be a short retention environment and may be considered as the initial creation environment or processing environment.

A design specification, or similar document, must describe the file structure(s) in which the e-records are stored, the capacity requirements of the storage, and how the security scheme is implemented. The file structure and security are tested during the qualification.

In a typical manufacturing environment (Figure 13.1), data is collected directly from equipment. To ensure the integrity of raw data, control signals between computers and equipment should be checked by verification

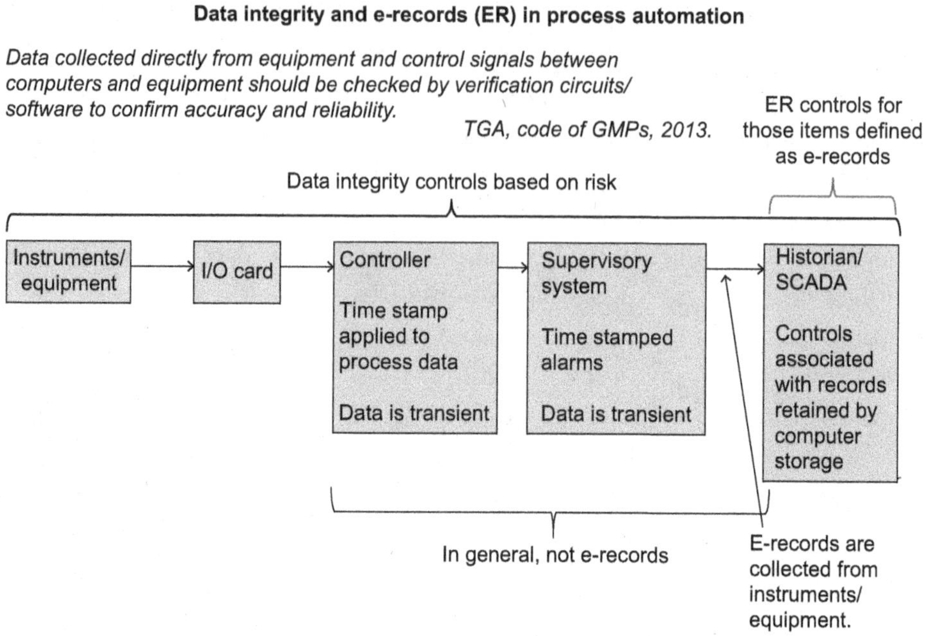

Figure 13.1 I/Os verification.

circuits/software to confirm accuracy and reliability. Refer to Chapter 5, "Data Input/Output Principles," and the EMA Annex 11 p5.

Logical security is addressed in Chapter 12.

When the e-records are in the storage device, the physical protection of the e-records must be adequate. This comprises the protection of e-records storage as well as the environmental impacts influencing the respective e-records storage devices.

Media can deteriorate as a result of their environment. Copying information without changing it offers a short-term solution for preserving access to digital material by ensuring that information is stored on newer media before the old media deteriorates beyond the point where the information can be retrieved.

As applicable, web and database servers should be separated in terms of their physical location. Database servers should be isolated from a website's demilitarized zone (DMZ).* These servers can locate them on a physically separate network segment from the web and other Internet-accessible

* A DMZ is a physical or logical subnetwork that contains and exposes an organization's external-facing services to a larger and untrusted network, usually the Internet. The purpose of a DMZ is to add an additional layer of security to an organization's local area network (LAN); an external network node only has direct access to equipment in the DMZ, rather than any other part of the network.

servers that support the business. Preferably, the database server should be partitioned off from the web servers by a dedicated firewall. This firewall should only allow database traffic between the web server and the database server. The firewall should also deny and log all traffic from any other location, or other types of traffic from the web server.

As an element of the e-records integrity in storage, there must be a record of any e-records change made that includes the previous entry, who made the change, and when the change was made.*

To reduce the risk of losing e-records in storage, and to guarantee e-records readiness for the users, periodic back ups must be performed. The back up must be stored separately from the primary storage location, and at a frequency that is based on an analysis of the risk to the good manufacturing practice (GMP) of e-records and the capacity of the storage device.

The efficacy of the back up and restore processes must be verified as part of the qualification process. In addition, the capacity level of the storage must be monitored.

As with archived e-records, the e-records in storage need to be verified periodically for accessibility, readability, and integrity. If changes are implemented to the computer infrastructure and/or application, then it is required to ensure and test the ability to retrieve e-records.

One critical element to consider, as part of the implementation of e-records retained by computer storage, is the legal hold to the e-records. These are records in which the regulated entity is involved in litigation. These records cannot be destroyed, even if the retention period has expired. The regulated entity is under a legal obligation to retain all records involving or related to legal matters. A mechanism must be implemented to tag the e-records that are impacted by a legal hold.

File Integrity Checking†

Periodically, e-records and the associated file(s) should be checked for integrity.

File integrity checkers provide a way to identify system files that have been changed by computing while storing a checksum for every guarded

* Health Canada, Good Manufacturing Practices (GMP) guidelines for Active Pharmaceutical Ingredients (APIs), GUI-0104, C.02.05, Interpretation #15, December 2013.

† NIST, *Technical Guide to Information Security Testing and Assessment*, Special Publication 800-115, September 2008.

file and establishing a file checksum database. Stored checksums are later recomputed to compare their current value with their stored value, which identifies file modifications. A file integrity checker is usually included with any commercial host-based intrusion detection system, and is also available as a stand-alone utility.

Although an integrity checker does not require a high degree of human interaction, it must be used carefully to ensure its effectiveness. File integrity checking is most effective when system files are compared with a reference database created using a system that is known to be secure—this helps ensure that the reference database was not built with compromised files. The reference database should be stored off-line to prevent attackers from compromising the system and covering their tracks by modifying the database. In addition, because patches and other updates change files, the checksum database should be kept up-to-date. For file integrity checking, strong cryptographic checksums such as Secure Hash Algorithm 1 (SHA-1) should be used to ensure the integrity of the e-records stored in the checksum database.

E-Records Handling

The controls and security associated with archived and stored e-records can be summarized as follows:

- Adequate assignment and maintenance of access rights. Access by authorized personnel only—including the use of individual user accounts and passwords (check for leavers, changers, and so on).
- Validation of systems and maintenance of the validated state.
- Audit trails established, activated, and periodically monitored. Is the audit trail functionality implemented/activated? Are online clock adjustments protected? Which is the source of the time stamp?
- Controlled and defined processes for any modification/change, and so on, to e-records. Is there an independent check of critical e-records (including a review of audit trail data)? Safe storage of e-records, for example, correct file system setup or database protection. Does the file saving procedure save into a protected environment?
- Electronic signatures that are specific to authorized personnel.
- Data backup and verification. How about the creation of backup copies? Are the backup copies monitored periodically for accessibility,

readability, and accuracy? Are data generally protected against loss, damage, or overwriting?

- Archival and record retention.
- Recovery and contingency plans.

Additional Readings

GAMP5, Anticipating Archiving and Migration Needs, (Section 8.8) in *A Risk-based Approach to Compliant GxP Computerized Systems*, 2008.

MHRA, Good laboratory practice: guidance on archiving, March 2006.

Chapter 14

Electronic Record Controls: During Processing*

The validation/qualification process for the functionality of the applications, components, and/or interfaces handling e-records is the foundation to achieving the integrity of the e-records during processing. After deployment, these applications, components and/or interfaces are maintained following all good manufacturing practice (GMP)-related controls applicable to computer systems during the operational and maintenance phases of the service-level commitment (SLC).

Archiving

Refer to Chapter 13.

Audit Trails†

As part of the reliability of e-records, audit trails refer to a journal, paper based or computer based, or version control that can trace the records modifications to the records.‡

* López, O., A computer data integrity compliance model, *Pharmaceutical Engineering* 35, 2, March/April 2015.

† US FDA, *Guidance for Industry Computerized Systems Used in Clinical Investigations*, Section IV.D.2, May 2007.

‡ Perez, R., Reid, C., and Wyn, S., A risk-based approach to audit trails, *Pharmaceutical Engineering*, 35, 2, March/April 2015.

Computer-generated, time-stamped electronic audits trails are the preferred method for tracking changes to electronic source records.

The audit trails mechanism provides the capability to reconstruct modified e-records and, consequently, does not obscure previously recorded e-records. The use of electronic audit trails or alternative methods that fulfill the audit trail requirements, help to confirm that only authorized additions, deletions, or alterations of GMP-relevant e-records have occurred and allow a means to reconstruct significant details about manufacturing activities and data collection. This is necessary to verify the quality and data integrity pertinent with GMP-relevant e-records.

The need for audit trails should be determined based on a justified and documented risk assessment that takes into consideration the circumstances surrounding system use, the likelihood that the information might be compromised, and any system vulnerabilities. Should it be decided that audit trails or other appropriate methods are needed to ensure e-records integrity, personnel who create, modify, or delete e-records should not be able to modify the documents or security measures used to track e-record changes. Audit trails, or other appropriate methods used to capture e-record activities

- As with any GMP-relevant e-records, are subject to all requirements regarding e-records integrity.
- Should describe when, by whom, and the reason changes were made to the e-record. Original information should not be hidden though the use of audit trails or other measures used to capture e-record activities.
- Must be available and, if necessary, convertible to a readable form.
- Must be regularly reviewed.
- Should be retained as long as the associated e-records.
- Changes to audit trail data should be prevented by the system.

The audit trail tracking mechanism includes a time stamp that indicates the time of the entry. The date and time of an audit trail should be synchronized to a trusted date–time service. Computer-generated, time-stamped audit trails, or other appropriate methods, can also capture information related to the creation, modification, or deletion of current good manufacturing practice (cGMP)-relevant e-records and may be useful to ensure compliance with the appropriate regulations. For more information on time stamps regulatory expectations, refer to Chapter 12, "Timestamping Controls."

*What shall be done in the case of legacy systems without audit trail?**
First of all, it must be clarified whether the data can be changed at all (e.g., electronic recorders or standard practice statement). If not, this should be the reasoning within the risk assessment for the audit trail not being necessary. Define in a standard operating procedure (SOP) that each change has to be documented, for example, in a logbook, and verified by a second person.

Built-In Checks

Refer to Chapter 11.

Electronic Signature†

Annex 11 sees the formalization of electronic signatures in European Medical Agency (EMA) GMPs. Many computer systems have implemented electronic signatures based on the US Food and Drug Administration (FDA) 21 Code of Federal Regulations (CFR) Part 11, but the European regulation does not appear as stringent as the US regulation. The requirements for electronic signatures have the same impact as handwritten signatures within the boundaries of the company, being permanently linked to the respective record and including the time and date that a signature was applied. There is not the stated bureaucracy and formality of 21 CFR 11 to send letters the US FDA, have no repudiation of an electronic signature requirements or the different types of signatures. However, many of the same requirements are implicit, as the European legislation simply states that electronic signatures have the same impact as handwritten signatures and hence all of the nonrepudiation requirements apply immediately.

Operational Checks

The objective of operational checks is to enforce the sequencing of steps and events as applicable to the process managed by the computer system. The application-dependent algorithms, sequencing of operations,

* Mangel, A., Q&A on Annex 11, *GMP Journal* 8, April/May 2012.

† McDowall, R.D., ECA, The new GMP Annex 11 and Chapter 4 is Europe's answer to Part 11, *GMP News*, January 2011.

instructions to the operator, critical embedded requirements, and safety-related precautions to be followed within the computer system are encompassed in the computer program(s) that drive the computer system. These application-dependent and predicate rule requirements are defined in the requirements document, implemented as part of the project phase and executed during the operational phase.

The controls applicable to e-records processing are established, as appropriate, during the implementation of the computer system and each control is reevaluated during periodic reviews.

Printouts/Reports

Even with the increased use of computer systems in GMP-regulated activities and subsequently e-records, it is very common to see regulated users rely on printouts as hardcopies attached to the batch records and/or rely on printouts to perform regulated activities.

REGULATORY EXPECTATION

All data defined as critical data and associated metadata should be printable.

Aide Memoire (Ref. #: 07121202) of the German ZLG
Central Authority of the Laender for Health Protection

The following concepts are applicable to displayed reports. Displayed reports are often used for real-time decision-making.

If printouts are used as quality records, then the design, qualification, and controls of these printouts are critical. The reports are validated as per applicable procedural control.

In cases of internal audits (e.g., self-inspections [Eudralex Volume 4, Chapter 9]) or external audits (e.g., inspections by regulatory agencies or competent authorities), it must be possible to obtain printed reports of e-records that were not specified or validated during the implementation of the normal required reports. These reports can be considered ad hoc reports.

In the case of ad hoc reports, a report generator can be utilized to take data from a source such as a database or a spreadsheet, and use it to produce a document in a format that satisfies a particular human readership.

If the printout is created by a report generator, then verification of the printout must be performed before providing the printout to the auditor/ inspector.

In any case, the printout functionality must provide the capability to print audit trails. In case a system is not capable to generate printouts indicating if any of the e-records have been changed since the original entry, it may be acceptable to describe in a procedure the fact that a print-out of the related audit trail report must be generated and linked manually to the record supporting batch release.*

The printout must also be clear. "Clearly printed" means printouts in which, apart from the values themselves, the units and the respective context can also be seen.† Units and the respective context are considered metadata.

There must be a procedure to ensure that the data contained in the final report matches original observations. This procedure may apply to raw data, data in case-report forms (in hard copy or electronic form), computer printouts, statistical analyses, and tables.

Section 1.8 in the EMA Annex 15‡ established that "appropriate checks should be incorporated into qualification and validation work to ensure the integrity of all data obtained."

The expectation of the competent authorities is that the regulated user doesn't just accept the data contained in a validation report. This report must be verified with the raw data confirming such a report. "It is important that data is complete and accurate. We would expect you to do some checks of data integrity when you are preparing validation documents. It is not just checking that there are no typing errors in the document. It is drilling down into the data. You may want to look at the audit trails."§

---

* European Medicines Agency (EMA): GMP/GDP compliance, questions and answers: Good manufacturing practice: Annex 11 Computerised Systems, Question 10, http://www.ema.europa.eu/ema/index.jsp?curl=pages/regulation/q_and_a/q_and_a_detail_000027.jsp&mid=WC0b01ac05800296ca#section9.

† Mangel, A., Q&As on Annex 11, *Journal for GMP and Regulatory Affairs*, 8, April/May 2012.

‡ EudraLex, *The Rules Governing Medicinal Products in the European Union Volume 4, EU Guidelines for Good Manufacturing Practice for Medicinal Products for Human and Veterinary Use*, Annex 15, March 2015.

§ Eglovitch, J., EU inspectors to focus on integrity of process validation data, *The Gold Sheet*, November 2015.

Printouts must be verified before hardware and/or software is exchanged. As part of the validation/qualification of the software/hardware, regression testing can be used to check that the data concerned can also be printed in the new configuration.

Security

Refer to Chapter 12.

Chapter 15

Electronic Record Controls: While in Transit*

For various reasons, e-records may be moved between systems. The controls associated with moving e-records must verify that e-records have remained unaltered in transit. This principle is also applicable to e-records from creation to reception.

The following are the controls associated with e-records while in transit.

Qualification of IT Infrastructure†

Computer infrastructure is considered as equipment.‡,§ All current good manufacturing practice (cGMP) controls associated with equipment are applicable to the computer infrastructure, including the location of the hardware, maintenance, the calibration of the sensors associated with the infrastructure, and the qualification.

* López, O., A computer data integrity compliance model, *Pharmaceutical Engineering* 35, 2, March/April 2015.

† López, O. *Computer Infrastructure Qualification for FDA Regulated Industries*, PDA and DHI Publishing, River Grove, IL, 2006.

‡ WHO, Technical Report Series No. 937, Annex 4, Appendix 5, Validation of computerized systems, Section 7.1.2, 2006.

§ US FDA, CPG Sec. 425.100 Computerized drug processing; CGMP applicability to hardware and software.

Qualification* of the hardware includes:

- Service design
- Service delivery, including installation and evaluation of the system
- Change control, maintenance and calibration, security, contingency planning, training, performance monitoring, and periodic reevaluation.

The computer infrastructure must be brought into conformance with the regulated entity's established standards through a planned verification process, building on acknowledged, good IT practices. Once in conformance, the infrastructure must be maintained by established processes and quality assurance (QA) controls, the effectiveness of which must be periodically verified.†

Built-In Checks

Computer systems exchanging data electronically with other systems should include, if technically feasible, appropriate built-in checks for the correct computer inputs and outputs (I/Os).

> *Why are built-in checks required for electronic interfaces if the interface has been validated?*‡ The question cannot be answered as such. The checks of data built into the interface are tested within the context of validation. Changes in a system can be problematic if they concern data that is transferred via that interface.

The correct I/Os ensures the secure exchange of data between systems and, furthermore, correct inputs on the processing of data. These built-in checks maximize the mitigation associated with I/Os errors.

The impact on network-based technologies is that insufficient error checking at the point of transaction entry can result in incorrect transaction processing and data integrity risks. Integrity can be lost when data is processed incorrectly, or when transactions are incorrectly handled due to errors or delayed processing.

---

* WHO, Technical Report Series No. 937, Annex 4, Appendix 5, Validation of computerized systems, Section 6.3, 2006.

† Cappucci, W.; Chris Clark, C.; Goossens, T.; Wyn, S., ISPE GAMP CoP Annex 11 interpretation, *Pharmaceutical Engineering*, July/August 2011.

‡ Mangel, A., Q&A on Annex 11, *GMP Journal* 8, April/May 2012.

The built-in check is the mechanism that can ensure the authenticity, integrity, and confidentiality of transmissions, and the mutual trust between communicating parties. It provides

- Shared node authentication to ensure each node of the others' identity
- Transmission integrity to guard against improper information modification or destruction while in transit
- Transmission confidentiality to ensure that information in transit is not disclosed to unauthorized individuals, entities, or processes

This built-in check mechanism can support both application and machine credentials, and user machines (user nodes).

Critical to the security of information exchange is a method at the point of transaction entry that guarantees receiving exactly what the sender intended between computer system interfaces. For this case, it is suggested that a "checksum" be utilized to ensure file integrity.* A checksum, or hash sum, is a fixed-size datum computed from an arbitrary block of digital data for the purpose of detecting errors that may have been introduced during a file's transmission or storage. The integrity of the data can be checked at any later time by recomputing the checksum for the file and comparing it with the stored checksum value. If the checksum values do not match, the data was almost certainly altered (either intentionally or unintentionally).

The use of a checksum for transmitting files provides a number of benefits, including

- The integrity of each file, which can be verified by comparing the checksum submitted with the file and the computed checksum calculated on receipt.
- The ability to verify that the file has not been altered in the historical archive. This is particularly useful as files are migrated from one storage medium to another (e.g., when files are backed up to magnetic tape storage).

In addition to all of the foregoing controls, computer, network, and interface components must be verified periodically to ensure correct communication between components.†

---

* ICH, *Electronic Standards for the Transfer of Regulatory Information*, June 2015, http://www.ich.org/products/electronic-standards.html.

† US FDA CPG Sec. 425.400 Computerized drug processing; input/output checking.

Accuracy Checks

Critical data* entered manually by an authorized person into the computer system requires input verification to prevent incorrect data entry. The intent of the accuracy check is to confirm that there is an independent verification record to show that the data entered manually was, in fact, entered accurately.

The independent verification of the manually entered critical data can be performed by a second authorized person or a computer system.

For critical data that is transferred between computer systems, or from a computer system to paper, the verification of accuracy can be performed by a second person or, if the system is properly validated, by the computer system itself.

There should be no difference between the manual input by the user and the take-over of data from another system. In the same way, processing operations performed by the system should be checked by the system itself, or by a second person as appropriate.

The impact on network-based technologies is that insufficient error checking at the point of transaction entry can result in incorrect transaction processing and data integrity risks. Integrity can be lost when data is processed incorrectly, or when transactions are incorrectly handled due to errors or delayed processing.

In the context of a computer system check, verification is a check that is programmed to run in the background of data entry, and configured to ensure the accuracy of the data input. This could be specific checks on data format, ranges, or values.

As the system automatically compares data on input with predefined limits, for example, the user should be warned of potential errors when the data is entered manually or as an input from another computer system. For security purposes, the validity of the source of data input may be determined.

Faulty data entry can trigger a chain of events that could result in a serious production error and the possible distribution of an adulterated product. Thus, while increasingly sophisticated system safeguards and computer monitoring of essential equipment and programs help to protect data, no automated system exists that can completely substitute for human oversight and supervision.

---

* Critical Data: Data with high risk to product quality or patient safety, ISPE GAMP COP, Annex 11—Interpretation, July/August 2011.

Chapter 16

Electronic Records and Contract Manufacturers

Service providers are parties who provide any services irrespective of whether they belong to an independent (external) enterprise, to the same company group/structure, or to an internal service unit.

The service provider that is used as an example in this chapter is a contract manufacturer.

In a contract manufacturer setting, the owner of the drug or the contract giver engages an outside party or contract acceptor to complete the contracted manufacturing process.

The contract giver is responsible for ensuring that the drugs introduced are neither adulterated nor misbranded as a result of the actions of their selected contract acceptor facility. All contract acceptors must ensure compliance with applicable current good manufacturing practices (cGMPs) for all manufacturing, testing, or other support operations performed, to make a drug(s) for the contract giver.

> *During a May 27 to June 9 inspection, it was uncovered that Seattle Genetics also failed to retain electronic versions of the executed batch records of Adcetris bulk drug substance and finished drug product, leaving no means to verify that the printed version of the electronic records is an accurate representation of what was provided to Seattle Genetics by its contract manufacturers.*
>
> **QMN**
>
> *Vol. 7, No. 38, September 25th 2015.*

Before entering into a contract, the contract giver must make sure that the contract acceptor's standards are congruent with their own. The contract giver should evaluate the methods by which the contract taker tests products to make sure that the product is of good quality. There should be evidence that the contract giver has evaluated the contract acceptor with respect to such standards.

The relationship between the contract giver and the acceptor is established in a service-level agreement (SLA) or similar document. The SLA should appropriately define, agree, and control any activity covered by the cGMP regulations in order to avoid misinterpretations that could result in a product or operation of unsatisfactory quality.

The SLA establishes the duties of each party: the quality management system of the contract giver, how the records and documentation required by the applicable cGMP regulations will be made available for immediate retrieval, data integrity governance, and how copies will be made and maintained under certification or controlled copy procedure.

If it is decided that the method to collect the production system records is electronic, the SLA should indicate that all e-records will be stored in such a manner as to maintain their traceability, reliability, and integrity throughout the required record-keeping time frames, established in the applicable regulations.

As discussed in this book, all e-records integrity controls applicable to typical production systems are applicable to the contract acceptor's production systems. Of special interest between the contract giver and contract acceptor, is how the contract giver will receive the executed batch records.

Manufacturing e-records should be kept at the site where the manufacturing activity occurs, and should be readily available. A true copy of the manufacturing e-records must be sent to the contract giver. Using this true copy of the manufacturing e-records, the contract giver verifies that the contract acceptor adhered to the manufacturing formula, including the applicable instructions.

There are challenges to account for by sending the manufacturing e-records to the contract giver. Chapter 15 accounts for the controls associated with this transfer.

Contract givers should perform periodic audits as part of their vendor assurance program. These audits must take into account the management of e-records integrity as part of the overall contract acceptor's data integrity governance.

Additional Readings

EudraLex, *The Rule Governing Medicinal Products in the European Union, Volume 4 EU Good manufacturing practice (GMP) Medicinal Products for Human and Veterinary Use*, Chapter 7: Outsourced Activities, January 2013.

López, O., *EU Annex 11 Guide to Computer Validation Compliance for the Worldwide Health Agency*, CRC Press, Boca Raton, FL, 2015.

Parenteral Drug Association (PDA), Technical Report No. 32 Auditing of supplier providing computer products and services for regulated pharmaceutical operations, *PDA Journal of Pharmaceutical Science and Technology*, Release 2.0, 58, 5, September/October 2004.

Chapter 17

Electronic Records and Cloud Computing*

The National Institute of Standards and Technology (NIST) define cloud computing as the following:

> Cloud computing is a model for enabling convenient, on-demand network access to a shared pool of configurable computing resources (e.g., networks, servers, storage, applications, and services) that can be rapidly provisioned and released with minimal management effort or service provider interaction. This cloud model promotes availability and is composed of five essential characteristics, three service models, and four deployment models.

The cloud computing practice uses a network of remote servers hosted on the Internet to store, manage, and process e-records, rather than a local server or a personal computer.

A cloud service provider† is a company that offers some component of cloud computing, typically Infrastructure as a Service (IaaS), Software as a Service (SaaS), or Platform as a Service (PaaS), to other businesses or individuals.

The first sidebar in this chapter provides a view of the typical models in cloud environments. In each model, the shaded part relates to the elements controlled by the cloud service provider.

---

* López, O., Trustworthy computer systems, *Journal of GxP Compliance 19. 2*, July 2015.

† Service provider: An organization supplying services to one or more internal or external customers (ITIL Service Design, 2011 Edition).

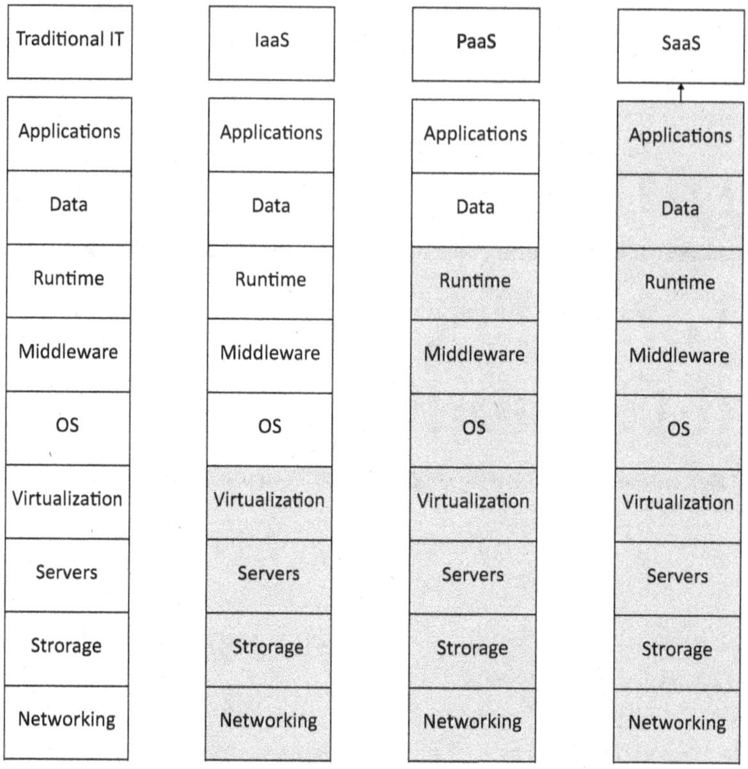

- IaaS: A virtual data center environment—including servers, databases, network, storage, and so on—hosted at the cloud service provider's facility.
- PaaS: A development environment for software applications hosted by the cloud service provider—who provides tools, programming codes, interface modules, and so on—that allows IT professionals to develop and integrate software applications in the cloud infrastructure environment, which is either hosted by the service provider or contracted to another provider.
- SaaS: A software application hosted by the cloud service provider in order to perform functions or processes. In this model, a regulated user uses a vendor's software application via a web browser or program interface. The regulated user does not manage or control the underlying cloud infrastructure—including the network, servers, operating systems, storage, or application capabilities—with the possible exception of the application's configuration settings.

Business Process as a Service (BPaaS) is a new but popular model for cloud services, where the cloud service provider takes full responsibility for not only the design, management and control of its software application, but also the operation of the business process on behalf of the client company.

From the perspective of the regulated user, the most complex scenario is the BPaaS model.

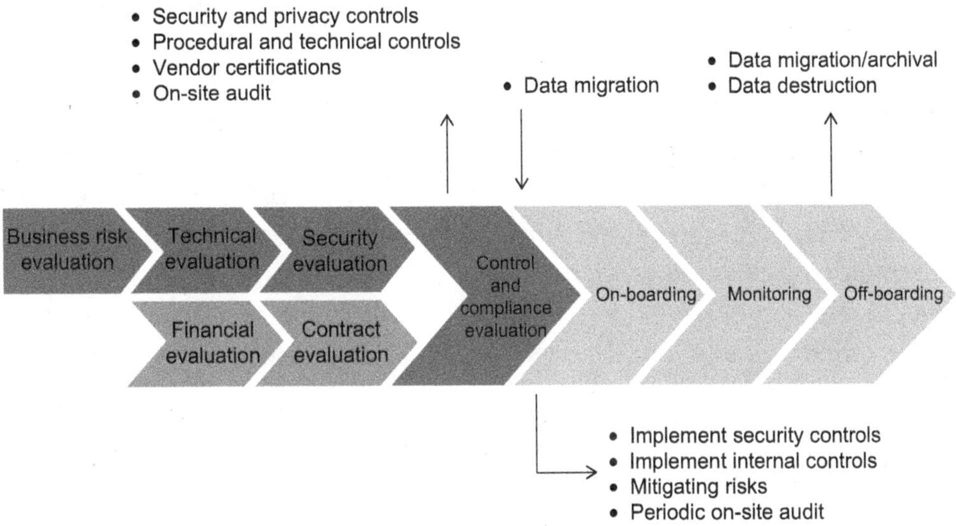

Where the regulated user chooses to outsource cloud computing, which can affect product conformity with requirements, the regulated user should ensure control and hold responsibility for the suitability and operability of those computer-related services. Control of such outsourced computer-related services should be identified within the quality management system* and a clear statement of the responsibilities of the cloud service provider should be given. The statement of responsibilities is defined in a formal quality agreement (e.g., a service-level agreement [SLA]).

The way to achieve such regulated user controls over the cloud service provider is established by the regulated user defining clear requirements for the service, a careful selection of the cloud service provider, an all-inclusive quality agreement between the regulated user and the cloud service provider, and periodic evaluation of the cloud service provider.

It is important to implement a cloud governance policy to establish a standard and effective cloud system life cycle (SLC). This SLC contains your approach to the selection, integration, ongoing management, and subsequent decommissioning of cloud-based services.

* NSAI, ISO 9001, Quality Management Systems—Requirements, Section 4.1.

The cloud governance policy points to the procedures and records that indicate how and on what basis (e.g., risk assessments and requirements) the cloud service provider is evaluated and selected (PIC/S PI-011-3-11.2); the tools for assessing its fitness for purpose against predetermined requirements, specifications, and anticipated risks; as well as periodic reviews to assess if the cloud service is maintained and operated in accordance with the specified requirements and quality agreements. Additionally, how to add new services and how these services are developed, qualified/validated, and deployed must be part of this evaluation.

The overall evaluation may consist of technical capabilities and security-related criteria, as well as procedural and technical control. Other critical evaluations are financial and contractual.

Specifically applicable to security, the selection criteria to be considered for the capabilities of a cloud service provider are as follows*:

- Data Center Security
  - Hardware security
  - Software security
  - Web vulnerability scans and reports
  - Penetration testing
- E-records Protection and Compliance
  - E-records protection (encryption)
  - Backup and restore
  - Data center location
  - E-records ownership declarations
- Network Security
  - Connection security
- Reliability
  - Disaster recovery
- Trustworthiness
  - Auditing

As part of this evaluation, the cloud service e-records integrity governance is assessed.

* ECA IT Compliance Working Group, SOP: Selection Process for Cloud Service Providers, Rev 1.0, Draft.

The tools for assessing fitness for purpose against predetermined requirements can take the form of a history report of previous deliveries or service provisions, the transfer and assessment of questionnaires (postal audits), or supplier/vendor audits.

The evaluation and audit reports should be made available for review to provide an understanding of the audit processes.*

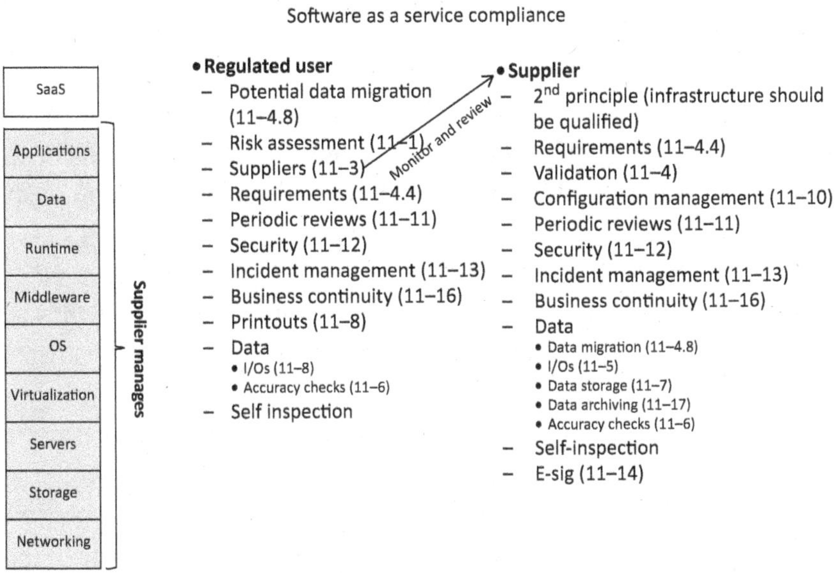

In the context of EMA Annex 11, the third sidebar provides a pictorial view of the items that the regulated user and the supplier need to comply with in a cloud environment. Note that during the operation of the system, periodic audits to the cloud computing environment supplier act as an interface between the regulated user and the supplier

The regulated entity must perform periodic audits as part of their vendor assurance program. These audits must take into account the management of e-records integrity as part of the overall cloud service provider's e-records integrity governance.

As the reader may have noticed, no matter the selected model (traditional or cloud), the requirements for trustworthy and compliant computer systems to be able to perform regulated activities are the same. Additionally, the responsibility of a computer system's performance of regulated activities always belongs to the regulated user.

* Aide-mémoire of German ZLG regarding EU GMP Annex 11, September 2013.

From the point of view of the cloud service providers and the regulated users, the applicable e-records controls are contained in Chapters 10 through 15.

From the point of view of the regulated users, there are additional controls and requirements to consider.

E-records migration is the process of transferring e-records between storage types, formats, or computer systems. It is a key consideration for any system implementation, upgrade, or consolidation. E-records migration is usually performed programmatically to achieve automated migration, freeing up human resources from tedious tasks. E-records migration occurs for a variety of reasons, including server or storage equipment replacements or upgrades, website consolidation, server maintenance, and data center relocation.*

If e-records are transferred to another format or system, the verification of the e-records migration should include corroboration that e-records are not altered in value, meaning, structure, context, or links (e.g., audit trails) during this migration process.

Accessibility and readability of the e-records (11 p7.1) must be maintained in their migration.

Of special interest to the regulated user and the cloud service provider is how the e-records will be accessed and, when necessary, sent to the regulated user.

The controls associated with sending and receiving e-records are discussed in Chapter 15.

In general, e-records transfer is ensured by the commonly used network protocols. The integrity of e-records stored in the cloud must be ensured by

- Proper assignment of access permissions by the cloud customer and cloud service provider based on "need to have," "need to know," and "minimum possible access level" principles.
- Cloud service provider running technical infrastructure in line with good IT practice. The cloud environment must be properly secured and that includes professional patch management, malware protection, intrusion detection and prevention, and so on.

---

* Janssen, C., Data migration, http://www.techopedia.com/definition/1180/data-migration.

All of the critical elements that are important for the cloud customer must be part of the SLA and understood by the cloud service provider. The cloud service provider must commit to complying with these requirements.

Additional Readings

Cloud Service Alliance, Cloud controls matrix, Rev 3.0.1, July 2014.

Cloud Service Alliance, Security guidance for critical areas of focus in cloud computing, Rev 3.0, November 2011.

ECA, ECA IT compliance working group, shared platform and cloud services implications for information governance and records management, http://www.it-compliance-group.org/icg_downloads.html.

Chapter 18

Self-Inspections

Introduction

A quality systems approach calls for self-inspections or internal audits. These are independent assessments that are used by management to verify compliance with the principles of good manufacturing practice (GMP). The self-inspection program covers the service provider's performance of regulated functions and offers an opportunity to use external resources for this assessment.

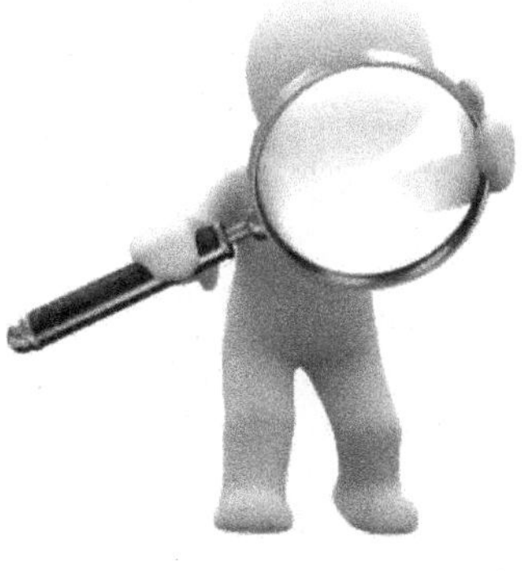

Self-inspections should be performed frequently enough to identify problems and to prevent noncompliances from arising, while ensuring the overall health of the quality system.*

In January 2014, the Medical and Health Products Regulatory Agency (MHRA) confirmed that as of that year pharmaceutical facilities would be

* EduQuest, How often should you audit your suppliers?, EduQuest-ions & Answers, February 2016.

expected to verify their e-records' integrity in the context of self-inspection. The performance of periodic self-inspection is required by Chapter 9 of the European Commission (EC)'s GMP Guide.*

Self-inspections are performed and documented to ensure that the planned audit schedule takes into account the relative risks of the various quality system activities, the results of previous audits and corrective actions, and the need to audit the complete system. Procedures should describe how the auditors are trained in objective evidence gathering, their responsibilities and auditing procedures. Procedures should also define auditing activities such as the scope and methodology of the audit, the selection of auditors, and the audit conduct (audit plans, opening meetings, interviews, closing meetings, and reports).

The self-inspections' findings and corrective actions should be documented and brought to the attention of the responsible management of the regulated firm. Approved corrective actions should be finished in a timely and effective manner.

Two examples of self-inspections on service providers performing regulated services in relation to e-records integrity are described in Chapters 16 and 17.

E-Records Self-Inspections

In the context of e-records integrity, the electronic records' governance must be examined. All the requisite procedures referenced in the governance document are defined, documented, and implemented.

There is no need to have distinct e-records integrity governance. The e-records related to worldwide regulations and guidelines recognize that the same regulations are applicable whether the data is recorded on paper or electronically.

The main activity of the person performing the inspection is to look up the identification of the critical e-records used by the regulated user, and to identify how the regulated user manages critical e-records.

Self-inspections should identify and inform management of opportunities to improve systems and processes that have an impact on the reliability of

* EudraLex, The rule governing medicinal products in the European Union, Volume 4 EU Good manufacturing practice (GMP) medicinal products for human and veterinary use, Chapter 9: Self inspections, 2001.

e-records, including e-records integrity. The allocation of resources to these improvements effectively reduces e-records integrity risks. For example, identifying and addressing the technical difficulties encountered with equipment that is used to perform multiple regulated operations may greatly improve the reliability of e-records for all of those operations; identifying security conflicts and allocating independent IT personnel to perform system administration for computer systems—including the management of security, backup, and archival resources—may reduce potential conflicts of interest, and may greatly streamline and improve e-records management efficiencies.

The International Pharmaceutical Excipients Council (IPEC)'s "Good Manufacturing Practices Audit Guideline for Pharmaceutical Excipients" 2008, provides a questionnaire in Section 6.3.2.3 that can be used to perform the initial assessment of computer systems. Some of the items addressed in this questionnaire are related to e-records integrity.

- If computerized systems are used in a manner that can impact excipient quality, have they been demonstrated to consistently function as expected?
- What process is used to control changes to systems and programs that can have an effect on the quality of the product, to assure that changes receive the proper review and approval with regard to potential effects before being instituted and that only authorized personnel can make such changes? Are personnel trained subsequent to changes?
- How is access to computerized systems limited in order to protect the e-records from tampering and to prevent e-records' alteration?
- If passwords are used as a security measure, are there provisions for periodic changes of those passwords? Are there designees for all critical system operations and emergencies?
- What is the procedure for reviewing and updating security access when a person leaves the department or company? Is their access to the system, or are their access codes for the system, revoked in a timely fashion?
- What backup systems are in place, such as copies of programs and files, duplicate tapes, or microfilm? Has the retrievability of information from master tapes and backup tapes been verified? Are there procedures in place for disaster recovery in the event of a power outage, loss of the server and computer system, and so on?

During the inspection, focus on change management. It must be confirm that approved changes applicable to e-records integrity are actually occurring. Verify that all e-records integrity–related changes are done in a controlled manner and documented.

If computer systems are involved in gathering, storing, or transmitting e-records these need to be identified and their capabilities established. The following are important:

- What is the source of the data entered into the computer?
- Who enters the data?
- When is the data entered?
- Who has access to the computer and to the security codes?
- How are e-records that were previously entered changed? An audit trail? By whom?
- How are e-records submitted to a sponsor (hard disk, floppy disk, fax, modern network, mail, messenger)?
- How are errors, omissions, and so on, in the e-records received, corrected, and documented?

Close attention should be paid if/when the following occurs:

- Audit trails are inactivated.
- Access to e-records is not controlled.
- Dates on printouts do not correlate with raw data.
- Systems ensuring full e-records integrity are inadequate.
- There are other discrepancies identified:
  - Back-dating.
  - Invalidation of e-records that is not justifiable.

Focus on raw e-records handling & e-records review/verification.

E-Records Remediation

If gaps are found during the self-inspections, it may be required to upgrade the control strategies and apply quality risk management and/or sound scientific principles to the current business models, as well as the current technologies that are in use.*

Refer to Chapter 19.

Additional Reading

ISO/IEC 12207, Systems and software engineering: Software lifecycle processes, 7.2.7 Software Audit Process, February 2008.

* WHO, Guidance on good data and record management practices, QAS/15.624, September 2015, (Draft).

Chapter 19

Electronic Records Remediation Project

A fundamental norm of computer systems that perform activities covered by medicine manufacturing practice regulations is the high level of security required to protect regulated e-records. Regulatory agencies or competent authorities make compulsory the issues related to security as the result of e-records integrity deviations having a potential impact on public health.

All computer systems performing activities covered by medicine manufacturing practices regulations must protect their e-records by means of the applicable controls discussed in this book. For those computer systems that implement electronic signatures, the security and control of electronic signatures must also be provided. The electronic signature is linked and saved as part of an additional e-record. As such, all of the requirements associated with e-records are also applicable to the e-record containing the electronic signature and the associated link(s).

> Organizations subject to medical product good practice requirements have been using computerized systems for many decades but fail to adequately review and manage original electronic records and instead often only review and manage incomplete and/or inappropriate printouts.*

* WHO, Guidance on good data and record management practices, QAS/15.624, September 2015 (Draft).

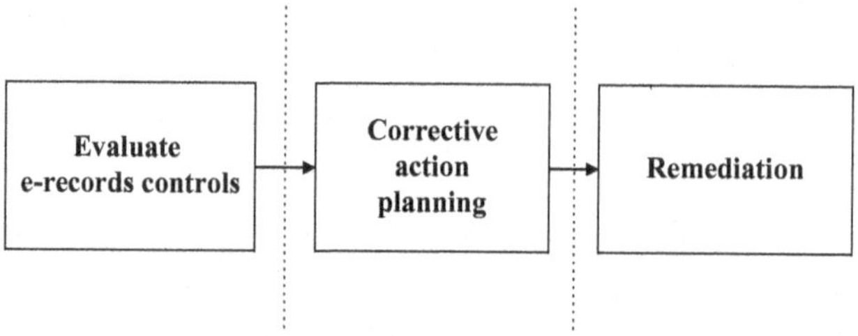

Figure 19.1 Complete remediation project.

Figure 19.1 illustrates a complete remediation project. Like any project, the schedule is based on priorities, risks, time, and the availability of resources.

This chapter identifies the key principles for remediating e-records with integrity–related issues. It is not intended to cover everything that an organization's management needs to do in order to achieve and maintain compliance with data integrity regulatory requirements and expectations.

Evaluate E-Records Controls

As part of the remediation process for e-records integrity–related requirements, a comprehensive investigation and evaluation must be performed on the actual controls to the e-records.

An evaluation plan is needed in order to define the nature, extent, schedule and responsibilities of the evaluation process. It should be described the methodology to evaluate the e-records. Results should include conclusions about the extent of data integrity deficiencies and their root cause.

The best guidance about data integrity remediation, is contained in the US FDA warning letters to USV Limited (February 2014).

The objective of this evaluation is to uncover the extent of the inaccuracies in the e-records, including the reliability of the computer systems managing these e-records, procedural controls, changes in management, e-records and system security, system backups, operator (user) training, as well as inaccuracies in the recorded e-records and reports themselves.

If the evaluation demonstrates that the e-records do not meet the applicable regulatory requirements, then the evaluation would not in itself support the integrity of the e-records.

This evaluation is the first phase to achieving an organized, prioritized, and balanced remediation project approach. The results of the evaluation will determine whether the e-records management practices and security procedures specific to the system will provide a controlled environment ensuring the integrity of the e-records.

As part of the prioritization, a risk assessment of how the observed deficiencies may affect the reliability and completeness of the quality information available for the drug product should be conducted. The risk assessment also provides information on the effects of potentially compromised data on release decisions, which rely on data generated by an uncontrolled system.

Each critical e-record must be identified and well understood in order to prioritize the work. E-records and process flow diagrams are used as tools for reviewing the operation. Other factors to take into account during the prioritization process are the components and functions that have regulatory implications.

An evaluation report must be generated for each e-records repository and the computer system managing those records. The evaluation report summarizes the current operation of the computer system, allocates its priority, provides a reference to any supporting documentation, and identifies the compliance gaps in each repository and associated computer system managing those records.

The audit report also should include any discrepancies between data or information identified in approved applications, and the actual results, methods, or testing conditions. The report should include an explanation of the impact of all discrepancies.

Based on the information on each evaluation report, a corrective action plan can be generated describing. the specific procedures, actions and controls that regulated entity will implement.

Corrective Action Planning

The remediation action items identified in the e-records integrity evaluation should be documented in a detailed implementation plan.

The purpose of the corrective action plan is to investigate the extent of the deficient practices noted during the evaluation. The action plan must include an investigation into the root causes of the data integrity issue and the associated risk assessment.

The corrective action plan must define the overall activities, schedule, costs, and responsibilities necessary to guide the development and implementation of technological and procedural controls, in order to bring the e-records into compliance with data integrity–related expectations. The plan should identify any existing technological/procedural controls that may be modified or new technological/procedural controls that need to be implemented, in order to ensure that the data integrity–related regulatory requirements are completed in a consistent and uniform manner.

Using the evaluation reports, the remediation activities, available resources, project schedule, and the business cost of the remediation approach can be estimated. This will enable a business decision to be made regarding the remediation or replacement of the current system, or the components surrounding the e-records, based on the cost-effectiveness of the system/components and their operational feasibility.

The plan must contain the activities that place emphasis on achieving consistent, high-quality, sustainable compliance solutions.

For data integrity–related issues found on computer systems performing activities covered by medicine manufacturing practice regulations, the corrective action plan must describe the broad actions that will be taken to ensure product quality and the prevention of the recurrence of these breaches of e-records integrity.

Once the corrective action plan has been approved, it can then be executed.

Remediation

The remediation process consists of six major activities. These activities are the following.

- Interpretation
- Training
- Remediation execution
- New application assessments
- Application upgrade assessments
- Supplier qualification program

During the remediation phase, the e-records and the associated controls are brought into compliance by implementing the procedural and/or technological controls determined by the corrective action plan. In addition, the processes needed to sustain the compliance solutions are implemented.

Interpretation

The ability to evaluate the risks of a particular e-record in relationship to its integrity regulatory expectations requires a thorough understanding of the regulation and a consistent interpretation. The objective of the interpretation phase in this plan is to provide a current, consistent, competent, and authoritative interpretation of e-records integrity to IT and interested outside parties.

Training

In the context of e-records integrity, awareness and understanding of the applicable regulation(s) and guidelines is fundamental to the success of the remediation plan. The objective of e-records integrity training is to ensure that all systems containing e-records and e-records owners have an appropriate level of knowledge on how to preserve the integrity of such e-records.

Remediation Execution

Once the corrective action plan is approved, the computer technology suppliers and developers are requested to identify products in which deficiencies can be overcome. When appropriate, procedural controls need to be revised and/or developed in order to address the deficiencies that cannot be solved by technological controls.

It is probable that the implementation of technological controls will require a comprehensive service-level commitment (SLC)—including the recommendation, conceptualization, and implementation of the new technology; the release and early operation of the new technology; and the decommissioning and disposal of old technologies. If the technological implementation fails, the failure should be documented along with details of the corrective action taken. Once this action has been taken, the system must be reevaluated in the same way as any other system that has been subject to an upgrade or correction.

When all of the action items applicable to the affected e-records have been implemented, it can be formally released for operation and support under a maintenance agreement.

The corrective action plan should be periodically reviewed since the evolving technology requirements will need to be considered and the plan revised accordingly.

New Applications and Application Upgrade Assessments

The objective of e-records integrity assessments for new repositories, applications managing e-records, and for application upgrades, is to identify the e-records integrity gaps before releasing the system into production. All gaps must be corrected by technological controls and/or procedural controls.

New/upgrades to systems/components that are released into production must have the highest level of e-records integrity compliance.

Suppliers Qualification Program

A key business strategy has been the outsourcing of work to computer technology suppliers and developers. The objective of qualifying computer technology suppliers and developers is to evaluate and monitor these "strategic" partners for e-records integrity compliance, and to provide an input to partner selection and partner relationship management processes.

For each supplier qualification performed, a report must be prepared that describe the results of the qualification.

Remediation Project Report

The remediation project report provides evidence of successful project completion. It summarizes the findings, the technological and procedural controls, and the associated activities that were necessary to establish the computer technology's compliance with e-records integrity–related requirements. This report and all supporting documentation should be archived.

This report ensures that the data reported is complete, meaningful, and related to the specific acceptance criteria and/or specifications. The conclusions must be supported by documented evidence.

Once a legacy system has achieved a satisfactory, documented e-records integrity compliant state, any subsequent changes can be prospectively validated.

Additional Reading

Eglovitch, J., How to remedy data integrity failures: FDA's step-by-step approach, *The Gold Sheet*, October 2015.

Chapter 20

Summary

The higher the level of automated processes, the lower the risk for poor data integrity.

Markus Roemer
Appendix VII

Despite challenges that regulatory agencies or competent authorities face about data integrity, awareness of the issue has significantly increased the understanding and knowledge of the computer systems and quality control systems that are relevant to the manufacturing of medicinal products. Since e-records integrity deviations have a potential impact on public health, regulatory agencies or competent authorities are focusing on the integrity of e-records and training inspectors on this topic.

Throughout this book, the technological and procedural controls to preserve the integrity of e-records have been identified. The following figure depicts the key elements of data integrity.

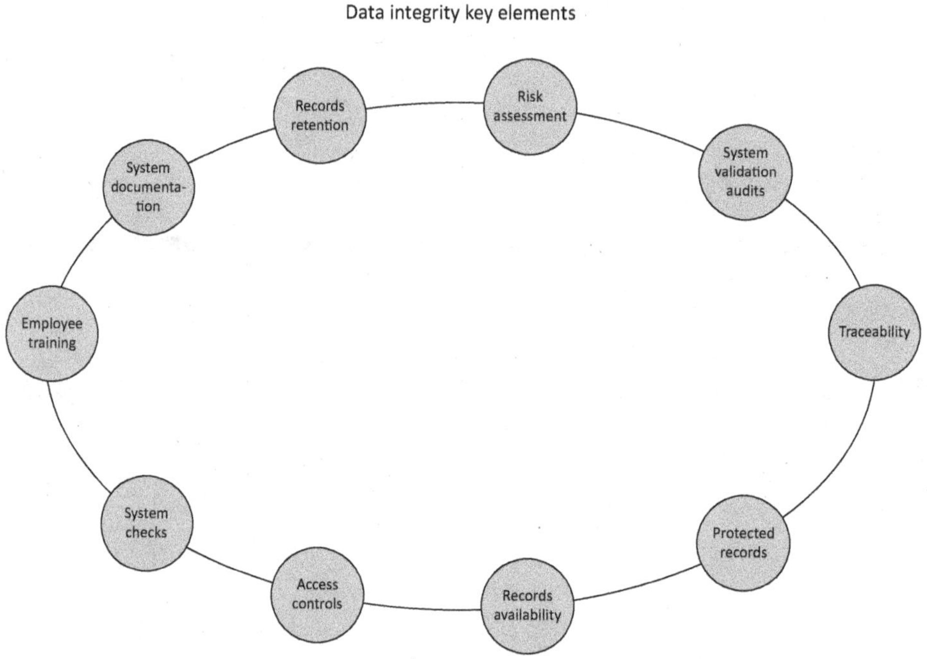

The good data integrity practices (GDIP) that are applicable to critical e-records can be summarized as the following:

- As part of a risk management system, decisions on the extent of the validation and e-records integrity controls should be based on a justified and documented risk assessment of the computer system (11 p1).
- When data is generated, recorded, processed, saved, and revised in the form of electronic documents, validated computer systems shall be used. All operations along with the users that are performing them and the associated times of those operations shall be recorded. The authenticity, validity, and traceability of data shall be ensured.
- Training for computer users must focus on the importance and principles of e-records integrity.
- The system owner is the person responsible for the availability and maintenance of a computer system and for the security of the e-records residing on that system. (Annex 11 Glossary) The owner of this role must be named and recorded.
- Raw data may be recorded by trustworthy computer systems and must be recorded at the time that the raw data is generated.

- Computer systems should be designed to increase the detection of errors/changes to e-records. In cases where the modification or deletion of an e-record has occurred, there should be a record accounting for that modification or deletion.
- The record accounting for the modification or deletion of e-records can be an automated audit trail or another adequate control to facilitate the traceability of the e-records' modification or deletion. A risk assessment establishes the method to be used.
- All e-records that keep track of modifications or deletions of other e-records (e.g., electronic audit trails) become e-records that are subject to the same e-records-related controls.
- E-records must be recorded at the time of performance to create a record (contemporaneously).
  - 21 CFR 211.100(b)
  - EUDRALEX Vol 4 Chapter 4 Section 4.8
  - WHO (draft) Data Integrity Guidance "Contemporaneous record"
  - MHRA Data Integrity Guidance - Definition "Computer system transactions"
- The recording of the e-record is not combined into a single computer system transaction with other operations (MHRA).
- Data recording
  - At the time of recording e-records, the accuracy of these e-records must be checked.
  - Appropriate built-in checks must be implemented for the correct computer inputs and outputs (I/Os).
  - Data entered manually into a computer must be independently checked.
- Security
  - Role-based security on all databases, data servers, networks, and applications must be established.
  - Only authorized persons should be able to enter or modify e-records in computer systems.
  - Access to e-records should be restricted by passwords or other means.
  - Security should also extend to devices used to store programs, such as tapes, disks, and magnetic strip cards. Access to these devices should be controlled.

- E-records should be protected by back-up transfer on magnetic tape, microfilm, paper printouts, or other means. As part of the back up procedure, back up intervals, retrievability, and storage must be established. In the case of paper printouts, or other means, the backup must be certified as a true copy of the initial e-record.
- 21 CFR 211.180(d) requires records to be retained "either as original e-records or true copies such as photocopies, microfilm, microfiche, or other accurate reproductions of the original records." Similarly, worldwide requirements are established in other good manufacturing practice (GMP)-related regulations.
- During the retention period of e-records, these must be readily available.
- Periodically, e-records retained by computer storage need to be verified for accessibility, readability, integrity, and the state of their security.
- The computer system documentation mostly covers the relevant steps associated with the handling of data integrity controls.
- Routine preventive maintenance shall be implemented for the system, an emergency response system for system failures shall be available, and measures for recovery after system disasters have occurred shall be prepared.
- Procedures are established and implemented covering the above items.

Overall, to protect the integrity of e-records the following must be considered:

- Confidentiality of e-records entry or collection
- Storage, transmission, and processing
- Access control, segregation of duties and audit trails

The regulated user will need evidence to demonstrate that quality attributes of the e-records are designed and built into the e-records life cycle. This evidence is obtained through validation, verification, analysis, and monitoring documentation. These attributes are controlled by way of operational and maintenance controls.

Finally, manufacturing systems must operate in a validated state; they must maintain standard operating procedures (SOPs) for use of the system, an audit trail of data changes ensuring that there is no deletion of the entered data, a security system to protect against unauthorized access, a list of the individuals authorized to make data changes, and adequate backup of the data. If data is transformed during processing, it should always be possible to compare the original data and observations with the processed data. There should be no loss of quality when an electronic system is used in place of a paper system.*

* EMA, Reflection Paper on the expectations for electronic source documents used in clinical trials, August 2010.

Appendix I: Glossary of Terms

For additional terms, refer to the *Glossary of Computerized System and Software Development Terminology**; *A Globally Harmonized Glossary of Terms for Communicating Computer Validation Key Practices*,† EudraLex—Volume 4 Good manufacturing practice (GMP) Guidelines—Glossary,‡ and the MHRA GMP Data Integrity Definitions and Guidance for Industry (March 2015).

For the purpose of this glossary, the terms and definitions given in 9000-3 and ISO 12207 are applicable. In the event of conflicting terms and definitions, the terms and definitions specified in this glossary and the references in the first paragraph above apply.

abstraction: This is a basic principle of software engineering, and enables understanding of the application and its design, and the management of complexity.

acceptance criteria: The criteria that a system or component must satisfy to be accepted by a user, customer, or other authorized entity. (IEEE)

acceptance test: Testing conducted to determine whether a system satisfies its acceptance criteria and to enable the customer to determine whether or not to accept the system. (IEEE)

access: The ability or opportunity to gain knowledge of stored information. (DOD 5015.2-STD)

---

* FDA, *Glossary of Computerized System and Software Development Terminology*, Division of Field Investigations, Office of Regional Operations, Office of Regulatory Affairs, Food and Drug Administration, August 1995.

† Herr, Robert R. and Wyrick, Michael L., A globally harmonized glossary of terms for communicating computer validation key practices, *PDA Journal of Pharmaceutical Science and Technology*, March/April 1999.

‡ http://ec.europa.eu/health/files/eudralex/vol-4/pdfs-en/glos4en200408_en.pdf.

accuracy: Refers to whether the data values stored for an object are the correct values. To be correct, data values must be accurate and must be represented in a consistent and unambiguous form.

acquirer: An organization that acquires a system, software product or software service from a supplier. (ISO 12207:1995*)

application: Software installed on a defined platform/hardware providing specific functionality. (EMA Annex 11)

application developer: See "software developer."

approver(s): In the context of configuration management, the approver is the person(s) responsible for evaluating the recommendations made by the reviewers, and for rendering a decision on whether or not to proceed with a proposed change and initiate a change request.

archive: Long-term, permanent retention of completed data and relevant metadata in its final form with the purpose of reconstructing the process or activity.

assessment: Investigation of processes, systems, or platforms by a subject matter expert or by IT Quality and Compliance. An assessment does not need to be independently conducted, in contrast to an audit.

audit: An independent examination of a software product, software process, or set of software processes to assess their compliance with specifications, standards, contractual agreements, or other criteria. (IEEE)

auditor: In the context of configuration management, the auditor is the person responsible for reviewing the steps taken during a development or change management process to ensure that the appropriate procedures have been followed.

audit trail: An electronic means of auditing the interactions with records within an electronic system so that any access to the system can be documented as it occurs so that unauthorized actions to the e-records can be identified; for example, their modification, deletion, or addition. (DOD 5015.2-STD) (2) GMP audit trails are metadata that are a record of GMP critical information (for example the change or deletion of GMP relevant data). (MHRA)

authentication: Verifying the identity of a user, process, or device, often as a prerequisite for allowing access to the resources in an information system. (NIST Special Publication 800-18)

authenticity: The property of being genuine and being able to be verified and trusted; confidence in the validity of a transmission, a message,

* Note: The 1995 revision is not the most recent version.

or message originator. See "authentication." (NIST Special Publication 800-18)

automated systems: Includes a broad range of systems including, but not limited to, automated manufacturing equipment, automated laboratory equipment, process control, manufacturing execution, clinical trials data management, and document management systems. The automated system consists of the hardware, software, and network components, together with the controlled functions and associated documentation. Automated systems are sometimes referred to as computerized systems. (PICS CSV PI 011-3*)

availability: Ensuring the timely and reliable access to and use of information. (44 U.S.C., SEC. 3542)

backup: A copy of current (editable) data, metadata and system configuration settings (variable settings that relate to an analytical run), maintained for the purpose of disaster recovery. (MHRA)

baseline: An agreed description of the attributes of a product, at a point in time, which serves as a basis for defining change. A "change" is a movement from this baseline state to a next state.

bespoke computerized system: A computerized system individually designed to suit a specific business process. (EMA Annex 11)

best practices: Practices established by experience and common sense.

biometrics: Methods of identifying a person's identity based on physical measurements of that individual's physical characteristics or repeatable actions. Some examples of biometrics include identifying a user based on their physical signature, fingerprints, and so on.

calibration: A set of operations that establish, under specified conditions, the relationship between values of quantities indicated by a measuring instrument or measuring system, or values represented by a material measure or reference material, and the corresponding values realized by standards. (PICS CSV PI 011-3)

certificate: Certificates are used to verify the identity of an individual, organization, Web server, or hardware device. They are also used to ensure non-repudiation in business transactions, as well as to enable confidentiality through the use of public-key encryption.

certification authority: As part of a public key infrastructure, an authority in a network that issues and manages from a Certificate Server

---

* PI 011-3. Good practices for computerised systems in regulated "GXP" Environments, Pharmaceutical Inspection Co-operation Scheme (PIC/S), September 2007.

security credentials and public key for message encryption and decryption. (NARA)

certified copy: (1) A copy of original information that has been verified, as indicated by a dated signature, as an exact copy having all of the same attributes and information as the original. (Source: FDA, Electronic Source Data in Clinical Investigations, September 2013) (2) A copy of original information that has been verified as an exact (accurate and complete) copy having all of the same attributes and information as the original. The copy may be verified by a dated signature or by a validated electronic process. (Source: CDISC (Clinical Data Interchange Standards Consortium) Clinical Research Glossary Version 8.0, December 2009)

change: Any variation or alteration in form, state or quality. This includes additions, deletions, or modifications that impact the hardware or software components used, affecting operational integrity—service level agreements, or the validated status of applications on the system.

change control: A formal system by which qualified representatives of appropriate disciplines review proposed or actual changes that might affect the validated status of facilities, systems, equipment or processes. The intent is to determine the need for action that would ensure, and document, that the system is maintained in a validated state. (EMA Annex 15, Qualification and Validation)

cipher: A series of transformations that converts plaintext to cipher text using the cipher key.

cipher key: A secret cryptography key that is used by the key expansion routine to generate a set of round keys.

cipher text: Data output from the cipher or input to the inverse cipher.

clear printed: Printouts that, apart from the values themselves, allow for the units and the respective contexts to also be seen. (*Journal for GMP and Regulatory Affairs*, Q&As on Annex 11, Issue 8, April/May 2012)

cloud computing: Is the practice of using a network of remote servers hosted on the Internet to store, manage, and process data, rather than a local server or a personal computer.

code audit: An independent review of source code by a person, team, or tool to verify compliance with software design documentation and programming standards. Correctness and efficiency may also be evaluated. (IEEE)

Code of Federal Regulations: The codification of the general and permanent rules published in the Federal Register by the executive departments and agencies of the Federal Government.

code inspection: A manual [formal] testing [error detection] technique where the programmer reads source code, statement by statement, to a group who ask questions analyzing the program logic, analyzing the code with respect to a checklist of historically common programming errors, and analyzing its compliance with coding standards. This technique can also be applied to other software and configuration items. (Myers/NBS)

code review: A meeting at which software code is presented to project personnel, managers, users, customers, or other interested parties for comment or approval. (IEEE)

code walkthrough: A manual testing [error detection] technique where program [source code] logic [structure] is traced manually [mentally] by a group with a small set of test cases, while the state of program variables is manually monitored, to analyze the programmer's logic and assumptions. (FDA Glossary of Computerized System and Software Development Technology (8/95), FDA)

commercial of the shelf software: Software commercially available, whose fitness for use is demonstrated by a broad spectrum of users. (EMA Annex 11)

commissioning: Refer to "site acceptance testing." (SAT)

competent: Having the necessary experience and/or training to adequately perform the job.

completeness: The property that all necessary parts of the entity in question are included. Completeness of a product is often used to express the fact that all requirements have been met by the product.

complexity: In the context of this book, complexity means the degree to which a system or component has a design or implementation that is difficult to understand and verify.

compliance: Compliance covers the adherence to application-related standards, conventions, or regulations in laws and similar prescriptions. It refers to the fulfillment of regulatory requirements.

compliant system: A system that meets applicable guidelines and predicated requirements.

computer: (1) A functional unit that can perform substantial computations, including numerous arithmetical and logical operations without human intervention. (2) The hardware components and associated software designed to perform specific functions.

computer system: (1) A system including the input of data, electronic processing, and output of information, to be used either for reporting or automated control (PICS CSV PI 011-3). (2) A functional unit, consisting of one or more computers, associated peripheral input and output devices, and associated software that uses common storage for all or part of a program, and all or part of the data necessary for the execution of the program. It executes user-written or user-designated programs; performs user-designated data manipulation, including arithmetic operations and logic operations; and can execute programs that modify themselves during their execution. A computer system may be a stand-alone unit or may consist of several interconnected units. (ANSI)

computer systems validation: (1) The *formal assessment and reporting* of quality and performance measures for all the life-cycle stages of software and system development, its implementation, qualification and acceptance, operation, modification, re-qualification, maintenance and retirement. This should enable both the regulated user and competent authority to have a high level of confidence in the integrity of the processes executed within the computer system(s) and the processes controlled by and/or linked to the computer system(s) within the prescribed operating environment(s) (PICS CSV PI 011-3*). (2) Documented evidence that provides a high degree of ensurance that a computerized system analyses, controls, and records data correctly, and that data processing complies with predetermined specifications. (WHO)

computerized process: A process where some or all of the actions are controlled by a computer.

computerized system: (1) A system controlled partially or totally by a computer. (2) See "automated systems."

computer validation: Refer to "computer systems validation."†

concurrent validation: In some cases, a drug product or medical device may be manufactured individually or on a one-time basis. The concept of prospective or retrospective validation as it relates to those situations may have limited applicability. The data obtained during the manufacturing and assembly process may be used in conjunction

* PI 011-3. Good practices for computerised systems in regulated "GXP" environments, Pharmaceutical Inspection Co-operation Scheme (PIC/S), September 2007.

† Ibid.

with product testing to demonstrate that the instant run yielded a finished product meeting all of its specifications and quality characteristics. (FDA)

confidentiality: Preserving authorized restrictions on information access and disclosure, including the means for protecting personal privacy and proprietary information. (44 U.S.C., SEC. 3542)

configurable software: Application software, sometimes general purpose, written for a variety of industries or users in a manner that permits users to modify the program to meet their individual needs. (FDA)

configuration item: Entity within a configuration that satisfies an end use function and that can be uniquely identified at a given reference point. (ISO 9000-3)

contemporaneous e-records: E-records recorded at the time they are generated.

control system: Included in this classification are supervisory control and data acquisition systems (SCADA), distributed control systems (DCS), statistical process control systems (SPC), programmable logic controllers (PLCs), intelligent electronic devices, and computer systems that control manufacturing equipment or receive data directly from manufacturing equipment PLCs.

consistency: The property of logical coherency among constituent parts. Consistency may also be expressed as adherence to a given set of rules.

correctness: The extent to which software is free from design and coding defects, that is, fault-free. It is also the extent to which software meets its specified requirements and user objectives.

criticality: In the context of this book, criticality means the regulatory impact to a system or component. See "critical system."

critical: Describes a process step, process condition, test requirement, or other relevant parameter or item that must be controlled within predetermined criteria to ensure that the product/process meets its specification.

critical electronic records: In this book critical e-records is interpreted as meaning e-records with high risk to product quality or patient safety. (ISPE GAMP COP Annex 11—Interpretation, July/August 2011)

critical data: In this book critical data is interpreted as meaning data with high risk to product quality or patient safety. (ISPE GAMP COP Annex 11 – Interpretation, July/August 2011)

critical requirement: A requirement that, if not met, has an adverse impact on any of the following: Patient safety, product quality, requirements satisfying health authority regulation, cGxP data integrity or security.

critical systems: Systems that directly or indirectly influence patient safety, product quality and data integrity.

custom built software: Also known as a bespoke system, custom-built software is software produced for a customer, specifically to order, to meet a defined set of user requirements. (GAMP)

customized computerized system: See "bespoke computerized system."

data: The contents of the record; the basic unit of information that has a unique meaning and can be transmitted. Information derived or obtained from raw data (e.g., a reported analytical result). (MHRA)

database: In relation to electronic records, this is a set of data, consisting of at least one file or of a group of integrated files, usually stored in one location and made available to several users at the same time for various applications. (36 CFR 1234.2, reference (ii))

data base management system (DBMS): A software system used to access and retrieve data stored in a database. (36 CFR 1234.2, reference (ii))

data collection: The process of gathering and measuring information.

data governance: The sum of arrangements to ensure that data. Irrespective of the format in which it is generated, are recorded, processed, retained and used to ensure a complete, consistent and accurate record throughout the data lifecycle.

data handling: The process of ensuring that data is stored, archived or disposed of in a safe and secure manner during the data lifecycle.

data migration: The process of moving data from one computer system to another without converting the data.

data integrity: The property that data has not been altered in an unauthorized manner. Data integrity covers data in storage, being processed, and in transit (NIST SP 800-33). It refers to the extent to which all data is complete, consistent and accurate throughout the data lifecycle. (MHRA)

data lifecycle: All phases in the life of the data (including raw data) from their initial generation and recording through processing (including transformation or migration), use, data retention, archive/retrieval and destruction. (MHRA)

data ownership: It refers to the possession of information and the associated responsibilities.

data selection: The process of determining the appropriate data type, source, and suitable instruments for data collection.

data source: The origin where data is collected from.

data warehousing: An architected, periodic, and coordinated process of copying from numerous sources into an optimized environment capable of analytical and informational processing.

decommissioning: A planned, systematic process to disassemble and retire from service a facility system and equipment without altering the integrity (validation state) of any other facility, system or equipment previously connected to the facility, system or equipment being decommissioned. The decommissioning is done via inspection, testing and documentation.

decryption: The transformation of unintelligible data ("ciphertext") into original data ("clear text").

delete: The process of permanently removing, erasing, or obliterating recorded information from a medium, especially an electronic medium.

deliverable: A tangible or intangible object produced as a result of project execution, as part of an obligation. In validation projects, "deliverables" are usually documents.

design qualification: The documented verification that the proposed design of the facilities, systems and equipment is suitable for the intended purpose. Also known as "design verification." (EMA Annex 15, Validation and Qualification.

derived data: Data that was originally supplied in one form, but was converted to another form using some automated process.

developer: An organization that performs development activities (including requirements analysis, design, and testing through acceptance) during the software life cycle process.

development: Software life cycle process that contains the activities of requirements analysis, design, coding, integration, testing, installation and support for the acceptance of software products. (ISO 9000-3)

deviation: When a system does not act as expected.

digital certificate: A credential issued by a trusted authority. An entity can present a digital certificate to prove its identity or its right to access information. It links a public-key value to a set of information that identifies the associated entity with the use of the corresponding private key. Certificates are authenticated, issued, and managed by a trusted third party called a CA.

digital signature standard (DSS): A National Institute of Standards and Technology (NIST) standard for digital signatures, used to authenticate both a message and the signer. DSS has a security level comparable to RSA (Rivest-Shamir-Adleman) cryptography, having 1024-bit keys.

disaster recovery: The activities required to restore one or more computer systems to their valid state in response to a major hardware or software failure or the destruction of facilities.

discrepancy: Any problem or entry into the Problem Reporting System. Includes all bugs and may also include design issues.

destruction: In records management, this refers to the major type of disposal action. Methods of destroying records include selling or salvaging the record medium and burning, pulping, shredding, macerating, or discarding it with other waste materials.

disposition: Disposition means those actions taken regarding records after they are no longer in office space, to conduct current business. These action include: (41 CFR 201-4 and RM Handbook, references (kk) and (w))

documentation: (1) Manuals, written procedures or policies, records or reports, that provide information concerning the uses, maintenance, or validation of a process or system involving either hardware or software. This material may be presented in electronic media. Documents include, but are not limited to standard operating procedures (SOPs), technical operating procedures (TOPs), manuals, logs, system development documents, test plans, scripts and results, plans, protocols, and reports. Refer to "Documentation" and "Documentation, level of" in the *Glossary of Computerized System and Software Development Terminology,* August 1995. (2) Any written or pictorial information describing, defining, specifying, reporting or certifying activities, requirements, procedures, or results. (ANSI N45.2.10-1973)

electronic record: Information recorded in electronic form that requires a computer system to access or process (SAG, "A Guide to Archiving of Electronic Records," February 2014). In this book, based on the MHRA definitions, raw data and data are considered e-records. When refering to both electronic raw data and data, the term "e-records" will be used.

electronic record life cycle: All phases in the life of the electronic record from initial generation and recording through processing (including transformation or migration), use, electronic records retention, archive/retrieval and destruction.

electronic source data: Data initially recorded in electronic format. (Source: FDA, Electronic Source Data in Clinical Investigations, September 2013)

end user: Personnel who use the validated computer system.

emergency change: A change to a validated system that is determined to be necessary to eliminate an error condition that prevents the use of the system and interrupts the business function.

emulation: Refers to the process of mimicking, in software, a piece of hardware or software so that other processes think that the original equipment/function is still available in its original form. Emulation is essentially a way of preserving the functionality of and access to digital information that might otherwise be lost due to technological obsolescence.

encryption: (1) The process of converting information into a code or cipher so that people will be unable to read it. A secret key, or password, is required to decrypt (decode) the information. (2) Transformation of confidential plaintext into ciphertext to protect it. An encryption algorithm combines plaintext with other values called keys, or ciphers, so the data becomes unintelligible. [45 CFR 142.304]

entity: A software or hardware product that can be individually qualified or validated.

establish: As defined in this book, it means to define, document, and implement.

evaluation: A systematic determination of the extent to which an entity meets its specified criteria.

expected result: What a system should do when a particular action is performed.

factory acceptance test: An acceptance test in the supplier's factory, usually involving the customer. (IEEE)

failure analysis: Is the process of collecting and analyzing data to determine the cause of a failure. One of the software-based fault location techniques is automatic test pattern generation.

FDA guidance documents: FDA guidance documents represent the FDA's current thinking on a particular subject. These documents do not create or confer any rights for or on any person and do not operate to bind FDA or the public. An alternative approach may be used if such an approach satisfies the requirements of the applicable statutes, regulations, or both.

federal register: A daily issuance of the US government which provides a uniform system for making available to the public regulations and legal notices issued by Federal agencies.

field devices: Hardware devices that are typically located in the field at or near the process, and which are needed to bring information to the computer or to implement a computer-driven control action. Devices include sensors, analytical instruments, transducers, and valves.

File: An arrangement of records. The term is used to denote papers, photographs, photographic copies, maps, machine-readable information, or other recorded information, regardless of physical form or characteristics, accumulated or maintained in filing equipment, boxes, machine-readable media, or on shelves and occupying office or storage space. (Noun) (41 CFR 201-4 and 36 CFR 1220.14, references (kk)) and (11))

final rule: The regulation finalized for implementation, published in the US Federal Register (FR)—preamble and codified—and codified in the Code of Federal Regulation (CFR).

format: For electronic records, the format refers to the computer file format described by a formal or vender standard or specification. For non-electronic records, the format refers to its physical form; for example, paper, microfilm, video, and so on.

function: A set of specified, ordered actions that are part of a process.

functional testing: Application of test data derived from the specified functional requirements without regard to the final program structure.

GMP: Good manufacturing practice means the part of quality assurance that ensures that products are consistently produced and controlled in accordance with the quality standards appropriate to their intended use. (Commission Directive 2003/94/EC)

GMP controls: A set of controls that provide ensurance of consistently continued process performance and product quality.

GMP regulated activities: The manufacturing-related activities established in the basic legislation compiled in Volume 1 and Volume 5 of the publication The rules governing medicinal products in the European Union, US FDA 21 CFR Part 211, "Current Good Manufacturing Practice In Manufacturing, Processing, Packing or Holding of Drugs; General and Current Good Manufacturing Practice For Finished Pharmaceuticals" or any predicate rule applicable to medicinal products for the referenced country.

GxP application: Software entities that have a specific user-defined business purpose that must meet the requirements of a GxP regulation.

GXP computerized systems: A computer system that performs a regulated operation that is required to be formally controlled under a GXP international life science requirements.

GXP regulation: A global abbreviation intended to cover GMP, GCP, GLP, and other regulated applications in context. The underlying international life science requirements such as those set forth in the US FD&C Act, US PHS Act, FDA regulations, EU Directives, Japanese MHL.W regulations, Australia TGA, or other applicable national legislation or regulations under which a company operates. (GAMP Good Practice Guide, IT Infrastructure Control and Compliance, ISPE 2005)

human readable: An electronic record, data or signature that can be displayed in a viewable form, for example on paper or on a computer screen and that has meaning. (words in a written language)

hybrid systems: Hybrid computer systems include combinations of paper records (or other non-electronic media) and electronic records, paper records and electronic signatures, or handwritten signatures executed to electronic records.

information technology: Any equipment or interconnected system or subsystem of equipment that is used in the automatic acquisition, storage, manipulation, management, movement, control, display, switching, interchanging, transmission, or reception of data or information by the executive agency. For purposes of the preceding sentence, equipment is used by an executive agency if the equipment is used by the executive agency directly or is used by a contractor under a contract with the executive agency that: (i) Requires the use of such equipment; or (ii) requires the use, to a significant extent, of such equipment in the performance of a service or the furnishing of a product. The term "information technology" includes computers, ancillary equipment, software, firmware and similar procedures, services (including support services), and related resources. [40 U.S.C., SEC. 1401]

infrastructure: The hardware and software, such as networking software and operation systems, that makes it possible for the application to function. (EMA Annex 11)

integrity: Protection against unauthorized changes to information.

interface: A shared boundary that allows for interaction or communication with another system component. (ANSI/IEEE)

impact of change: The impact of change is the effect of the change on the GXP computer system. The components by which the impact of change is evaluated may include, but not be limited to, business considerations, resource requirements and availability, the application of appropriate regulatory agency requirements, and the criticality of the system.

inspection: (1) A manual testing technique in which program documents (design and requirement specifications, source codes or user manuals) are examined in a very formal and disciplined manner to discover any errors, violations of standards or other problems. Checklists are typically used in accomplishing this process. (2) A visual examination of a software product to detect and identify software anomalies, including errors and deviations in standards and specifications. Inspections are peer examinations led by impartial facilitators who are trained in inspection techniques. Determination of remedial or investigative action for an anomaly is a mandatory element of software inspection, although the solution should not be determined in the inspection meeting.

installation qualification: Establishing confidence that process equipment and ancillary systems are capable of consistently operating within established limits and tolerances. (FDA)

integration testing: Orderly progression of testing in which software elements, hardware elements, or both, are combined and tested, until all intermodule communication links have been integrated.

integrity: Guards against improper information modification or destruction, and includes ensuring information non-repudiation and authenticity. (44 U.S.C., Sec. 3542)

intended use: Use of a product, process or service in accordance with the specifications, instructions and information provided by the manufacturer (ANSI/AAMI/ISO 14971). (2) Refers to the objective intent of the persons legally responsible for the labeling of devices. The intent is determined by such persons' expressions or may be shown by the circumstances surrounding the distribution of the article. This objective intent may, for example, be shown by labeling claims, advertising matter, oral or written statements by such persons or their representatives. It may be shown by the circumstances that the article is, with the knowledge of such persons or their representatives, offered and used for a purpose for which it is neither labeled nor advertised. After it has been introduced into interstate commerce by its manufacturer, the intended uses of an article may change. If, for example, a packer, distributor, or seller intends an article for different uses than those intended by the person from whom he received the devices, US FDA Draft Guidance for Industry and Food and Drug Administration Staff - Mobile Medical Applications, July 2011.

IT infrastructure: The hardware and software, such as networking software and operation systems, that makes it possible for the application to function. (EMA Annex 11)

key practices: Processes that are essential for computer validation, consisting of tools, workflow, and people. (PDA)

legacy systems: (1) Production computer systems that are operating on older computer hardware or are based on older software applications. In some cases, the vendor may no longer support the hardware or software. (2) These are regarded as systems that have been established and in use for a considerable amount of time. For a variety of reasons, they may be generally characterized by a lack of adequate GMP compliance-related documentation or records pertaining to the development and commissioning stages of the system. Additionally, because of their age there may be no records of a formal approach for the validation of the system (PICS CSV PI 011-3*).

life cycle: All phases in the life of the system from initial requirements until retirement including design, specification, programming, testing, installation, operation, and maintenance. (EMA Annex 11)

life cycle model: A framework containing the processes, activities, and tasks involved in the development, operation, and maintenance of a software product, spanning the life of the system from the definition of its requirements to the termination of its use. (ISO 9000-3)

life cycle (record): The life span of a record from its creation to its final disposition is considered its lifecycle. There are four stages in a record lifecycle: Creation, maintenance, retention management and disposal.

living document: A document (or collection of documents) revised as needed throughout the life of a computer system. Only the most recent version(s) is (are) effective, and supersedes prior versions.

logically secure and controlled environment: A computing environment, controlled by policies, procedures, and technology, that deters

* PI 011-3. Good practices for computerised systems in regulated "GXP" environments, Pharmaceutical Inspection Co-operation Scheme (PIC/S), September 2007.

direct or remote unauthorized access that could damage computer components, production applications and/or data.

maintainer: An organization that performs maintenance activities. (ISO 12207:199^{5}4)

major change: A change to a validated system that is determined by reviewers and requires the execution of extensive validation activities.

manufacture: All operations involving the purchase of materials and products, production, quality control, release, storage, and the dispatch of medicinal products and related controls.

manufacturing: All operations involving the receipt of materials, production, packaging, repackaging, labeling, relabeling, quality control, release, storage and distribution of medicinal products and the related controls.

may: This word, or the adjective "optional," means that an item is truly optional. The word "may" is used for permissible actions.

metadata: The data that describes stored data: That is, data describing the structure, data elements, interrelationships, and other characteristics of electronic records (DOD 5015.2-STD). It refers to data that describes the attributes of other data, and provides context and meaning. Typically, these are data that describe the structure, data elements, interrelationships and other characteristics of data. This also permits data to be attributable to an individual. (MHRA)

migration: The periodic transfer of digital materials from one hardware/software configuration to another, or from one generation of computer technology to a subsequent generation.

minor change: A change to a validated system that is determined by reviewers to require the execution of only targeted qualifications and validation activities.

model: A model is an abstract representation of a given object.

module testing: Refer to *Testing, Unit* in the *Glossary of Computerized System and Software Development Terminology,* August 1995.

NEMA enclosure: Hardware enclosures (usually cabinets) that provide different levels of mechanical and environmental protection to the devices installed within it.

non-conformance: A departure from the minimum requirements specified in a contract, specification, drawing, or other approved product description or service.

non-custom purchased software package: A generally available, marketed software product that performs specific data collection, manipulation, output, or archiving functions. Refer *to Configurable, off-the-shelf software* in the *Glossary of Computerized System and Software Development Terminology,* August 1995.

non-repudiation: Strong and substantial evidence of the identity of the signer of a message and the message's integrity, sufficient enough to prevent a party from successfully denying the origin, submission or delivery of the message and the integrity of its contents.

objective evidence: Qualitative or quantitative information, records or statements of fact pertaining to the quality of an item or service, or to the existence of a quality system element, that is based on observation, measurement or tests and that can be verified.

operator: An organization that operates the system. (ISO 12207:1995[4])

operating environment: All outside influences that interface with the computer system. (GAMP)

ongoing evaluation: A term used to describe the dynamic process employed, after a system's initial validation, that can assist in maintaining the validated state of the computer system.

operational testing: Refer to *Operational Qualification* in the *Glossary of Computerized System and Software Development Terminology,* August 1995.

operating system: Software that controls the execution of programs and that provides services such as resource allocation, scheduling, input/output control, and data management. Usually, operating systems are predominantly software, but partial or complete hardware implementations are possible. (ISO)

original record: Data as the file or format in which it was originally generated, preserving the integrity (accuracy, completeness, content and meaning) of the record, for example, an original paper record of manual observation, or an electronic raw data file from a computerized system. (MHRA)

packaged software: Software provided and maintained by a vendor/supplier that can provide general business functionality or system services. Refer *to Configurable, off-the-shelf software* in the *Glossary of Computerized System and Software Development Terminology,* August 1995.

Part 11 records: Records that are required to be maintained under predicate rule requirements and that are maintained in electronic format in place of paper format, or, that are maintained in electronic format in addition to paper format, and that are relied upon to perform regulated activities. Part 11 records include records submitted to the FDA, under predicate rules (even if such records are not specifically identified in the agency's regulations) in electronic format (assuming the records have been identified in docket number 92S-0251 as the types of submissions that the agency accepts in electronic format) (FDA guidance: Part 11 Scope and Application).

password: A character string used to authenticate an identity. Knowledge of the password that is associated with a user ID is considered proof of authorization to use the capabilities associated with that user ID. (CSC-STD-002-85)

periodic review: A documented assessment of the documentation, procedures, records, and performance of a computer system to determine whether or not it is still in a validated state and what actions, if any, are necessary to restore its validated state (PDA). The review is performed at regular intervals. The timing of these intervals is left flexible.

person: "person," refers to an individual or an organization with legal rights and duties.

personal identification number: A PIN is an alphanumeric code or password used to authenticate the identity of an individual.

physical environment: The physical environment of a computer system comprises the physical location and the environmental parameters in which the system physically functions.

planned change: An intentional change to a validated system for which an implementation and evaluation program is predetermined.

policy: A directive which usually specifies what is to be accomplished.

preamble: Analysis preceding a proposed or final rule that clarifies the intention of the rulemaking and any ambiguities regarding the rule. Responses to comments made on a proposed rule are published in the preamble preceding the final rule. Preambles are published only in the FR and do not have a binding effect.

predicate regulations: The Federal Food, Drug, and Cosmetic Act, the Public Health Service Act or any FDA Regulation, with the exception of 21 CFR Part 11. Predicate regulations address the research, production, and control of FDA regulated articles.

primary record: The record which takes primacy in cases where those collected or retained concurrently by more than one method fail to concur. (MHRA)

procedural controls: (1) Written and approved procedures providing appropriate instructions for each aspect of the development, operations, maintenance, and security applicable to computer technologies. In the context of regulated operations, procedural controls should have QA/QC controls that are equivalent to the applicable predicate regulations. (2) A directive usually specifying how certain activities are to be accomplished. PMA CSVC.

process: (1) A set of specified, ordered actions required to achieve a defined result. (2) A set of interrelated or interacting activities that transform input into outputs. (ISO 9000-3)

process owner: The person responsible for the business process. (EMA Annex 11)

process system: The combination of the process equipment, support systems (such as utilities), and procedures used to execute a process.

production environment: The operational environment in which the system is being used for its intended purpose, that is, not in a test or development environment.

production verification (PV): Documented verification that the integrated system performs as intended in its production environment. PV is the execution of selected performance qualification (PQ) tests in the production environment using production data.

project: A project is an activity that achieves specific objectives through a set of defining tasks and the effective use of resources.

project management: Project management is the application of knowledge, skills, tools, and techniques to project activities in order to meet the project requirements. (ANSI)

prospective validation: Validation conducted prior to the distribution of either a new product, or a product made under a revised manufacturing process, where the revisions may affect the product's characteristics. (FDA)

qualification: (1) The action of proving that any equipment works correctly and actually leads to the expected results. The word validation is sometimes widened to incorporate the concept of qualification (PIC/S). (2) Qualification is the process of demonstrating whether a computer system and associated controlled process/operation, procedural controls, and documentation are capable of fulfilling specified requirements. (3) The process of demonstrating whether an entity is capable of fulfilling specified requirements. (ISO 8402: 1994, 2.13.1)

qualification protocol: A prospective experimental plan stating how qualification will be conducted, including test parameters, product characteristics, production equipment, and decision points on what constitutes an acceptable test. When executed, a protocol is intended to produce documented evidence that a system or subsystem performs as required.

qualification reports: These are test reports which evaluate the conduct and results of the qualification carried out on a computer system.

quality: The totality of features and characteristics of a product or service that bears on its ability to satisfy given needs.

quality assurance: All planned and systematic activities implemented within the quality system, and demonstrated as needed, to provide adequate confidence that an entity will fulfill its requirements for quality.

quality management: All activities of the overall management function that determine the quality policy, objectives, and responsibilities and implement them by such means as quality planning, quality control, quality assurance, and quality improvement within the quality system.

raw data: All data on which quality decisions are based should be defined as raw data. It includes data that is used to generate other records. (Source: Volume 4, EU Good Manufacturing Practice Medicinal Products for Human and Veterinary Use, Chapter 4: Documentation)

Original records and documentation, retained in the format in which they were originally generated (i.e., paper or electronic), or as a "true copy." Raw data must be contemporaneously and accurately recorded by permanent means. In the case of basic electronic equipment that does not store electronic data, or provides only a printed data output (e.g., balance or pH meter), the printout constitutes the raw data. (MHRA)

Any laboratory worksheets, records, memoranda, notes, or exact copies thereof that are the result of original observations and activities of and around a nonclinical laboratory study, and that are necessary for the reconstruction and evaluation of the report of that study. In the event that exact transcripts of raw data have been prepared (e.g., tapes that have been transcribed verbatim, dated, and verified as accurate by signature), the exact copy or exact transcript may be substituted for the original source as raw data. Raw data may include photographs, microfilm or microfiche copies, computer printouts, magnetic media, including dictated observations, and recorded data from automated instruments. (Source: US FDA 21 CFR 58.3(k))

record: Provides evidence of various actions taken to demonstrate compliance with instructions, for example, activities, events, investigations and, in the case of manufactured batches, a history of each batch of the product, including its distribution. Records include the raw data that is used to generate other records. For electronic records, regulated users should define which data is to be used as raw data. At least, all data on which quality decisions are based should be defined as raw data. (Eudralex Vol 4 Ch 4)

A record consists of information, regardless of the medium, detailing the transactions of business. Records include all books, papers, maps, photographs, machine-readable materials, and other documentary materials, regardless of physical form or characteristics, made or received by an agency of the United States Government under Federal law or in connection with the transaction of public business and preserved or appropriate for preservation by that Agency or its legitimate successor as evidence of the organization, functions, policies, decisions, procedures, operations, or other activities of the Government or because of the value of data in the record. (44 U.S.C. 3301, reference (bb))

record owner: "record owner" means a person or organization who can determine the contents and use of the data collected, stored, processed or disseminated by that party regardless of whether or not the data was acquired from another owner or collected directly from the provider.

records management: The field of management responsible for the efficient and systematic control of the creation, receipt, maintenance, use and disposition of records, including the processes for capturing and maintaining evidence of and information about business activities and transactions in the form of records. (ISO 15489: 2001)

record reliability: A reliable record is one whose contents can be trusted as a full and accurate representation of the transactions, activities, or facts to which they attest and can be depended upon in the course of subsequent transactions or activities. (NARA)

record retention period: Length of time that the electronic record is to be retained, as mandated by the requirement of the record type, based on regulations or documented policies.

record retention schedule: A list of record types with the required storage conditions and defined retention periods. The time (retention) periods are based upon regulatory, legal and tax compliance requirements as well as operational needs and historical value.

repository for electronic records: A direct access device on which the electronic records and metadata are stored.

reengineering: The process of examining and altering an existing system to reconstitute it in a new form. May include reverse engineering (analyzing a system and producing a representation at a higher level of abstraction, such as design from code), restructuring (transforming a system from one representation to another at the same level of abstraction), documentation (analyzing a system and producing user or support documentation), forward engineering (using software products derived from an existing system, together with new requirements, to produce a new system), retargeting (transforming a system to install it on a different target system), and translation (transforming source code from one language to another or from one version of a language to another). (DOD-STD-498)

regression testing: Regression testing is the process of testing changes to computer programs to make sure that the older programming still works with the new changes. Regression testing is a normal part of the program development process and, in larger companies, is done by code testing specialists. Test department coders develop code test scenarios and exercises that will test new units of code after they have been written. These test cases form what becomes the *test bucket.* Before a new version of a software product is released, the old test cases are run against the new version to make sure that all the old capabilities still work. The reason they might not work is because changing or adding new code to a program can easily introduce errors into code that is not intended to be changed.

regulated electronic records: A regulated record maintained in electronic format.

regulated operations: Process/business operations carried out on a regulated agency product that is covered in a predicated rule.

regulated record: A record required to be maintained or submitted by GxP regulations.

regulated user: The regulated good practice entity, that is responsible for the operation of a computerized system and the applications, files and data held therein (PIC/S PI 011-3) See also "user" and "operator."

regulatory requirements: Any part of a law, ordinance, decree, or other regulation that applies to the regulated article.

release: Particular version of a configuration item that is made available for a specific purpose. (ISO 9000-3)

reliability: The ability of a system or component to perform its required functions under stated conditions for a specified period of time. (American National Standards Institute/The Institute of Electrical and Electronics Engineers, Inc. (IEEE) Std 610.12-1990, IEEE Standard Glossary of Software Engineering Terminology)

reliable records: Records that are a full and accurate representations of the transactions, activities or facts to which they attest and can be depended upon in the course of subsequent transactions or activities.

remediate: In the context of this book, the software, hardware and/or procedural changes employed to bring a system into compliance with the applicable GXP rule.

remediation plan: A documented approach on bringing existing computer systems into compliance with the regulation/s.

replacement: The implementation of a new compliant system after the retirement of an existing system.

reports: Document the conduct of particular exercises, projects or investigations, together with results, conclusions and recommendations. (Eudralex Vol 4 Ch 4)

requirement: A condition or capability that must be met or possessed by a system or system component to satisfy a contract, standard, specification, or other formally imposed document. The set of all requirements forms the basis for a subsequent development of the system or system component. (ANSI/IEEE)

re-qualification: Repetition of the qualification process or a specific portion thereof.

retention period: The duration for which records are retained. Retention periods are defined in a retention schedule document. These retention schedules are based on business requirements, country-specific regulatory and legal requirements.

retirement phase: The period in the system life cycle (SLC) in which plans are made and executed to decommission or remove a computer technology from operational use.

retrospective evaluation: Establishing documented evidence that a system does what it purports to do based on an analysis of historical information. The process of evaluating a computer system, that is currently in operation, against standard validation practices and procedures. The evaluation determines the reliability, accuracy, and completeness of a system.

retrospective validation: See "retrospective evaluation."

revision: Different versions of the same document. Can also be used in reference to software, firmware and hardware boards. Implies a fully tested, fully functional and released unit/component/document.

risk: A measure of the extent to which an organization is threatened by a potential circumstance or event, and typically a function of the following:

a. The adverse impacts that would arise if the circumstance or event occurs; and
b. The likelihood of occurrence. Likelihood is influenced by the ease of exploit(s) required and the frequency with which an exploit or like-objects are being attacked at present. (K. Dempsey, P. Eavy and G. Moore, "Automation Support for Security Control Assessments Volume 1: Overview," Draft NISTIR 8011, February 2016.)

risk assessment: A comprehensive evaluation of the risk and its associated impact.

risk management: The tasks and plans that help avoid risk and helps minimize damage.

review: A process or meeting during which a software product is presented to project personnel, managers, users, customers, user representatives, or other interested parties for comment or approval. (IEEE)

site acceptance test (SAT): Inspection and/or dynamic testing of the systems, or major system components, to support the qualification of an equipment system conducted and documented at the manufacturing site.

security controls: The management, operational, and technical controls (i.e., safeguards or countermeasures) prescribed for an information system to protect the confidentiality, integrity, and availability of the system and its information.

self-inspection: An audit carried out by people from within the organization to ensure compliance with GMP and regulatory requirements.

segregation of duties: A process that divides roles and responsibilities so that a single individual cannot subvert a critical process.

service provider: An organization supplying services to one or more internal or external customers. (ITIL Service Design, 2011 Edition)

shall: Used to express a provision that is binding, per regulatory requirement. Statements that use "shall" can be traced to regulatory requirements and must be followed to comply with such requirements.

should: Used to express a non-mandatory provision. Statements that use "should" are best practices, recommended activities, or options to perform activities, to be considered in order to achieve quality project results. Other methods may be used if it can be demonstrated that they are equivalent.

signature, handwritten: The scripted name or legal mark of an individual handwritten by that individual and executed or adopted with the present intention to authenticate a writing in a permanent form. (21 CFR 11.3(8))

site acceptance test: An acceptance test at the customer's site, usually involving the customer. (IEEE)

software developer: Person or organization that designs software and writes programs. Software development includes the design of the user interface and the program architecture as well as programming the source code. (TechWeb Network, http://www.techweb.com/encyclopedia/)

software development standards: Written policies or procedures that describe practices that a programmer or software developer should follow in creating, debugging, and verifying software.

software item: Identifiable part of a software product. (ISO 9000-3)

software product: Set of computer programs, procedures, and possibly associated documentation and data. (ISO 9000-3)

source code: The human readable version of the list of instructions (programs) that enable a computer to perform a task.

source data: All of the information in original records, and certified copies of original records, of clinical findings, observations, or other activities in a clinical trial that are necessary for the reconstruction and evaluation of the trial. Source data is contained in source documents (original records or certified copies). (Source: EMA/INS/GCP/454280/2010 GCP Inspectors Working Group (GCP IWG). Reflection paper on expectations for electronic source data and data transcribed to electronic data collection)

All of the information found in original records, and in certified copies of the original records, of 120 clinical findings, observations, or other activities (in a clinical investigation) used for the 121 re-construction and evaluation of the trial. Source data is contained in source documents 122 (original records or certified copies). (Source: FDA, Electronic Source Data in Clinical Investigations, September 2013)

specification: A document that specifies, in a complete, precise, verifiable manner, the requirements, design, behavior, or other characteristics of a system or component, and often, the procedures for determining whether these provisions have been satisfied. (IEEE)

static analysis: (1) Analysis of a program that is performed without executing the program. (NBS) (2) The process of evaluating a system or component based on its form, structure, content, or documentation. (IEEE)

standard instrument software: These are driven by non user-programmable firmware. They are configurable. (GAMP)

standard operation procedures: See "procedural controls."

standard software packages: A complete and documented set of programs supplied to several users for a generic application or function. (ISO/IEC 2382-20:1990)

subject matter experts: Individuals with specific expertise and responsibility in a particular area or field. (ASTM, E 2500–07 Standard Guide for Specification, Design, and Verification of Pharmaceutical and Biopharmaceutical Manufacturing Systems and Equipment)

supplier: An organization that enters into a contract with the acquirer for the supply of a system, software product or software service under the terms of the contract. (ISO 12207:199[5]4)

system: (1) People, machines, and methods organized to accomplish a set of specific functions (ANSI). (2) A composite, at any level of complexity, of personnel, procedures, materials, tools, equipment, facilities, and software. The elements of this composite entity are used together in the intended operational or support environment to perform a given task or achieve a specific purpose, support, or mission requirement (DOD). (3) A group of related objects designed to perform or control a set of specified actions.

system backup: The storage of data and programs on separate media, stored separately from the originating system.

system documentation: The collection of documents that describe the requirements, capabilities, limitations, design, operation, and maintenance of an information processing system. See: "Specification," "Test documentation," in the user's guide. (ISO)

system integrity: The quality that a system has when it performs its intended function in an unimpaired manner, free from unauthorized manipulation. (NIST SP 800-33)

system life cycle: All phases in the life of the system from initial requirements until retirement; including design, specification, programming, testing, installation, operation, and maintenance. (EMA Annex 11)

system owner: The person responsible for the availability, and maintenance of a computerized system and for the security of the data residing on that system. (EMA Annex 11)

system retirement: The removal of a system from operational usage. The system may be replaced by another system or may be removed without being replaced.

system software: See "operating system."

system specification: In this book, system specification corresponds to requirements, functional and/or design specifications. Refer to "specification."

system test: The process of testing an integrated hardware and software system to verify that the system meets its specified requirements.

technological controls: Are program enforcing compliance rules.

templates: Guidelines that outline the basic information for a specific set of equipment. (JETT)

testing: Examining the behavior of a program by executing the program on sample data sets.

test non-conformance: A non-conformance occurs when the actual test result does not equal the expected result or an unexpected event (such as a loss of power) is encountered.

test report: Document that presents test results and other information relevant to a test. (ISO/IEC Guide 2:2004)

test script: A detailed set of instructions for the execution of the test. This typically includes the following:

- Specific identification of the test
- Prerequisites or dependencies
- Test objectives
- Test steps or actions
- Requirements or instructions for capturing data (e.g., screen prints, report printing)
- Pass/fail criteria for the entire script

- Instructions to follow in the event that a non-conformance is encountered
- Test execution date
- Person(s) executing the test
- Review date
- Person reviewing the test results

For each step of the test script, the item tested, the input to that step, and the expected result are indicated prior to execution of the test. The actual results obtained during the steps of the test are recorded on or attached to the test script. Test scripts and results may be managed through computer-based electronic tools. Refer to *Test case* in the *Glossary of Computerized System and Software Development Terminology*, August 1995.

third party: Parties not directly managed by the holder of the manufacturing and/or import authorization.

time-stamp: A record mathematically linking a piece of data to a time and date.

traceability: (1) The degree to which a relationship can be established between two or more products of the development process, especially products having a predecessor-successor or master-subordinate relationship to one another; for example, the degree to which the requirements and design of a given software component match. (IEEE) (2) The degree to which each element in a software development product establishes its reason for existing; for example, the degree to which each element in a bubble chart references the requirement that it satisfies.

traceability analysis: The tracing of (1) Software requirements specifications to system requirements in concept documentation, (2) Software design descriptions to software requirements specifications and vice versa, and (3) Source code to corresponding design specifications and design specifications to source code. Analyze identified relationships for correctness, consistency, completeness, and accuracy. (IEEE)

traceability matrix: A matrix that records the relationship between two or more products; for example, a matrix that records the relationship between the requirements and the design of a given software component. (IEEE)

training plan: Documentation describing the training required for an individual based on his or her job title or description.

training record: Documentation (electronic or paper) of the training received by an individual that includes, but is not limited to, the individual's name or identifier, the type of training received, the date that the training occurred, the trainer's name or identifier, and an indication of the effectiveness of the training (if applicable).

transfer: The act or process of moving records from one location to another.

transient nemory: Memory that must have a constant supply of power or the stored data will be lost.

true copy record: (1) An exact copy of an original record that may be retained in the same or in a different format than the original, for example, a paper copy of a paper record, an electronic scan of a paper record, or a paper record of electronically generated data (MHRA). (2) An accurate reproduction of the original record regardless of the technology used to create the reproduction (for example, printing, scanning, photocopying, microfilm, or microfiche). A true copy of an electronic record must contain the entire record, including all of the associated metadata, audit trails, and signatures, as applicable, to preserve the content and meaning.

trust: In the network security context, "trust" refers to privacy (the data is not viewable by unauthorized people), integrity (the data stays in its true form), non-repudiation (the publisher cannot say that they did not send it), and authentication (the publisher--and recipient--are who they say they are).

trustworthy computer systems: Trustworthy computer systems consists of computer infrastructure, applications, and procedures that.

- Are reasonably suited to performing their intended functions
- Provide a reasonably reliable level of availability, reliability and correct operation
- Are reasonably secure from intrusion and misuse
- Adhere to generally accepted security principles.

trustworthy records: Reliability, authenticity, integrity, and usability are the characteristics used to describe trustworthy records from a record management perspective. (NARA)

unplanned (emergency) change: An unanticipated necessary change to a validated system requiring rapid implementation.

usable records: Records that can be located, retrieved, presented and interpreted.

user: The company or group responsible for the operation of a system (GAMP) (see also "regulated user"). The GxP customer, or user organisation, who is contracting a supplier to provide a product. In the context of this document it is, therefore, not intended to apply only to individuals who use the system, and is synonymous with "customer." (EMA Annex 11)

user backup/alternative procedures: Procedures that describes the steps to be taken for the continued recording and control of the raw data in the event of a computer system interruption or failure.

unit: A separately testable element specified in the design of a computer software element. Synonymous with component, or module. (IEEE)

unit test: Test of a module for typographic, syntactic, and logical errors, for correct implementation of its design, and for satisfaction with its requirements.

user ID: A sequence of characters that is recognized by the computer and that uniquely identifies one person. The UserID is the first form of identification. A "UserID" is also known as a "PIN" or identification code.

users: People or processes accessing a computer system either by direct connections (i.e., via terminals) or indirect connections (i.e., preparing input data or receiving output that is not reviewed for content or classification by a responsible individual).

validated: Indicates a status that designates that a system or software complies with applicable GMP requirements.

validation: Action of proving, in accordance with the principles of good manufacturing practice, that any procedure, process, equipment, material, activity or system actually leads to the expected results (see also "qualification"). (PIC/S)

validation coordinator: A person or designee responsible for coordinating the validation activities for a specific project or task.

validation plan: A multidisciplinary strategy from which each phase of a validation process is planned, implemented, and documented to ensure that a facility, process, equipment, or system does what it is designed to do. May also be known as a system or software quality plan.

validation protocol: A written plan stating how validation will be conducted, including test parameters, product characteristics, production equipment, and decision points on what constitutes acceptable test results. (FDA)

validation summary report: Documents confirming that the entire project's planned activities have been completed. On acceptance of the validation summary report, the user releases the system for use, possibly with a requirement that continued monitoring should take place for a certain time. (GAMP)

verification: (1) The process of determining whether or not the products of a given phase of the SLC fulfil the requirements established during the previous phase. (2) A systematic approach, verifying that manufacturing systems, acting singly or in combination, are fit for their intended use, have been properly installed, and are operating correctly. This is an umbrella term that encompasses all types of approaches to ensuring that systems are fit for use, such as qualification, commissioning, verification, system validation, or other (ASTM 5200). (3) Confirmation by examination and the provision of objective evidence that specified requirements have been fulfilled (FDA Medical Devices). (4) In design and development, verification concerns the process of examining the results of a given activity to determine conformity with the stated requirement for that activity.

verification (validation) of data: The procedures carried out to ensure that the data contained in the final report match original observations. These procedures may apply to raw data, data in case-report forms (in hard copy or electronic form), computer printouts and statistical analysis and tables. (WHO)

walk-through: A static analysis technique in which a designer or programmer leads members of the development team and other interested parties through a software product, and the participants ask questions and make comments about possible errors, violation of development standards, and other problems. (IEEE)

warehouse: A facility or location where things are stored.

will: This word denotes a declaration of purpose or intent by one party, not a requirement.

work products: The intended result of activities or processes. (PDA)

worst case: A set of conditions encompassing upper and lower processing limits and circumstances, including those within standard operating procedures, that pose the greatest chance of process or product failure when compared to ideal conditions. Such conditions do not necessarily induce product or process failure. (FDA)

written: In the context of electronic records the term "written" means "recorded, or documented on media, paper, electronic or other substrate" from which data may be rendered in a human readable form. (EMA GMP Chapter 4, 2011)

Appendix II: Abbreviations and/or Acronyms

ABA	American Bar Association
ADP	Automated Data Processing
AKA	Also Known As
ANDAs	Abbreviated New Drug Applications
ANSI	American National Standard Institute
API	Active Pharmaceutical Ingredients
ASEAN	Association of Southeast Asian Nations
ASTM	American Society for Testing and Materials
CA	Certification Authority
CAPA	Corrective and Preventive Actions
CEFIC	Conseil Européen des Fédérations de l'Industrie Chimique
CFDA	China Food & Drug Administration
CFR	Code of Federal Regulation
cGMP	current Good Manufacturing Practices
CMC	Chemistry, Manufacturing, and Controls
CPG	FDA Compliance Policy Guide
CRC	Cyclic Redundancy Check
CRL	Certificate Revocation List
CROs	Contract Research Organizations
CSV	Computer Systems Validation
DCS	Distributed Control System
DES	Data Encryption Standard
DMR	Device Master Record
DQ	Design Qualification
DSA	Digital Signature Algorithm
DSHEA	Dietary Supplement Health and Education Act

DTS	Digital Timestamping Service
EC	European Commission
EDMS	Electronic Document Management System
EEA	European Economic Area
EEC	European Economic Community
EFS	Encrypting File System
EMA	European Medicines Agency
EMEA	European Medicines Agency
ERP	Enterprise Resource Planning
EU	European Union
EVM	Earned Value Management
FAT	Factory Acceptance Test
FD&C Act	US Food Drug and Cosmetic Act
FDA	Food and Drug Administration
FR	US Federal Register
FTP	File Transfer Protocol
GAMP	Good Automated Manufacturing Practices
GCP	Good Clinical Practices
GEIP	Good E-records Integrity Practices
GLP	Good Laboratory Practices
GMPs	United States Good Manufacturing Practices
GXP	A global abbreviation intended to cover GMP, GCP, GLP, and other regulated applications in context GXP can refer to one specific set of practices or to any combination of the three.
HMA	Heads of Medicines Agencies
HMI	Human Machine Interface
IaaS	Infrastructure as a Service
ICH	International Conference for Harmonization of Technical Requirements for Registration of Pharmaceuticals for Human Use
ICS	Industrial Control System
I/Os	Inputs and outputs
IEC	International Electrotechnical Commission
IEEE	Institute of Electrical & Electronic Engineers
IIS	Internet Information Services
IMDRF	International Medical Device Regulators Forum
ISA	International Society of Automation
ISO	International Organization for Standardization
ISPE	International Society for Pharmaceutical Engineering

IT Information Technologies
ITIL IT Infrastructure Library
KMS Key Management Service
LAN Local Area Network
LIMS Laboratory Information Management System
MA Marketing Authorization
MES Manufacturing Execution System
MHRA Medicines and Healthcare Products Regulatory Agency (United Kingdom medicines and medical devices regulatory agency)
MRA Mutual Recognition Agreements
MTBF Mean Time Between Failures
MTTR Mean Time to Repair or Mean Time To Recovery
NARA National Archives and Records Administration
NBS National Bureau of Standards
NDAs New Drug Applications
NEMA National Electrical Manufacturers Association
NIST National Institute of Standards and Technology
NTP Network Time Protocol
OECD Organization for Economic Co-operation and Development
OLAs Operational Level Agreements
OMCL Official Medicines Control Laboratories
OSHA US Occupational Safety & Health Administration
OTS Off-the-Shelf
P&ID Process and Instrumentation Drawings
PaaS Platform as a Service
PAI PreApproval Inspections
PAT Process Analytical Tools
PDA Parenteral Drug Association
PIC/S Pharmaceutical Inspection Co-Operation Scheme http://www.picscheme.org/
PIN Personal Identification Number
PKCS Public-Key Cryptography Standards
PKI Public Key Infrastructure
PLC Programmable Logic Controller
PQS Pharmaceutical Quality System
QA Quality Assurance
QbD Quality by Design
QC Quality Control
QMS Quality Management System

QP	Qualified Person
R&D	Research and Development
RFP	Request for Proposal
RTU	Remote Terminal Unit
SaaS	Software as a Service
SAP	Systems, Applications and Products
SAS	The Statistical Analysis System licensed by the SAS Institute, Inc.
SAT	Site Acceptance Test
SCADA	Supervisory Control and Data Acquisition
SDLC	Software Development Life Cycle
SHA-1	Secure Hash Algorithm 1
SLA	Service-Level Agreement
SLC	System Life Cycle
SME	Subject Matter Experts
SOPs	Standard Operating Procedures
SPC	Statistical Process Control
SQA	Software Quality Assurance
SQE	Software Quality Engineering
SSA	US Social Security Administration
SSL	Secure Sockets Layer
SWEBOK	Software Engineering Body of Knowledge
TGA	Therapeutic Goods Administration
TLS	Transport Layer Security
UCs	Underpinning Contracts
UK	United Kingdom
UPS	Uninterruptable Power Supply
US	United States
US FDA	United States Food and Drugs Administration
VPN	Virtual Privates Network
WAN	Wide Area Network
WBS	Work Breakdown Structure
WHO	World Health Organization

Appendix III: Regulatory Cross Match

	References				
	Old Annex 11	*211*	*820*	*11*	*Others/Guidelines*
Principle					GAMP 5 –Management Appendix M3
a. This annex applies to all forms of computerized systems used as part of GMP-regulated activities. A computerized system is a set of software and hardware components that together fulfill certain functionalities.		211.68[1]	820.70(i)	11.2(b)	EU Directives 2003/94/EC and 91/412/EECPIC/S PI 011-3 ISO 13485 7.5.2 Article 1 draft Annex 2 CFDA GMP
b. The application should be validated; the IT infrastructure should be qualified.	11-3	211.68	820.70(i) 820.30(g) 820.170	11.10(a)	Eudralex Volume IV, Glossary PIC/S PI 011-3 ICH Q7A Good Manufacturing Practice Guidance for Active Pharmaceutical Ingredients, Sections 5.40 and 5.41 WHO—Technical Report Series, No. 937, 2006. Annex 4. Appendix 5, Section 7.1 (Hardware) ISO 13485 7.5.2; 7.3.6; 7.2; 7.2.1; 7.2.2 Article 10 draft Annex 2 CFDA GMP GAMP GPG: IT Infrastructure Control and Compliance, 2005 Draft OECD Guidance Document, Sections 1.1 and 1.4 ICH E6 Guideline for GCP (June 1996), Section 5.5.3(a) ANMAT (Argentina) 5.21 US FDA General Principles of Software Validation, Section 5.2.6

c. Where a computerised system replaces a manual operation, there should be no resultant decrease in product quality, process control, or quality assurance. There should be no increase in the overall risk of the process.	Principle				PIC/S PI 011-3 US FDA CPG 7348.810—Sponsors, CROs, and Monitors Brazilian GMPs Title VII Art 570 Thailandia CSV GMPs Article 2 draft Annex 2 CFDA GMP
General					
1. Risk Management Risk management should be applied throughout the life cycle of the computerized system, taking into account patient safety, *data integrity*, and product quality. As part of a risk management system, decisions on the extent of validation and *data integrity controls* should be based on a justified and documented risk assessment of the computerized system.		211.68(b)[2]	820.30(g)		812.66[3] ICH Q9 Quality Risk Management ICH Q7 5.40 NIST, Risk Management Guide for Information Technology Systems, Special Publication 800- 30 GHTF, Implementation of risk management principles and activities within a Quality Management System ISO 14971:2007, Medical devices—Application of risk management to medical devices GAMP Forum, Risk Assessment for Use of Automated Systems Supporting Manufacturing Process—Risk to Record, Pharmaceutical Engineering, Nov/Dec 2002 GAMP/ISPE, Risk Assessment for Use of Automated Systems Supporting Manufacturing Process—Functional Risk, Pharmaceutical Engineering, May/Jun 2003 EU Annex 20 US FDA Guidance for the Content of Pre Market Submission for Software Contained in Medical Devices, May 2005 Pressman, Roger S., Software Engineering—A Practitioner's Approach, McGraw-Hill GAMP 5 –Management Appendices M3 and M4; Operational Appendices O2, O6, O8, O9. Brazilian GMPs Title VII Art 572. ISO 13485 7.3.6

(Continued)

	References				
	Old Annex 11	*211*	*820*	*11*	*Others/Guidelines*
					WHO, Technical Report Series No. 281, 2013 Health Canada API, C.02.05, Interpretation #12 Articles 3. 6, 12 draft Annex 2 CFDA GMP Draft OECD Guidance Document, Section 1.2 ANMAT (Argentina) 5.21 US FDA General Principles of Software Validation Section 4.8 PIC/S Guidance PI 011-3, Sections 4.5 and 4.6
2. Personnel There should be close cooperation between all relevant personnel such as process owner, system owner, qualified persons, and IT. All personnel should have appropriate qualifications, level of access, and defined responsibilities to carry out their assigned duties.	11-1	Sub Part B	820.20(b) (1) and (2) 820.25	11.10(i)	EudraLex, The Rule Governing Medicinal Products in the European Union, Volume 4, EU Guidelines for Good Manufacturing Practices for Medicinal Products for Human and Veterinary Use, Part 1, Chapter 2—Personnel, February 2014 21 CFR 110(c) 21 CFR 606.160(b)(5)(v) ICH E6 GCP 4.1; 4.2.3, 4.2.4; 5.4.1; 5.5.1; 5.6.1 21 CFR Part 312.53(a) and .53(d). 21 CFR 58.29 WHO—Technical Report Series, No. 937, 2006. Annex 4, Section 13 GAMP 5 6.2.3.1, 6.2.3.3, 6.2.3.3. 6.2.3.5 and Operational Appendix O12 Brazilian GMPs Title VII Art 571. ISO 13485 5.5; 5.5.1; 5.5.3; 6.2; 6.2.1; 6.2.2 Japan CSV Guideline (Guideline on Management of Computerized Systems for Marketing Authorization Holder and Manufacturing of Drugs and Quasi-drugs, October 2010), Section 6.8

					Thailandia CSV GMPs, Clause 510. Health Canada API, C.02.006 Draft OECD Guidance Document, Section 1.3 Brazil API (RDC Resolution #69 Chapter VI Section VI Art. 258))
3. Suppliers and Service Providers 3.1 When third parties (e.g., suppliers, service providers) are used, for example, to provide, install, configure, integrate, validate, maintain (e.g., via remote access), modify, or retain a computerized system or related service or for data processing, formal agreements must exist between the manufacturer and the third parties, and these agreements should include clear statements of the responsibilities of the third party. IT-departments should be considered analogous. 3.2 The competence and reliability of a supplier are key factors when selecting a product or service provider. The need for an audit should be based on a risk assessment. 3.3 Documentation supplied with commercial off-the-shelf products should be reviewed by regulated users to check that user requirements are fulfilled. 3.4 Quality system and audit information relating to suppliers or developers of software and implemented systems should be made available to inspectors on request. 3.5 The supplier should be assessed appropriately.	11-18	Sub Part B 211.34	820.20(b) (1) and (2) 820.50		EudraLex, The Rules Governing Medicinal Products in the European Union Volume 4, Good Manufacturing Practice, Medicinal Products for Human and Veterinary Use, Chapter 7: Outsourced Activities, January 2013 21 CFR 110(c) ICH Q7 Good Manufacturing Practice Guidance for Active Pharmaceutical Ingredients ICH Q10 Section 2.7 Management of Outsourced Activities and Purchased Materials ICH E6 Section 5.2.1. WHO—Technical Report Series, No. 937, 2006. Annex 4. Appendix 5, Section 6.2 GAMP 5 Section 6.1.4 GAMP 5 –Management Appendices M2 and M6 Brazilian GMPs Title VII Art 589. ISO 13485 5.5; 5.5.1; 5.5.3; 6.2; 6.2.1; 6.2.2' 7.4; 7.4.1 China GMPs, Section 7 Thailandia CSV GMPs, Clause 527 PDA, Technical Report No. 32 Auditing of Supplier Providing Computer Products and Services for Regulated Pharmaceutical Operations, *PDA Journal of Pharmaceutical Science and Technology*, Sep/Oct 2004, Release 2.0, Vol 58 No 5

(*Continued*)

	References				
	Old Annex 11	*211*	*820*	*11*	*Others/Guidelines*
					CEFIC CSV Guide, Section 7.4.6. Article 4 draft Annex 2 CFDA GMP Draft OECD Guidance Document, Sections 1.5 and 1.6. PIC/S Guidance PI 011-3 Sections 5.1, 5.2, 11
Project Phase					
4. Validation 4.1 The validation documentation and reports should cover the relevant steps of the life cycle. Manufacturers should be able to justify their standards, protocols, acceptance criteria, procedures, and records based on their risk assessment. 4.2 Validation documentation should include change control records (if applicable) and reports on any deviations observed during the validation process. 4.3 An up-to-date listing of all relevant systems and their GMP functionality (inventory) should be available. For critical systems, an up-to-date system description detailing the physical and logical arrangements, data flows, and interfaces with other systems or processes, any hardware and software prerequisites, and security measures should be available.	11-2; 11-4; 11-5; 11-7	211.68 211.100(a) and (b)	820.3(z) 803.17 820.40 820.170 820.30(g) 820.70(g) 820.70(i) 820.70(i) 820.30(c) 820.3(z) and (aa) 820.30(f) and (g) 820.30 820.50	11.10(a); 11.10(k); 11.10(h).	Article 9 Section 2, Commission Directives 2003/94/EC ISO 90003:2004, Sections 7.3.2; 7.3.3; 7.3.4; 7.3.5; 7.3.6.2a; 7.3.6.2.b; 7.3.6.2.c; 7.5.1.5; 7.5.1.6; 7.3.6.2d; 7.3.7; 7.5.3.2 ISO-27000, Sections 12.1, 12.2 Medicines and Healthcare products Regulatory Agency (MHRA) (UK). IEEE PIC/S PI 011-3 Sections 6.3, 7, 9, 10, 13.2, 14.3, 23.8, 23.10 21 CFR 606.160(b)(5)(ii) and 606.100(b)(15) ICH Q7 Good Manufacturing Practice Guidance for Active Pharmaceutical Ingredients, Sections 5.41, 12.2 ICH Q9 Quality Risk Management. 11-1 ICH E6 GCP 2.10, 2.11, 5.5.3(a) and (b), 5.5.4

4.4 User requirements specifications should describe the required functions of the computerised system and be based on documented risk assessment and GMP impact. User requirements should be traceable throughout the life cycle.[4] 4.5 The regulated user should take all reasonable steps to ensure that the system has been developed in accordance with an appropriate quality management system. The supplier should be assessed appropriately. 4.6 For the validation of bespoke or customized computerized systems, there should be a process in place that ensures the formal assessment and reporting of quality and performance measures for all the life-cycle stages of the system and formal assessment and reporting of quality and performance measures for all life-cycle stages of the system. 4.7 Evidence of appropriate test methods[5] and test scenarios should be demonstrated. *in particular, system (process) parameter limits, data limits, and error handling should be considered.*[6] Automated testing tools and test environments should have documented assessments for their adequacy. 4.8 *If data are transferred to another data format or system, validation should include checks that the data are not altered in value and/or meaning during this migration process.*[7]					21 CFR 58.61; 63(a) and (c); 58.81(c) and (d); 58.33 21 CFR 59.190 Blood Establishment Computer System Validation in the User's Facility, April 2013 US FDA General Principles of SoftwareValidation WHO—Technical Report Series, No. 937, 2006. Annex 4. Appendix 5 GAMP 5 Sections 4.2.1, 4.2.3, 4.2.4, 5.2.3, 5.2.5, 6.1.5, 6.1.6, 6.2.6, 6.2.8, 6.2.9, 6.2.10 GAMP 5 Development Appendices: D1–D7; Management Appendices M1–M10; Operational Appendix O1 21 CFR 1271.160(d) 21 CFR 803.17; 21 CFR 803.18 EU Annex 15 Brazilian GMPs Title VII Art 573, 574, 575, 576, 578 Brazilian Medical Devices (RDC No 16) Sections 1.2.4, 4.1.8, 4.2.1.1, 5.4.6, 5.5.2 and 5.5.3, 5.6 ISO 13485 2.3; 7.2; 7.2.1; 7.2.2; 7.5.1.2.2; 7.3.6; 6.3; 7.5.2 ISO/TR 14969:2004 7.5.2 ISO 27000 Section 7.1 Japan CSV Guideline (Guideline on Management of Computerized Systems for Marketing Authorization Holder and Manufacturing of Drugs and Quasi- drugs, October 2010), Sections 4, 5 and 9

(*Continued*)

	References				
	Old Annex 11	*211*	*820*	*11*	*Others/Guidelines*
					China GMPs Article 109 Thailandia CSV GMPs, Clauses 511, 512, 513, 514, 516 Health Canada API, C.02.05 Interpretation #12; #13; #14; 17. C.02.015 Interpretation #3; #13.5 Articles 5, 7, 8, 9, 11, 13 draft Annex 2 CFDA GMP Draft OECD Guidance Document, Section 1.1 Item 3, Sections 2.1, 2.2, 2.3, 2.4, 2.5, 2.6, 2.7. 2.8, 2.9 ANMAT (Argentina) 5.25 US FDA General Principles of Software Validation 4.1, 4.5, 5.1, 5.2, 5.2.1, 5.2.2, 5.2.3, 5.2.4, 5.2.5, 5.2.6, 23.10 Brazil API (RDC Resolution #69 Chapter VI Section VI) WHO Technical Report 986 Annex 2 (Section 15.9) ITIL Service Design (Section 5.2.8)
Operational Phase					GAMP 5 –Operational Appendix O12 Draft OECD Guidance, Section 3 Item 85 ANMAT (Argentina) 5.22 and 5.23
5. Data *Computerized systems exchanging data electronically with other systems should include appropriate built-in checks for the correct and secure entry and processing of data, in order to minimize risks.*[8]	11-6	211.68(b) 211.194(d)	806.1 820.25 820.70(a) 820.180 820.184	11.10(a) 11.10(b) 11.10(e) 11.10(f) 11.10(g) 11.10(h) 11.30	US FDA 425.400; 803.1; 803.10; 803.14; 806.10; 806.30; 58.15; 58.33; 58.35; 59.190 EudraLex—Volume 4 Good manufacturing practice (GMP) Guidelines, Part I—Basic Requirements for Medicinal Products, Chapter 4—Documentation GAMP 5 –Operational Appendix O9

					Brazilian GMPs Title VII Art 577. ISO 134854 6.2; 6.2.1; 6.2.2 7.5; 7.5.1; 7.5.1.1; 4.2.4; 7.5.1 Thailandia CSV GMPs, Clause 515 Draft OECD Guidance, Section 3.1 ICH E6 Section 2.10 ICH Q7 Section 5.45 ITIL, Service Design (Chapter 5.2.10)
6. Accuracy Checks For critical data[9] entered manually, there should be an additional check on the accuracy of the data. This check may be done by a second operator or by validated electronic means. The criticality and the potential consequences of erroneous or incorrectly entered data to a system should be covered by risk management.[10]	11-9	211.68(c)	820.25 820.70	11.10(f)	The APV Guideline "Computerized Systems" based on Annex 11 of the EU-GMP Guideline EudraLex—Volume 4 Good manufacturing practice (GMP) Guidelines, Part I—Basic Requirements for Medicinal Products, Chapter 4—Documentation PIC/S PI 011-3 EU Annex 11-1 WHO—Technical Report Series, No. 937, 2006. Annex 4. Appendix 5, Section 4.5 Brazilian GMPs Title VII Art 577, 580 ISO 13485 6.2; 6.2.1; 6.2.2; 7.5 Thailandia CSV GMPs, Clause 518 Health Canada API, C.02.015 Interpretation #18 Article 15 draft Annex 2 CFDA GMP Draft OECD Guidance, Section 3.2 ANMAT (Argentina) 5.26 and 5.30 Brazil API (RDC Resolution #69 Chapter VI Section VI Article 265) ITIL, Service Design (Chapter 5.2.10)

(*Continued*)

	References				
	Old Annex 11	*211*	*820*	*11*	*Others/Guidelines*
7. Data Storage 7.1 Data should be secured against damage by both physical and electronic means. Stored data should be checked for accessibility, readability, and accuracy. Access to data should be ensured throughout the retention period. 7.2 Regular backups of all relevant data should be done. Integrity and accuracy of backup data and the ability to restore the data should be checked during validation and monitored periodically.[11]	11-13 11-14	211.68(b)	803.1 820.20 820.40 820.180 806.1	11.10(c) 11.10(d) 11.10(e) 11.10(g) 11.10(h) 11.30	812.38 Chapter II Article 9 Section 2, Commission Directives 2003/94/EC PIC/S PI 011-3 EudraLex—Volume 4 Good manufacturing practice (GMP) Guidelines, Part I—Basic Requirements for Medicinal Products, Chapter 4—Documentation ICH E6 GCP 5.5.3(d) and (f) ICH Q7 5.48 21 CFR 58.33; .190(d); .35; .195 Specific records retention requirements are found in applicable predicate rule, for example, 21 CFR 211.180(c), (d), 108.25(g), and 108.35(h), and 58.195 812.140(a) and (b). WHO—Technical Report Series, No. 937, 2006. Annex 4. Appendix 5, Sections 5 and 7.2.2 21 CFR 123.9(f) GAMP Appendix O9 and O11Brazilian GMPs Title VII Art 585. ISO 13485 6.2; 6.2.1; 6.2.2; 7.5 Japan CSV Guideline (Guideline on Management of Computerized Systems for Marketing Authorization Holder and Manufacturing of Drugs and Quasi-drugs, October 2010), Section 6.3 Japan's Pharmaceutical and Food Safety Bureau "Using electromagnetic records and electronic signatures for application for approval or licensing of drugs," Section 3, April 2005

					Thailandia CSV GMPs, Clause 517, 522, 523 Health Canada API, C.02.05, Interpretation #16 Article 19 draft Annex 2 CFDA GMP. Draft OECD Guidance, Section 3.3 GAMP 5, Section 4.3.6.1 ISO 27000, Section 10.5 Brazil API (RDC Resolution #69 Chapter VI Section VI Article 269) WHO Technical Report 986 Annex 2 (Section 15.9) ITIL, Service Design (Chapter 5.2.11)
8. Printouts 8.1 It should be possible to obtain clear printed copies of electronically stored e-records. 8.2 For records supporting batch release, it should be possible to generate printouts indicating if any part of the e-record has been changed since the original entry.[12]	11-12	211.180(c)	43 FR 31508, July 21, 1978 803.1 803.10 803.14 806.30 820.40 820.180 806.1	11.10(b)	812.150, 58.15 Directive 1999/93/EC of the European Parliament and of the Council of 13 December 1999 on a Community framework for electronic signatures PIC/S PI 011-3 FDA, Guidance for Industry Part 11, Electronic Records; Electronic Signatures — Scope and Application, August 2003 The APV Guideline, "Computerized Systems" based on Annex 11 of the EU-GMP Guideline US FDA CPG Sec. 130.400 Use of Microfiche and/or Microfilm for Method of Records Retention Brazilian GMPs Title VII Art 583. ISO 13485 4.2.3; 4.2.4 Thailandia CSV GMPs, Clause 521 Draft OECD Guidance Document, Section 3.4

(Continued)

	References				
	Old Annex 11	*211*	*820*	*11*	*Others/Guidelines*
9. Audit Trails Consideration should be given, based on a risk assessment, to building into the system the creation of a record of all GMP- relevant changes and deletions (a system-generated "audit trail"). The reason for any changes to or deletions of GMP-relevant data should be documented. Audit trails need to be available and convertible to a generally intelligible form and regularly reviewed.[13] Note: In addition to the system-generated audit trail, some implementations included documentation that allow reconstruction of the course of events. Implicitly, this approach does not require a computer system–generated audit trail.	11-10		803.18 820.40	11.10(e) 11.10(k)(2) 11.50(a)(2)	1978 US CGMP rev. Comment paragraph 186 FDA, Guidance for Industry Part 11, Electronic Records; Electronic Signatures—Scope and Application, August 2003 The APV Guideline "Computerized Systems" based on Annex 11 of the EU-GMP Guideline PIC/S PI 011-3 ICH Q7 Good Manufacturing Practice Guidance for Active Pharmaceutical Ingredients. ICH E6 GCP 4.9.3; 5.5.3(c); 5.5.4 21 CFR 58.130(d). Glossary of the Note for Guidance on Good Clinical Practice (CPMP/ICH/135/95) Brazilian GMPs Title VII Art 581 ISO 13485 4.2.3 Thailandia CSV GMPs, Clause 519 Health Canada API, C.02.05, Interpretation #15 Draft OECD Guidance Document, Section 3.5 WHO Technical Report 986 Annex 2 (Section 15.9)
10. Change and Configuration Management Any changes to a computerized system including system configurations should only be made in a controlled manner in accordance with a defined procedure.	11-11	211.68	820.30(i) 820.70(i) 820.40	11.10(d) 11.10(e)	SO 90003, 2004, Sections 7.3.7 and 7.5.3.2 PIC/S PI 011-3 The APV Guideline "Computerized Systems" based on Annex 11 of the EU-GMP Guideline WHO—Technical Report Series, No. 937, 2006. Annex 4. Section 12 Pressman, Roger S., *Software Engineering—A Practitioner's Approach*, McGraw-Hill GAMP 5 –Management Appendix M3; GAMP 5 –Operational Appendices O6 and O7

					GAMP 5 Section 4.3.4.1. Brazilian GMPs Title VII Art 582. ISO 13485 7.3.7; 7.5.2; 4.2.3 Japan CSV Guideline (Guideline on Management of Computerized Systems for Marketing Authorization Holder and Manufacturing of Drugs and Quasi-drugs, October 2010), Section 6.6 China GMP, Articles 240–246. Thailandia CSV GMPs, Clause 520 Health Canada API, C.02.015 Interpretation #20 Article 17 draft Annex 2 CFDA GMP Draft OECD Guidance Document, Sections 1.7 and 3.6 ANMAT (Argentina) 5.28 ICH E6 Section 5.5.4 ICH Q7 Section 5.47 General Principles of Software Validation Sections 4.7 and 5.2.7
11. Periodic Evaluation Computerized systems should be evaluated periodically to confirm that they remain in a valid state and are compliant with GMP. Such evaluations should include, where appropriate, the current range of functionality, deviation records, incidents, problems, upgrade history, performance, reliability, security, and validation status report(s).		211.68 211.180(e)	820.20(c)	11.10(k) 11.300(b) and (e)	US FDA CPG 7132a.07, Computerized Drug Processing; Input/Output Checking ICH Q7, 12.60 WHO—Technical Report Series, No. 937, 2006. Annex 4. Appendix 5, Section 1.5 GAMP 5 Section 4.3.5 GAMP 5 –Management Appendix M3; GAMP 5 –Operational Appendices O3 and O8 58.35; 58.190; 58.195 Annex 15 clauses 23 and 45 ISO 13485 5.6; 5.6.1; 5.6.2; 5.6.3; 8.2.2; 8.5; 8.5.1 China GMPs Section 8. Draft OECD Guidance Document, Section 3.7 ITIL, Service Design (Chapter 5.2.13)

(*Continued*)

	References				
	Old Annex 11	*211*	*820*	*11*	*Others/Guidelines*
12. Security 12.1 Physical and/or logical controls should be in place to restrict access to computerized system to authorized persons. Suitable methods of preventing unauthorized entry to the system may include the use of keys, pass cards, personal codes with passwords, biometrics, and restricted access to computer equipment and data storage areas. 12.2 The extent of security controls depends on the criticality of the computerized system. 12.3 The creation, change, and cancellation of access authorizations should be recorded. 12.4 Management systems for data and documents should be designed to record the identity of the operator entering, changing, confirming or deleting data including date and time.[14]	11-8	211.68(b)		11.10(c) 11.10(d) 11.10(e) 11.10(g) 11.300	PIC/S PI 011-3, Sections 19.2; 19.3. ICH E6 GCP 4.1.5; 5.5.3(c), (d) and (e) ICH Q7 Section 5.4. 21 CFR Part 58.51; 58.190(d) WHO—Technical Report Series, No. 937, 2006. Annex 4. Appendix 5 Section 4 GAMP 5, Section 4.3.7.1 GAMP 5 –Management Appendix M9; GAMP 5 –Operational Appendix O11 Brazilian GMPs Title VII Art 579 Japan CSV Guideline (Guideline on Management of Computerized Systems for Marketing Authorization Holder and Manufacturing of Drugs and Quasi-drugs, October 2010), Section 6.4 Thailandia CSV GMPs, Clause 517 Health Canada API, C.02.05, Interpretation #15 Articles 14, 16 draft Annex 2 CFDA GMP Draft OECD Guidance Document, Section 3.8 ANMAT (Argentina) 5.24 ISO-27000, Sections 12.1 and 11.2 Brazil API (RDC Resolution #69 Chapter VI Art. 106 Paragraph 2) WHO Technical Report 986 Annex 2 (Section 15.9) ITIL, Service Design (Chapter 5.2.13)
13. Incident Management All incidents, not only system failures and data errors, should be reported and assessed. The root cause of a critical incident should be identified and should form the basis of corrective and preventive actions.	11-17	211.100(b)	820.100		ICH Q7A Good Manufacturing Practice Guidance for Active Pharmaceutical Ingredients, Section 5.46 ICH E6, Section 5.1.3 GAMP 5—Operational Appendices O4. O5, and O7

					Brazilian GMPs Title VII Art 588. ISO 13485 8.5; 8.5.1; 8.5.2; 8.5.3 Japan CSV Guideline (Guideline on Management of Computerized Systems for Marketing Authorization Holder and Manufacturing of Drugs and Quasi-drugs, October 2010), Sections 6.7 and 7.2 China GMPs, Sections 5 and 6 Thailandia CSV GMPs, Clause 526 Health Canada API, C.02.015 Interpretation #19 Articles 20 and 21 draft Annex 2 CFDA GMP Draft OECD Guidance Document, Section 3.9 ANMAT (Argentina) 5.27 US FDA General Principles of Software Validation, Section 5.2.7
14. Electronic Signature Electronic records may be signed electronically. Electronic signatures are expected to • Have the same impact as hand written signatures within the he boundaries of the company[15] • Be permanently linked to their respective record • Include the time and date that they were applied				11.3(b)(7) 11.10(e) 11.50; .70, .100, .200, .300	EU GMP Chapter 4 Principle Annex 11-8.1, 9, 12.4, 17 ICH Q7A Good Manufacturing Practice Guidance for Active Pharmaceutical Ingredients, Section 5.43 Electronic Signatures in Global and National Commerce (E-Sign), a US federal law. (available at: http://thomas.loc.gov/cgi-bin/query/z?c106:S.761:) 21 CFR 58.33; .81; .35; .120; .185 Japan's Pharmaceutical and Food Safety Bureau "Using electromagnetic records and electronic signatures for application for approval or licensing of drugs," Section 4, April 2005 Article 22 draft Annex 2 CFDA GMP Draft OECD Guidance Document, Section 3.10 ICH E6 Sections 2.8, 2.10, 2.11, 4.9.1, 4.9.7, 5.5.1, 5.5.3 (a)–(g), 5.5.4, 5.5.5, 5.5.6, 5.23.4

(Continued)

	References				
	Old Annex 11	*211*	*820*	*11*	*Others/Guidelines*
15. Batch Release When a computerized system is used for recording certification and batch release, the system should allow only qualified persons to certify the release of the batches, and it should clearly identify and record the person releasing or certifying the batches. This should be performed using an electronic signature.	11-19	211.68 211.186 211.192 211.188(b) (11) 211.188(a)		11.70; Sub Part C	21 CFR 211.68 The APV Guideline "Computerized Systems" based on Annex 11 of the EU-GMP Guideline 11-9; 11-14 EC Directive 2001/83 Brazilian GMPs Title VII Art 590 Thailandia CSV GMPs, Clause 528 Article 21 draft Annex 2 CFDA GMP Draft OECD Guidance Document, Section 3.11
16. Business Continuity For the availability of computerized systems supporting critical processes, provisions should be made to ensure the continuity of support for those processes in the event of a system breakdown (e.g., a manual or alternative system). The time required to bring the alternative arrangements into use should be based on risk and be appropriate for a particular system and the business process it supports. These arrangements should be adequately documented and tested.[16]	11-15 11-16				PIC/S PI 011-3 GAMP 5, Sections 4.3.6.2 and 4.3.6.3 GAMP 5 –Operational Appendix O10 Brazilian GMPs Title VII Art 586, 587 Thailandia CSV GMPs, Clause 524, 525 Draft OECD Guidance Document, Section 3.13 ANMAT (Argentina) 5.29 ICH Q7, Section 5.48 Brazil API (RDC Resolution #69 Chapter VI Section VI Articles 271 and 272)
17. Archiving Data may be archived. These data should be checked for accessibility, readability, and integrity. If relevant changes are to be made to the system (e.g., computer equipment or programs), then the ability to retrieve the data should be ensured and tested.[17]		211.68(b)		11.10(c)	Scientific Archivists Group, A Guide to Archiving of Electronic Records, 2014 www.sagroup.org.uk/images/documents/AGuidetoArchivingElectronicRecordsv1.pdf DOD 5015.2-STD, Design Criteria Standard for E-records Management Software Applications. GAMP 5 –Operational Appendix O13

					GAMP GPG: Electronic Data Archiving, 2007 Brazilian GMPs Title VII Art 584 Draft OECD Guidance Document, Section 3.12 Scientific Archivists Group, "A Guide to Archiving of Electronic Records" ITIL, Service Design (Chapter 5.2.13)

1 O. López, "A Historical View of 21 CFR Part 211.68," *Journal of GXP Compliance*, Vol. 15, No. 2, Spring 2011.

2 Federal Register, Vol 60 No. 13, 4087–4091, January 20, 1995.

3 All 21 CFR Part 812 regulations apply equally to both paper records and electronic records. The use of computer systems in clinical investigations does not exempt IDEs from any Part 812 regulatory requirement.

4 O. López, "Requirements Management," *Journal of Validation Technology*, Vol. 17, No. 2, Spring 2011.

5 Test methods—With the black-box test, the test cases are derived solely from the description of the test object, and the inner structure of the object is thus not considered when creating the test plan. With the white-box test, the test cases are derived solely from the structure of the test object. With the source-code review, the source code is checked against the documentation describing the system by one or several professionals. The APV Guideline "Computerized Systems," is based on Annex 11 of the EU-GMP Guideline, April 1996.

6 This sentence is related to the additional checks covered in Accuracy Checks (11-6).

7 Annex 11-4.8 is complemented with 11-7.1.

8 Annex 11-5 is fundamental in erecs integrity and it is related with Annex 11-4.7.

9 The term *critical data* in this context is interpreted as meaning data with high risk to product quality or patient safety. ISPE GAMP COP Annex 11—Interpretation, July/August 2011.

10 Annex 11-6 is another fundamental section related to erecs integrity.

11 Annex 11-7 is another fundamental section related with erecs integrity.

12 Annex 11-8 is another fundamental section related with erecs integrity.

13 Annex 11-9 is another fundamental section related with erecs integrity.

14 Annex 11-12 is another fundamental section related with erecs integrity.

15 The phase "within the boundaries of the company" clarifies that such signatures applied to records maintained by the regulated company are not subject to Directive 1999/93/EC on a company framework for esigs or the 2000/31/EC directive on electronic commerce, or any associated national regulations of EU member states on such topics.

16 Annex 11-16 is another fundamental section related with erecs integrity.

17 Annex 11-17 is another fundamental section related with erecs integrity.

Appendix IV: MHRA GMP Data Integrity Definitions and Guidance for Industry March 2015

Introduction

Data integrity is fundamental in a pharmaceutical quality system, which ensures that medicines are of the required quality. This document provides MHRA guidance on GMP data integrity expectations for the pharmaceutical industry. This guidance is intended to complement existing EU GMP relating to active substances and dosage forms, and should be read in conjunction with national medicines legislation and the GMP standards published in Eudralex volume 4.

The data governance system should be integral to the pharmaceutical quality system described in EU GMP Chapter 1. The effort and resources assigned to data governance should be commensurate with the risk to product quality and should also be balanced with other quality assurance (QA) resource demands. As such, manufacturers and analytical laboratories are not expected to implement a forensic approach to data checking on a routine basis, but instead design and operate a system that provides an acceptable state of control based on the data integrity risk and is fully documented with supporting rationale.

Data integrity requirements apply equally to manual (paper) and electronic data. Manufacturers and analytical laboratories should be aware that reverting from automated/computerized to manual/paper-based systems will not in itself remove the need for data integrity controls. This may also constitute a failure to comply with Article 23 of Directive 2001/83/EC, which requires an authorization holder to take account of scientific and technical progress and enable the medicinal product to be manufactured and checked by means of generally accepted scientific methods.

Throughout this guidance, associated definitions are shown as hyperlinks.

Establishing Data Criticality and Inherent Integrity Risk

In addition to an overarching data governance system, which should include relevant policies and staff training in the importance of data integrity, consideration should be given to the organizational (e.g., procedures) and technical (e.g., computer system access) controls applied to different areas of the quality system. The degree of effort and resources applied to the organizational and technical control of data life cycle elements should be commensurate with their criticality in terms of impact to product quality attributes.

Data may be generated by (i) a paper-based record of a manual observation, or (ii) in terms of equipment, a spectrum of simple machines through to complex highly configurable computerized systems. The inherent risks to data integrity may differ depending on the degree to which data (or the system generating or using the data) can be configured, and therefore potentially manipulated (see Figure A4.1).

With reference to Figure A4.1, simple systems (such as pH meters and balances) may only require calibration, whereas complex systems require validation for intended purpose. Validation effort increases from left to right

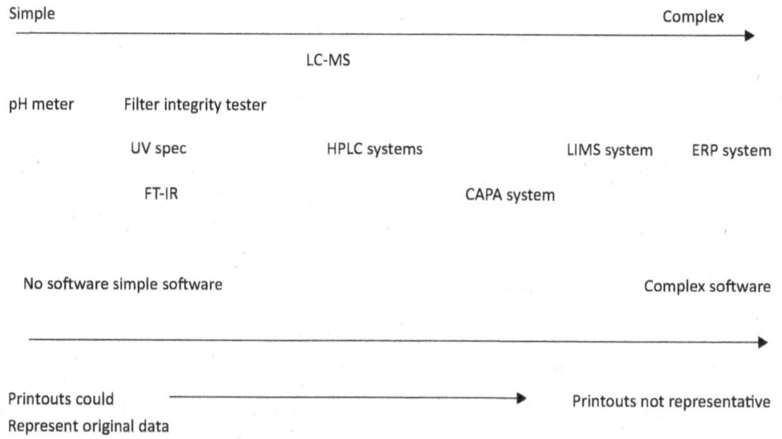

Figure A4.1 Diagram to illustrate the spectrum of simple machine (left) to complex computerized system (right), and relevance of printouts as "original data." (From Green Mountain QA LLC.)

in the figure. However, it is common for companies to overlook systems of apparent lower complexity. Within these systems, it may be possible to manipulate data or repeat testing to achieve a desired outcome with limited opportunity of detection (e.g., stand-alone systems with a user configurable output such as FT-IR, UV spectrophotometers).

Designing Systems to Ensure Data Quality and Integrity

Systems should be designed in a way that encourages compliance with the principles of data integrity. Examples include

- Access to clocks for recording timed events
- Accessibility of batch records at locations where activities take place so that ad hoc data recording and later transcription to official records are not necessary
- Control over blank paper templates for data recording
- User access rights that prevent (or audit trail) data amendments
- Automated data capture or printers attached to equipment such as balances
- Proximity of printers to relevant activities
- Access to sampling points (e.g., for water systems)
- Access to raw data for staff performing data checking activities

The use of scribes to record activity on behalf of another operator should be considered "exceptional," and only take place where

- The act of recording places the product or activity at risk, for example, documenting line interventions by sterile operators
- To accommodate cultural or staff literacy/language limitations, for instance, where an activity is performed by an operator but witnessed and recorded by a supervisor or officer

In both situations, the supervisory recording must be contemporaneous with the task being performed, and it must identify both the person performing the observed task and the person completing the record. The person performing the observed task should countersign the record wherever possible, although it is accepted that this countersigning step will be retrospective. The process for supervisory (scribe) documentation completion should be described in an approved procedure, which should also specify the activities to which the process applies.

Term	*Definition*	*Expectation/Guidance (Where Relevant)*
Data	Information derived or obtained from raw data (e.g., a reported analytical result)	Data must be A: Attributable to the person generating the data L: Legible and permanent C: Contemporaneous O: Original record (or true copy) A: Accurate
Raw data	Original records and documentation, retained in the format in which they were originally generated (i.e., paper or electronic), or as a true copy. Raw data must be contemporaneously and accurately recorded by permanent means. In the case of basic electronic equipment that does not store electronic data, or provides only a printed data output (e.g., balance or pH meter), the printout constitutes the raw data.	Raw data must • Be legible and accessible throughout the data life cycle. • Permit the full reconstruction of the activities resulting in the generation of the data.
In the following definitions, the term "data" includes raw data.		
Metadata	Metadata is data that describes the attributes of other data and provides context and meaning. Typically, this is data that describes the structure, data elements, interrelationships, and other characteristics of data. It also permits data to be attributable to an individual.	Example: data (bold text) **3.5** and metadata, giving context and meaning, (italic text) are *sodium chloride batch 1234,* **3.5** *mg. J Smith 01/07/14* Metadata form an integral part of the original record. Without metadata, the data have no meaning.

Data integrity	The extent to which all data is complete, consistent, and accurate throughout the data life cycle.	Data integrity arrangements must ensure that the accuracy, completeness, content, and meaning of data is retained throughout the data life cycle.
Data governance	The sum total of arrangements to ensure that data, irrespective of the format in which they are generated, are recorded, processed, retained, and used to ensure a complete, consistent, and accurate record throughout the data life cycle.	Data governance should address data ownership throughout the life cycle, and consider the design, operation, and monitoring of processes/systems in order to comply with the principles of data integrity including control over intentional and unintentional changes to information. Data governance systems should include staff training in the importance of data integrity principles and the creation of a working environment that encourages an open reporting culture for errors, omissions, and aberrant results. Senior management is responsible for the implementation of systems and procedures to minimize the potential risk to data integrity, and for identifying the residual risk, using the principles of ICH Q9. Contract givers should perform a similar review as part of their vendor assurance program.
Data life cycle	All phases in the life of the data (including raw data) from initial generation and recording through processing (including transformation or migration), use, data retention, archive/retrieval, and destruction.	The procedures for destroying data should consider data criticality and legislative retention requirements. Archival arrangements should be in place for long-term retention (in some cases, periods up to 30 years) for records such as batch documents, marketing authorization application data, traceability data for human-derived starting materials (not an exhaustive list). Additionally, at least 2 years of data must be retrievable in a timely manner for the purposes of regulatory inspection.

Primary record	The record that takes primacy in cases where <u>data</u> that are collected and retained concurrently by more than one method fail to concur.	In situations where the same information is recorded concurrently by more than one system, the data owner should define which system generates and retains the primary record, in case of discrepancy. The "primary record" attribute should be defined in the quality system, and should not be changed on a case-by-case basis. Risk management principles should be used to ensure that the assigned "primary record" provides the greatest accuracy, completeness, content, and meaning. For instance, it is not appropriate for low-resolution or static (printed/manual) data to be designated as a primary record in preference to high-resolution or dynamic (electronic) data. All data should be considered when performing a risk-based investigation into data anomalies (e.g., out of specification results).
Original record:/true copy	<u>Original record</u>: <u>Data</u> as the file or format in which they was originally generated, preserving the *integrity* (accuracy, completeness, content, and meaning) of the record, for example, original paper record of manual observation, or electronic raw data file from a computerized system.	Original records and true copies must preserve the integrity (accuracy, completeness, content, and meaning) of the record. Exact (true) copies of original records may be retained in place of the original record (e.g., scan of a paper record), provided that a documented system is in place to verify and record the integrity of the copy.

	True Copy: An exact verified copy of an original record. Data may be static (e.g., a "fixed" record such as paper or pdf) or dynamic (e.g., an electronic record which the user/reviewer can interact with). Example 1: A group of still images (photographs—the static "paper copy" example) may not provide the full content and meaning of the same event as a recorded moving image (video—the dynamic "electronic record" example). Example 2: Once printed or converted to static pdfs, chromatography records lose the capability of being reprocessed and do not enable more detailed viewing of baselines or any hidden fields. By comparison, the same dynamic electronic records in database format provide the ability to track, trend, and query data, allowing the reviewer (with proper access permissions) to reprocess, view hidden fields, and expand the baseline to view the integration more clearly.	It is conceivable for raw data generated by electronic means to be retained in an acceptable paper or pdf format, where it can be justified that a static record maintains the integrity of the original data. However, the data retention process must be shown to include verified copies of all raw data, metadata, relevant audit trail and result files, software/system configuration settings specific to each analytical run,* and all data processing runs (including methods and audit trails) necessary for the reconstruction of a given raw data set. It would also require a documented means to verify that the printed records were an accurate representation. This approach is likely to be onerous in its administration to enable a GMP-compliant record. Many electronic records are important to retain in their dynamic (electronic) format, to enable interaction with the data. Data must be retained in a dynamic form when it is critical to their integrity or later verification. This should be justified based on risk. * Computerized system configuration settings should be defined, tested, "locked," and protected from unauthorized access as part of computer system validation. Only those variable settings which relate to an analytical run would be considered as electronic raw data.

Computer system transactions	A computer system transaction is a single operation or sequence of operations performed as a single logical "unit of work." The operation(s) that make up a transaction may not be saved as a permanent record on durable storage until the user commits the transaction through a deliberate act (e.g., pressing a save button), or until the system forces the saving of data. The metadata (i.e., user name, date, and time) is not captured in the system audit trail until the user commits the transaction. In Manufacturing Execution Systems (MES), an electronic signature is often required by the system in order for the record to be saved and become permanent.	Computer systems should be designed to ensure that the executions of critical operations are recorded contemporaneously by the user and are not combined into a single computer system transaction with other operations. A critical processing step is a parameter that must be within an appropriate limit, range, or distribution to ensure the desired product quality. These should be reflected in the process control strategy. Examples of "units of work": • Weighing of individual materials • Entry of process critical manufacturing/analytical parameters • Verification of the identity of each component or material that will be used in a batch • Verification of the addition of each individual raw material to a batch (e.g., when the sequence of addition is considered critical to process control: see Figure A4.2) • Addition of multiple preweighed raw materials to bulk vessel when required as a single manufacturing step (e.g., when the sequence of addition is not considered critical to process control: see Figure A4.3)

Allows for contemporaneous recording of the material addition by the operator and verifier.

Material additions		
Step	Instructions	Data
1.	Scan barcode of material ABC123.	ABC123 <Barcode>
2.	Add material ABC123 to the blender.	Operator signature Verifier signature

Next step

Figure A4.2 Logical design permitting contemporaneous recording of addition of a single material in a manufacturing "unit of work." This record is permanently recorded (Step 2), with audit trail, before progressing to next "unit of work."

Does not allow for contemporaneous recording of the material addition by the operator and verifier.

Material additions		
Step	Instructions	Data
1.	Scan barcode of material ABC123.	ABC123 <Barcode>
2.	Add material ABC123 to the blender.	
3.	Scan barcode of material DEF456.	DEF456 <Barcode>
4.	Add material DEF456 to the blender.	
5.	Scan barcode of material GHI789.	GHI789 <Barcode>
6.	Add material GHI789 to the blender.	Operator signature Verifier signature

Next step

Figure A4.3 Logical design permitting the addition of multiple materials in a manufacturing "unit of work" before committing the record to durable media. Steps 1, 3, and 5 are contemporaneous entries (barcode), but are not permanently recorded with audit trail until Step 6.

Audit trail	GMP audit trails are metadata that are a record of GMP critical information (e.g., the change or deletion of GMP-relevant *data*) that permits the reconstruction of GMP activities.	Where computerized systems are used to capture, process, report, or store raw data electronically, system design should always provide for the retention of full audit trails to show all changes to the data while retaining previous and original data. It should be possible to associate all changes to data with the persons making those changes, and changes should be time stamped and a reason given. Users should not have the ability to amend or switch off the audit trail. The relevance of data retained in audit trails should be considered by the company to permit robust data review/verification. The items included in an audit trail should be those of relevance to permit reconstruction of the process or activity. It is not necessary for audit trail review to include every system activity (e.g., user logon/off, keystrokes, etc.), and may be achieved by review of designed and validated system reports. Audit trail review should be part of the routine data review/approval process, usually performed by the operational area that generated the data (e.g., laboratory). There should be evidence available to confirm that review of the relevant audit trails has taken place. When designing a system for review of audit trails, this may be limited to those with GMP relevance (e.g., relating to data creation, processing, modification and deletion, etc). Audit trails may be reviewed as a list of relevant data, or by a validated "exception reporting" process. QA should also review a sample of relevant audit trails, raw data, and metadata as part of self inspection to ensure ongoing compliance with the data governance policy/procedures.

		If no audit trailed system exists, a paper-based audit trail to demonstrate changes to data will be permitted until a full audit trail (integrated system or independent audit software using a validated interface) system becomes available. These hybrid systems are currently permitted, where they achieve equivalence to integrated audit trail described in Annex 11 of the GMP Guide. If such equivalence cannot be demonstrated, it is expected that facilities should upgrade to an audit trailed system by the end of 2017.
Data review		There should be a procedure that describes the process for the review and approval of data, including raw data. Data review must also include a review of relevant metadata, including audit trails. Data review must be documented. A procedure should describe the actions to be taken if the data review identifies an error or omission. This procedure should enable data corrections or clarifications to be made in a GMP-compliant manner, providing visibility of the original record and audit trailed traceability of the correction, using ALCOA principles (see data definition).

Computerized system user access/ system administrator roles		Full use should be made of access controls to ensure that people have access only to functionality that is appropriate for their job role, and that actions are attributable to a specific individual. Companies must be able to demonstrate the access levels granted to individual staff members and ensure that historical information regarding user access level is available. Shared logins or generic user access should not be used. Where the computerized system design supports individual user access, this function must be used. This may require the purchase of additional licenses. It is acknowledged that some computerized systems support only a single user login or a limited numbers of user logins. Where alternative computerized systems have the ability to provide the required number of unique logins, facilities should upgrade to an appropriate system by the end of 2017. Where no suitable alternative computerized system is available, a paper-based method of providing traceability will be permitted. The lack of suitability of alternative systems should be justified based on a review of system design, and documented. System administrator access should be restricted to the minimum number of people possible taking into account the size and nature of the organization. The generic system administrator account should not be available for use. Personnel with system administrator access should log in under unique logins that allow actions in the audit trail(s) to be attributed to a specific individual.

		System administrator rights (permitting activities such as data deletion, database amendment, or system configuration changes) should not be assigned to individuals with a direct interest in the data (data generation, data review or approval). Where this is unavoidable in the organizational structure, a similar level of control may be achieved by the use of dual user accounts with different privileges. All changes performed under system administrator access must be visible to, and approved within, the quality system. The individual should log in using the account with the appropriate access rights for the given task, e.g., a laboratory manager performing data checking should not log in as system administrator where a more appropriate level of access exists for that task.
Data retention		Raw data (or a true copy thereof) generated in paper format may be retained for example by scanning, provided that there is a process in place to ensure that the copy is verified to ensure its completeness. Data retention may be classified as archive or backup. Data and document retention arrangements should ensure the protection of records from deliberate or inadvertent alteration or loss. Secure controls must be in place to ensure the data integrity of the record throughout the retention period, and validated where appropriate.

		Where <u>data</u> and document retention are contracted to a third party, particular attention should be paid to understanding the ownership and retrieval of data held under this arrangement. The physical location in which the data is held, including the impact of any laws applicable to that geographic location, should also be considered. The responsibilities of the contract giver and acceptor must be defined in a contract as described in Chapter 7 of the GMP Guide.
• Archive	Long-term, permanent retention of completed <u>data</u> and relevant <u>metadata</u> in its final form for the purposes of reconstruction of the process or activity.	Archive records should be locked such that they cannot be altered or deleted without detection and <u>audit trail</u>. The archive arrangements must be designed to permit recovery and readability of the data and metadata throughout the required retention period.
• Backup	A copy of current (editable) <u>data</u>, <u>metadata</u>, and system configuration settings (variable settings which relate to an analytical run) maintained for the purpose of disaster recovery.	Backup and recovery processes must be <u>validated</u>.
File structure		File structure has a significant impact on the inherent <u>data integrity</u> risks. The ability to manipulate or delete <u>flat files</u> requires a higher level of logical and procedural control over data generation, <u>review</u> and storage.

• Flat files	A "flat file" is an individual record that may not carry with it all relevant metadata (e.g., pdf, dat, doc).	Flat files may carry basic metadata relating to file creation and date of last amendment, but may not audit trail the type and sequence of amendments. When creating flat file reports from electronic data, the metadata and audit trails relating to the generation of the raw data may be lost, unless these are retained as a true copy. Consideration also needs to be given to the "dynamic" nature of the data, where appropriate (see true copy definition). There is an inherently greater data integrity risk with flat files (e.g., when compared with data contained within a relational database), in that these are easier to manipulate and delete as a single file.
Relational database	A relational database stores different components of associated data and metadata in different places. Each individual record is created and retrieved by compiling the data and metadata for review.	This file structure is inherently more secure, as the data is held in a large file format that preserves the relationship between the data and metadata. This is more resilient to attempts to selectively delete, amend, or recreate data and the metadata trail of actions, compared with a flat file system. Retrieval of information from a relational database requires a database search tool, or the original application that created the record.

Validation: For intended purpose (See also Annex 15 and GAMP 5)		Computerized systems should comply with the requirements of EU GMP Annex 11 and be validated for their intended purpose. This requires an understanding of the computerized system's function within a process. For this reason, the acceptance of vendor-supplied validation data in isolation of system configuration and intended use is not acceptable. In isolation from the intended process or end user IT infrastructure, vendor testing is likely to be limited to functional verification only, and may not fulfill the requirements for performance qualification. For example: Validation of computerized system audit trail • A custom report generated from a relational database may be used as a GMP system audit trail. • SOPs should be drafted during OQ to describe the process for audit trail verification, including definition of the data to be reviewed. • "Validation for intended use" would include testing during PQ to confirm that the required data is correctly extracted by the custom report, and presented in a manner which is aligned with the data review process described in the SOP.

Revision History

Revision	**Publication Month**	**Reason for Changes**
Revision 1	January 2015	None. First issue.
Revision 1.1	March 2015	Added clarifications in response to stakeholder questions.

Appendix V: Relevant Worldwide GCP and GLP Regulations and Guidelines

Introduction

The following are relevant good clinical practice (GCP) and good laboratory practice (GLP) regulations and guidelines containing references associated with the integrity of e-records.

> *The regulatory requirements for the clinical data do not change whether clinical data are captured on paper, electronically, or using a hybrid approach.*
>
> **US FDA CPG 7348.810**
> *December 2008.*

Consistent with the globalization of the clinical and nonclinical laboratories regulatory requirements, the reader may agree that the principles of data integrity are contained in all major regulations and guidelines.

GCP

Title: Annex VI to Guidance for the Conduct of Good Clinical Practice Inspections: Record Keeping and Archiving of Documents, March 2010.
Regulation/Guideline: GCP
Organization: EC
Country: EU
E-Records Integrity Items:

If documents are to be archived using electronical or optical media, the methods for transferring the data to these media should be validated. A suitable backup strategy must be implemented to prevent loss or destruction of data. There must be a possibility to generate hard copies throughout the period of retention.

Title: Guidelines for Good Clinical Practices (Draft E6 (R2))
Guideline: GCP
Organization: EMA
Country: EU
E-Records Integrity Items:
Sponsor: Section 5.5.3

When using electronic trial data handling and/or remote electronic trial data systems, the sponsor should:

- Ensure that the systems are designed to permit data changes in such a way that the data changes are documented and that there is no deletion of entered data (i.e., maintain an audit trail, data trail, edit trail).
- Maintain a security system that prevents unauthorized access to the data. (e) Maintain a list of individuals who are authorized to make data changes (see 4.1.5 and 4.9.3).
- Maintain adequate backup of the data.
- Ensure the integrity of the data, including any data that describes the context, content, and structure of the data. This is particularly important when making changes to computerized systems, such as software upgrades or migration of data.
- Sponsor: Section 5.5.4
- If data is transformed during processing, it should always be possible to compare the original data and observations with the processed data.

Title: Annex III Guidance for the Conduct of Good Clinical Practice Inspections, Computer Systems*

Regulation/Guideline: GCP

Organization: EC

Country: EU

E-Records Integrity Items:

The EU GCP inspectors agreed in November 2007 to use PIC/S PI 011-3† as the reference for inspection of computer systems in clinical.

Title: Annex VI to Guidance for the Conduct of Good Clinical Practice Inspections: Record Keeping and Archiving of Documents,‡ March 2010

Regulation/Guideline: GCP

Organization: EC

Country: EU

E-Records Integrity Items:

If documents are to be archived using electronic or optical media, the methods for transferring the data to these media should be validated. A suitable backup strategy must be implemented to prevent loss or destruction of data. There must be a possibility to generate hard copies throughout the period of retention.

Title: Reflection Paper on Guidance for Laboratories That Perform the Analysis or Evaluation of Clinical Trial Samples, EMA/INS/GCP/532137/2010, February 2012

Regulation/Guideline: GCP

Organization: European Medicines Agency

Country: EU

E-records Integrity Items:

5.0 Definitions

Source data is equivalent to the term *raw data* used by many GLP-compliant laboratories. Both terms mean all information in original records and certified copies of original records of clinical findings, observations, or other activities in a clinical trial necessary for the reconstruction and evaluation of the

---

* EudraLex: Volume 10 Clinical Trials Guidelines, Chapter IV—Inspections.

† PI 011-3. Good practices for computerised systems in regulated "GXP" environments, Pharmaceutical Inspection Co-operation Scheme (PIC/S), September 2007.

‡ EudraLex: Volume 10 Clinical Trials Guidelines, Chapter IV—Inspections.

trial. Source data is contained in source documents (original records or certified copies).

6.12 Data recording

Any change to the data should be made so as not to obscure the previous entry. If data is generated, recorded, modified, corrected, and stored or archived electronically, it is recommended that an audit trail be electronically maintained rather than manually, whenever possible. The reason for any changes to the data should be justified and the justification documented. It should be possible to determine who made the change, when the change was made, and for what reason.

6.16 Computerized systems

Access to computerized systems should be controlled. The identity of those with specific access rights to computerized systems should be documented and subject to periodic review to ensure that the access restrictions remain current and appropriate.

6.21 Retention of data

Requirements for the archiving of electronic records are the same as those for other record types. However, there are a number of specific issues that should be considered, such as

- Long-term access to, and readability of, electronic information (data format)
- The shelf life of the storage medium where appropriate (CD-ROM, DVD, server, etc.)
- Quality control (QC) checks following data migration to a secure server or other storage medium

Title: CPG 7348.810—Sponsors, CROs, and Monitors and EMEA Procedure, December 2008

Regulation/Guideline: GCP

Organization: US FDA

Country: US

E-Records Integrity Items:

CPG 7348.810 provides instructions to Field and Center US FDA personnel for conducting inspections of sponsors, contract research organizations (CROs), and monitors, and recommending associated administrative/enforcement actions.

One area of advice to the field inspectors in this CPG is basic principles on e-records: the regulatory requirements for the clinical data do not change whether the clinical data is captured on paper, electronically, or using a hybrid approach.

Section I refers to the quality of the e-records. Specifically, Sections I-3 and I-4 refer to data collection and security, respectively.

3. Data Collection:
   a. Is the clinical investigator able to ensure accurate and complete electronic and human readable copies of electronic records, suitable for review and copying? (If you are unable to access records from the computerized system, contact the center immediately.)
   b. Determine whether electronic records and data meet the requirements applicable to paper records. For example, are electronic records used to meet case history requirements attributable, legible, contemporaneous, original, and accurate (ALCOA)?
   c. Describe how data is transmitted to the sponsor or contract research organization.
   d. Determine whether original data entries and changes can be made by anyone other than the clinical investigator.
   e. Determine how the electronic data was reviewed during monitoring visits. Document unauthorized changes or modifications made to original data and by whom.
4. Security
   a. Determine who is authorized to access the system.
   b. Describe how the computerized systems are accessed (e.g., password protected, access privileges, user identification).
   c. How is information captured related to the creation, modification, or deletion of electronic records (e.g., audit trails, date/time stamps)?
   d. Describe whether there are backup, disaster recovery, and/or contingency plans to protect against data loss. Were there any software upgrades, security or performance patches, or new instrumentation during the clinical trial? Could the data have been affected?
   e. Describe how error messages or system failures are reported to the sponsor, CRO, or study site and the corrective actions, if any, that are taken.

f. How were the system and data handled during site closure?

Title: Guidance for Industry—Computerized Systems Used in Clinical Investigations, Mat 2007

Regulation/Guideline: GCP

Organization: US FDA

Country: US

E-Records Integrity Items:

Section I: Because the source data is necessary for the reconstruction and evaluation of the study to determine the safety of food and color additives and the safety and effectiveness of new human and animal drugs and medical devices, this guidance is intended to assist in ensuring confidence in the reliability, quality, and *integrity* of the electronic source data and source documentation (i.e., electronic records).

Section II: The FDA's acceptance of data from clinical trials for decision-making purposes depends on the FDA's ability to verify the quality and *integrity* of the data during FDA on-site inspections and audits (21 CFR 312, 511.1(b), and 812).

Section IV.D.2: It is important to keep track of all changes made to information in the electronic records that document activities related to the conduct of the trial (audit trails). The use of audit trails or other security measures helps to ensure that only authorized additions, deletions, or alterations of information in the electronic record have occurred and allows a means to reconstruct significant details about study conduct and source data collection necessary to verify the quality and integrity of data.

Section IV.D.4: When electronic formats are the only ones used to create and preserve electronic records, sufficient backup and recovery procedures should be designed to protect against data loss. Records should regularly be backed up in a procedure that would prevent a catastrophic loss and ensure the quality and integrity of the data. Records should be stored at a secure location specified in the SOP. Storage should typically be off-site or in a building separate from the original records.

Section IV.D5: The integrity of the data and the integrity of the protocols should be maintained when making changes to the computerized system, such as software upgrades, including security and performance patches, equipment, and component replacement, and new instrumentation. The effects of any changes to the system should be evaluated, and some should be validated depending on risk. Changes that exceed previously established operational limits or design specifications should be validated. Finally, all changes to the system should be documented.

Section IV.F.1: We recommend that you incorporate prompts, flags, or other help features into your computerized system to encourage consistent use of clinical terminology and to alert the user to data that is out of acceptable range.

GLP

Title: Good Laboratory Practice for Nonclinical Laboratory Studies

Regulation/Guideline: GLP

Organization: US FDA

Country: US

E-Records Integrity Items:

21 CFR Part 58.81 (b) Standard operating procedures shall be established for, but not limited to, the following: (10) Data handling, storage, and retrieval.

Title: The Organization for Economic Co-operation and Development (OECD) DRAFT Advisory Document #16—The Application of the GLP Principles to Computerized Systems, September 2014.

Regulation/Guideline: GLP

Organization: OECD

Country: 34 Member countries span the globe, from North and South America to Europe and Asia-Pacific. They include the United States, Canada, Mexico, Chile, Turkey, and over 18 European countries.

E-Records Integrity Items:

12. Risk assessment should be applied throughout the life cycle of a computerized system taking into account data integrity and the quality of the study results. Decisions on the extent of validation and data integrity controls should be based on a justified and documented risk assessment.
24. Potential incompatibilities of roles and responsibilities should be considered to avoid risks to data integrity (if the system owner

and process owner are the same person, the control of the audit trail might be in the hands of a person using the system).

33. Hosted services (e.g., platform, software, archiving, backup, or processes as a service) should be treated like any other third-party service and require written agreements. It is the responsibility of the regulated user to evaluate the relevant service and to estimate risks to data integrity and data availability.
77. Qualification testing (e.g., DQ [Design Qualification]; IQ [Installation Qualification]; OQ [Operational Qualification]; and PQ [Performance Qualification]) should be carried out to ensure that a system meets its requirements. Such testing should check those areas where GLP data integrity is at risk.
94. It is the regulated user's responsibility to adequately control any electronic data entry systems regardless of their complexity, and to consider the impact of such systems on data quality and data integrity.
124. Documented security procedures should be in place for the protection of hardware, software, and data from corruption or unauthorized modification, or loss.
127. The potential for corruption of data by malignant code or other agents should also be addressed. Security measures should also be taken to ensure data integrity in the event of both short-term and long-term system failures.
128. Since maintaining data integrity is a primary objective of the GLP principles, it is important that everyone associated with a computerized system be aware of the necessity for the above security considerations. Management should ensure that personnel are aware of the importance of data security, the procedures and system features that are available to provide appropriate security, and the consequences of security breaches.
130. Appropriate and well-maintained authorization concepts should specify logical access rights to domains, computers, applications, and data.
159. Relevant data formats and hosting systems should be evaluated regarding accessibility, readability, and influences on data integrity during the archiving period.
165. All contingency plans need to be well documented and validated, and they should ensure continued data integrity and that the study is not compromised in any way.

Title: Validation of Computerized Systems—Core Document, PA/PH/OMCL (08) 69 3R, July 2009

Regulation/Guideline: GLP

Organization: Official Medicines Control Laboratories Network of the Council of Europe

Country: EU

E-Records Integrity Items:

Backup

Traceability must be ensured from raw data to results. If all or part of the traceability of parameters relevant for the quality of the results is available only in electronic form, a backup process must be implemented to allow for recovery of the system following any failure that compromises its integrity. Backup frequency depends on data criticality, amount of stored data, and frequency of data generation.

A procedure for regular testing of backup data (restore test), to verify the proper integrity and accuracy of data, should also be in place.

Protection of the software

Software must also be protected against any external interference that could change the data and affect the final results.

Selection of software and computer equipment (Annex 2)

The user requirements specification should contain all relevant functional, technical, and organizational specifications. It should also cover the aspects of information security and data protection.

Title: WHO Good Practices for Pharmaceutical Quality Control Laboratories, Technical Report Series, No. 957, 2010, Annex 1, 2010.

Regulation/Guideline: GLP

Organization: WHO

Country: All countries that are Members of the United Nations may become members of WHO by accepting its Constitution, a total of 194 Member states (http://www.who.int/countries/en/).

E-Records Integrity Items:

4.2 All original observations, including calculations and derived data, calibration, validation and verification records, and final results, should be retained on record for an appropriate period of time in accordance with national regulations and, if applicable, contractual arrangements, whichever is longer. The records should include the data recorded in the analytical worksheet by the technician or analyst on consecutively numbered pages with references to the appendices containing the relevant recordings, for example, chromatograms and spectra. The records for each test should contain sufficient information to permit the tests to be repeated and/or the results to be recalculated, if necessary. The records should include the identity of the personnel involved in the sampling, preparation, and testing of the samples. The records of samples to be used in legal proceedings should be kept according to the legal requirements applicable to them.

5.2 For computers, automated tests, or calibration equipment, and the collection, processing, recording, reporting, storage, or retrieval of test and/or calibration data, the laboratory should ensure that:

(b) Procedures are established and implemented for protecting the integrity of data. Such procedures should include, but are not limited to, measures to ensure the integrity and confidentiality of data entry or collection and the storage, transmission, and processing of data. In particular, electronic data should be protected from unauthorized access and an audit trail of any amendments should be maintained.

(d) Procedures are established and implemented for making, documenting, and controlling changes to information stored in computerized systems.

(e) Electronic data should be backed up at appropriate regular intervals according to a documented procedure. Backed-up data should be retrievable and stored in such a manner as to prevent data loss.

Additional Readings

GAMP CoP, Validation and data integrity in eClinical platforms, ISPE, June 2014.
Schmitt, S., Data integrity: FDA and global regulatory guidance, IVT, October 2014.

Appendix VI: Electronic Records Integrity in Non-Clinical Laboratories

R. D. McDowall, Director, R.D. McDowall Ltd.

Introduction

Data integrity is the current major regulatory topic. The subject has been at the centre of an increasing number of regulatory citations for laboratory data not just from the US Food and Drug Administration (FDA) but also other regulatory agencies such as the European Medicines Agency (EMA), Health Canada and the World Health Organisation (WHO). The focus has typically been centred on Quality Control (QC) laboratories operating to Good Manufacturing Practice (GMP) but there have also been issues with laboratories operating to Good Laboratory Practice (GLP) involved in the analysis of biological samples from non-clinical and clinical studies conducted during drug development. Data integrity is not just a single country or single continent problem but a global issue. The large proportion of data integrity problems are based on poor and/or outdated working practices rather than a minority of cases involving data falsification.

Data integrity it is not a new problem. Testing into compliance was the topic of the first case where the FDA took a pharmaceutical company, Barr Laboratories, to a contested court case in the early 1990s [1]. Laboratory analysis and resampling was undertaken until a passing result was obtained and the batch released. This case resulted in the writing of an FDA guidance on the Inspection of Pharmaceutical Quality Control Laboratories [2];

although the publication is over 20 years old it is still relevant now as many of the practices in QC laboratories worldwide have not changed radically. In addition, it resulted in the publication of United States Pharmacopoeia <1010> on outlier testing [3], a direct requirement from the court judgement, and also an FDA guidance for industry on Out of Specification (OOS) results [4].

Cases of fraud and falsification have occurred in the United States with Able Laboratories [5] and Leiner Health Products [6] in 2005 and 2006 respectively. In the case of Able Laboratories, the FDA had performed 7 pre-approval inspections (PAIs) with no major observations. It was an internal whistle-blower who alerted the Agency to the falsification that was occurring. As a result, the FDA have reviewed their approaches to inspections:

- Rewrote their Compliance Program Guide 7346.832 [7] which has objective 3 covering a data integrity audit for the laboratory data in the regulatory dossier.
- Trained their inspectors in data integrity which means that there is now a focus on computerised systems and the data contained therein rather than paper output.
- Produced a level 2 guidance on the FDA web site on aspects of data integrity: shared user log-ins, why paper cannot be raw data from a computerised system and using samples as system suitability test (SST) injections [8].

The European Medicines Agency is posting GMP non-compliances on line [9] where many cases of data integrity have been noted. As has Health Canada, interestingly, at the end of 2015, 86% of the companies listed on the Health Canada inspection tracker web site with compliance issues involved data integrity [10]. The Canadian authority has stated that GMP inspections will be unannounced due to the problems with data integrity issues it has found. Moreover, some companies cited in the web site have not been inspected by Health Canada but by another regulatory agency and this is a direct consequence of sharing inspection findings between regulators.

Data integrity is not a new problem and is not confined to one country or continent. Data integrity is a now global issue. In this Appendix we will take a holistic approach to laboratory data integrity, review the regulations and regulatory guidance impacting data integrity and then look at three ways of generating and recording laboratory data. The first is recording results by observation. The second discusses a chromatography data system used in hybrid mode where peak areas are input into a spreadsheet for calculation of the reportable result. The third and final example to be discussed is again a chromatography data system but used in electronic mode with electronic signatures. The advantage of discussing a chromatography data system as an example as these last two examples is that the application can be either as a standalone workstation or in networked architecture as well as hybrid or electronic mode.

Data Integrity Is More than Just Numbers

In the regulated analytical laboratory data integrity is not how a sample is analysed and a reportable result or results are obtained. Furthermore, it is not only about assessing how laboratory data have been interpreted, although that conclusion could be drawn when FDA warning letters are read.

It is important to understand that laboratory data integrity must be thought of in the context of analysis of samples within an analytical process that is operating under the auspices of a pharmaceutical quality system [11]. Data integrity does not exist in a vacuum.

The foundation of this approach under the umbrella of a pharmaceutical quality system there must be management leadership, corporate data integrity policies that lead to laboratory data integrity procedures, staff initial and on-going data integrity training and other areas within the context of a data governance system. These aspects are covered in the main chapters of this book.

Next, the analytical instruments and computerized systems used in the laboratory must be qualified for the specified operating range and validated for their intended purpose respectively. After this analytical procedures (covering sampling to generation of the reportable result) must be developed and validated under actual conditions of use. This includes analytical methods from a pharmacopoeia.

Finally, the analysis of sample will be undertaken using the right method and right data system, data will be generated, interpreted and the reportable result will be calculated. Although this will be the focus of this Appendix, it is important not to forget the importance of the quality system and well as instrument, qualification, computerized system validation and method development and validation.

GXP Regulations Summary for the Laboratory

Good Manufacturing Practice (GMP) Regulations and Guidance

In this section we will cover the GMP regulations from the USA and Europe along with regulatory guidance from the FDA, MHRA (Medicines and Healthcare Products Regulatory Agency) the UK regulator and the WHO (World Health Organisation) as shown in Figure A6.1. Figure A6.1 also shows, in the lowest level, that the data integrity guidance that is due to be published by the FDA and PIC/S (Pharmaceutical Inspection Convention/ Pharmaceutical Inspection Cooperation Scheme) and a Question and Answer on data integrity that the European Medicines Agency will issue. The dates for publication of these documents are not known but the reader is advised to be aware that further guidance is due and that this is a rapidly evolving field.

GMP regulations from the FDA and European Union contain the requirements for data integrity within the regulations:

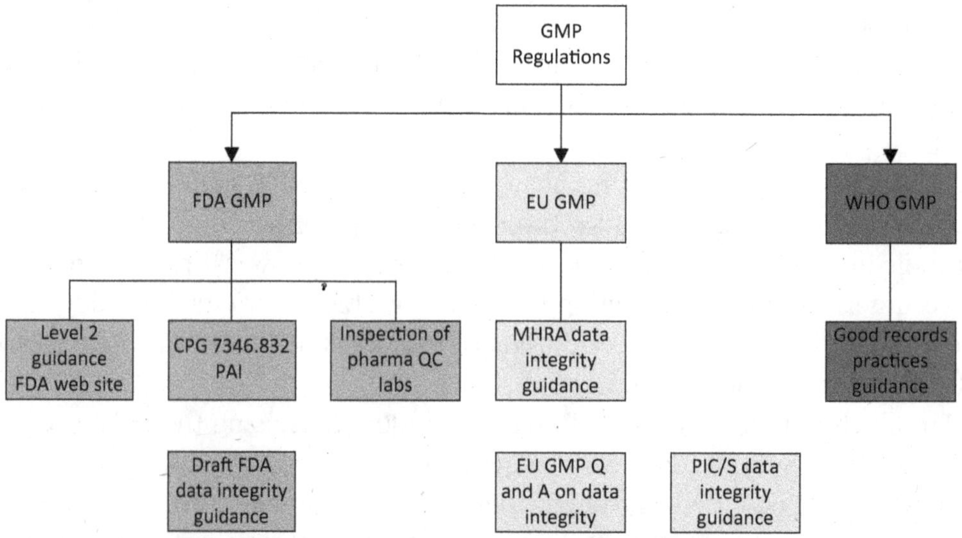

Figure A6.1 GMP Regulations and Regulatory Guidance for Data Integrity.

Good Laboratory Practice Regulations and Guidance

Currently the both US and OECD GLP regulations refer to raw data as original observations from which the study can be reconstructed. However, the term raw data was coined in the 1970s when there were few computerized systems available for non-clinical studies and the main record medium was paper. In the electronic world raw data is not a useful term as data and meta data are preferred terms. Perhaps in the context of GLP raw data used in conjunction with processed data is better.

There is little in both US and OECD GLP regulations [12,13] specifically about data integrity. However, the replacement for the out of date OECD guidance document 10 on the Application of GLP Principles for Computerised Systems [14] (which is 20 years old and out of date in many respects) is being replaced by OECD guidance document 17 [15] which is based on EU GMP Annex 11 but much expanded. This document has been discussed in the main body of this book and will not be repeated here.

Illustrating Laboratory Data Integrity Issues

To focus on the regulatory non-compliances that have occurred an analysis of FDA warning letters involving laboratory data integrity is instructive. Owing to the wide applicability of chromatography in the pharmaceutical industry, there has been an increasing trend to inspect chromatography data systems (CDS) operating in GMP regulated laboratories and this focus has discovered cases of poor management of data and cases of data falsification. The inspection focus has changed. Instead of wading through reams of paper printouts, regulatory inspections focus on the electronic records in the CDS. This change in this approach was triggered by the Able Laboratories fraud case [5] as the inspections only focused on paper printouts from the system. Some of the innovative analytical techniques employed by Able were a combination of:

- Copy and pasting chromatograms from passing batches to failing ones
- Extensive reintegration of chromatograms to ensure passing results
- Adjustments of weights, purity factors, calculations of ensure acceptable results

This was how an original result of 29% that would fail a specification of >85% was falsified to a passing result of 91% [5]. At the heart of the fraud was a CDS, which when investigated by the FDA following the alert by the whistle blower had an audit trail that identified the individuals responsible for the falsification of data. Identification of the problems in the laboratory led to the closing of the company in 2005 and the criminal prosecution of four individuals in 2007.

An analysis of the regulatory citations contained in FDA warning letters for laboratory data systems (mainly CDS) between 2013 and 2015 can be seen in Figure A6.2 [16]. Here the citations are grouped into four main areas: QMS failures and specific citations against equipment in §211.68(b), laboratory controls in §211.160–165 and laboratory records in §211.194. The focus in this Appendix is on the equipment (specifically analytical instruments), laboratory controls and records.

Equipment Citations

A frequent citation in the CDS warning letters, shown in Figure A6.2, is §211.68(b) in the section on automatic, mechanical, and electronic equipment [17] which requires that:

- Access is restricted to authorised individuals
- Changes are only instituted by authorised individuals
- The accuracy of calculations must be verified
- Backups must be exact and complete
- Backups must be secure from alteration, erasure or loss

Non-compliances in this area involve:

- Sharing of user identities between two or more users, so making it impossible to identify the individual who was responsible for a particular action within the CDS. Therefore, ensure that there are enough user licences for each user to have one for their job. Sharing user accounts may seem to be a smart way to save money but, if you get caught, the cost of rectifying the non-compliance makes the saving pale into insignificance. A list of current and historical users is essential for compliance with both Part 11 [18] and Annex 11 [19].
- Access privileges must be appropriate to a user's job function. Thus, not everyone can be a system administrator (with the possible exception of a standalone system with only two or three users). Usually there will need to be three or more user types or roles with corresponding access

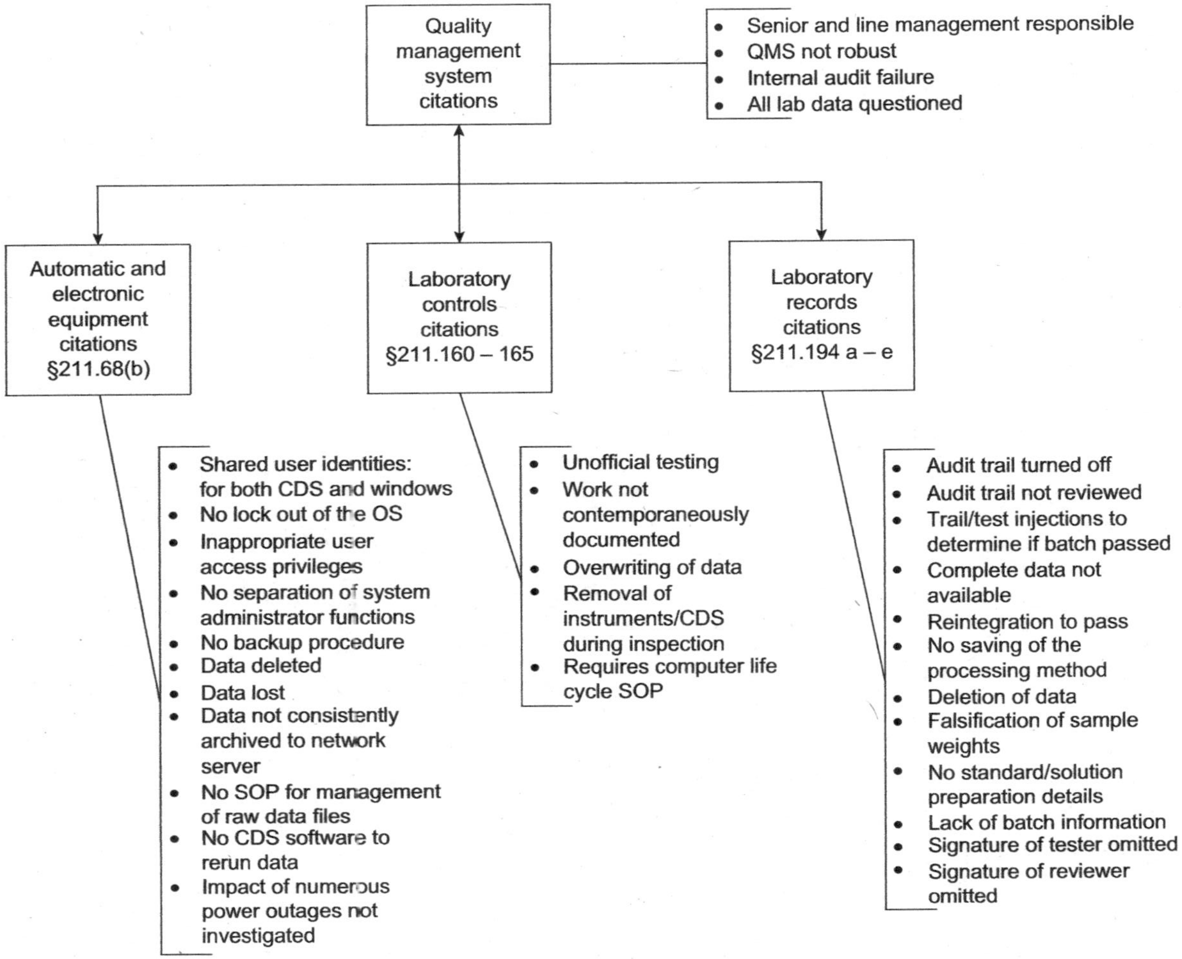

Figure A6.2 Data Integrity GMP Citations for Laboratory Data Systems in FDA Warning Letters 2013–2015 [16].

privileges which need to be documented outside of the system either in a configuration specification or an SOP. In this also consider a service engineer who may require access to service the attached instrument or perform an operational qualification.

- Ideally the system administrator needs to be independent of the function of the laboratory so that configuration settings cannot be changed and the audit trail turned on and off to hide falsification activities. Therefore, the system administration activities such as configuration of the software including controlled changes to it and user account management and access privileges need to use IT rather than laboratory staff.
- Limit access to both the CDS application software and the workstation operating system, as there are many citations for deletion of data in some file based CDS.
- Failing to backup data, incomplete backup of data, just being incompetent and loosing data when upgrading the CDS software or not having the CDS software to interpret the data files are just some of the ways companies have been cited under this section of the regulations. The simplest way to avoid this citation is to give the job of backup to the IT professionals who will do the job for you. There are a few catches here, are the IT staff trained, is there a backup SOP with evidence of actions, is recovery is tested regularly and has the backup process and software been validated? This is fine for a networked CDS but if there are standalone workstations then data may be located on the local workstation drive. This is not acceptable and, in my view, a CDS must be networked to avoid the backup problem.

The majority of citations above are where laboratories have standalone workstations.

Citations for Lack of Laboratory Controls

Human inventiveness knows no bounds when it comes to data falsification. One enterprising company [20] actually removed some of their chromatographs and workstations from site to hide data manipulation from inspectors. Other CDS non-compliance citations include:

- Unofficial testing—which we discuss in more detail in the next section under complete data

- Failing to document work contemporaneously. One way this can be achieved is by waiting until the chromatography has been performed, then working out the sample weight required and then falsifying the sample weights [5,6,20,21].
- Overwriting data is possible with some file based systems and this was used by a number of companies that used older and less compliant CDS applications.

Failure to Have Complete Laboratory Records

Here's where compliance failures become very interesting. Audit trails in some CDS were found to be turned off which is a poor approach to compliance in a regulated environment [5,6,20,21]. It is imperative that the audit trail is turned on and kept turned on otherwise changes are made to data cannot be attributed to the individual who made it and the old and new values are not recorded. Designers of CDS audit trails must embed them in the basic operation of the system so that they cannot be turned off and the only issue is if the laboratory wants to turn on the reason for change.

When the audit trail in the system was turned on, nobody reviewed the entries (except the inspectors) [5] but the audit trail is part of complete data that the second person reviewer needs to check.

Further non-compliance citations, outlined in Figure A6.2, are reintegration to pass and not saving the integration method—here there need to be technical controls in the CDS software and well as an SOP and training on when it is permissible to reintegrate and when it is not.

A common theme with many of the warning letters was the use of trial or test injections or unofficial testing [8]. This practice is a test injection of samples to check if a batch is going to pass or not, furthermore, the test injections are either conveniently forgotten or, worse, deleted from the CDS as if the test never occurred. The failure to document and/or delete the test injections brings a citation under 211.194(a) for not have complete data for the analysis [22] or raw data [23]. In one case there was the deletion of 5,301 data files from a data system.

Is the System Ready to Run?

However, let us look at the issue of "test" injections from another perspective. As chromatographers do we want to commit samples for analysis when a chromatographic system is not equilibrated? No should be the answer, we want to have a chromatograph ready especially for complex separations or where we analyse at or near the limits of detection/quantification. Therefore, we have a choice do we commit samples for analysis and if the SST samples fail resolve the problem and start again or do we have an independent solution to evaluate if a system is ready for the analysis at hand? Plainly the first option of hope for the best is not optimal and can lead to a waste of time, especially if the results are required for batch release. However, it keeps the regulators off your back as failing SST results mean that any results generated are not OOS by definition [4].

However, let us explore the evaluation injection(s) in a little detail. Let me be very clear here I am NOT advocating injecting aliquots from the vials for the samples under test—this is the quickest way to a warning letter as noted on the FDA web site [8]. I would argue that under scientifically soundness in §211.160(a) [17] the approach for evaluating if a chromatographic system needs a number of criteria that can be outlined as follows:

- All chromatographic systems need to equilibrate before they are ready for analysis. The time taken will typically depend on factors such as the complexity of the analysis, the age and condition of the column, detector lamp warm up time. Generally, there will be an idea of how long this will be from the method development/validation/verification/transfer work carried out in the laboratory and this should be documented in the analytical procedure.
- Prepare an independent reference solution of analyte(s) that will be used for the sole purpose of system evaluation. The solution container label needs to be documented to GMP standards and clearly identified for the explicit purpose of evaluating if a chromatograph is ready for a specific analysis.
- The analytical procedure needs to allow the use of system evaluation injections and also staff need to be trained in the procedure.
- Inject one aliquot from the evaluation solution and compare with the SST criteria. Clearly label the vial in the sequence file as a system evaluation injection. If the SST criteria are met then the system is ready for the analysis.
- At completion of the analysis, document the number of system evaluation injections as part of the analytical report for the run.

Using these regulatory citations as examples, to avoid such issues during an inspection, readers can see the nature of the controls required to operate their laboratory systems in compliance with the regulations and ensure data integrity.

Example Laboratory Data Generation and Reporting

Observation, Instruments, Spreadsheets and Systems

In this section we will discuss how laboratory data can be generated and this will be exemplified with three examples. The first example is recording a test result by observation. The second example is a hybrid chromatography data system (CDS) where observations generate electronic records and the metadata are written as well as contained within the software. Peak areas and chromatograms are printed out and are manually typed into a spreadsheet for calculation of the reportable result. We will discuss the issues with both the hybrid analytical computerized system and the spreadsheet. The last example is also a CDS but used as an electronic system where all activities from data acquisition to calculation of the reportable result are contained within the application and underlying database. The reportable result is electronically signed by the tester and the reviewer. These three examples are shown in Figure A6.3.

Recording a Result by Observation

The first example of data generation is by observation that is documented by writing the result into a laboratory notebook or on a controlled worksheet. In this instance, an analyst conducts a test and records the observed result, the typical tests are for the color and odor of a sample. Although the observed result cannot be independently checked, as the test is non-destructive, the sample is available for the test to be conducted again, if required. In the case of a color, a test may be made more objective by comparing the test substance against a color palette but this typically is only used for a finished product not for raw materials or active pharmaceutical ingredient (API) testing.

However, recording results by observation may also involve an analytical instrument such as a pH meter or an analytical balance. Here we enter the realm of risk assessment—how critical is the observed test result?

If the test is involves checking the pH value of a reagent or the aqueous portion of a mobile phase and documenting the result, then the risk

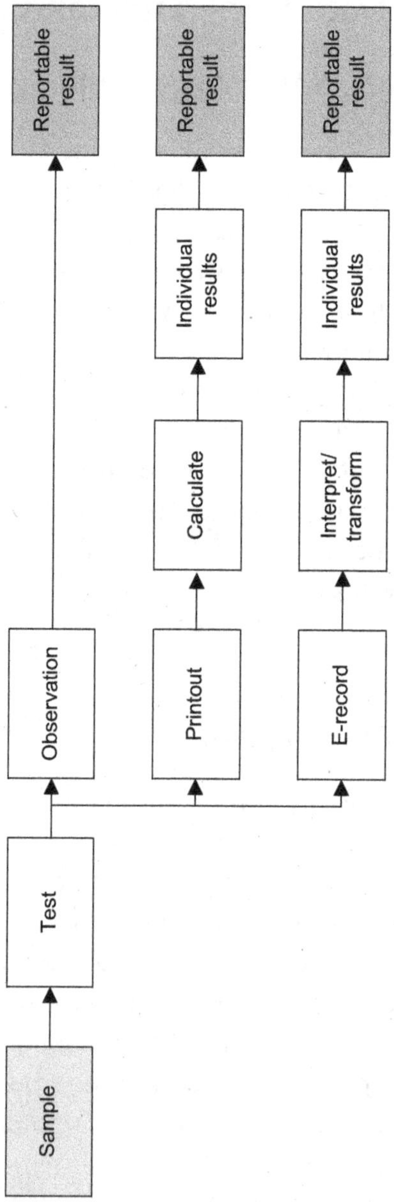

Figure A6.3 Three Options for Data Generation in a Regulated Laboratory.

is relatively low. The separation may not pass system suitability test (SST) criteria in the case of the mobile phase if the pH value is wrong and the SST failure minimizes the impact of the error. However, if the recording of results by observation involves an analytical balance where a user records the weight of the reference substance or sample displayed by the balance and records the weight, we enter a different level of risk. However, as shown in Table A6.1 the data integrity issue is that there is no independent evidence to verify that the value or result recorded is correct, has suffered from a transcription error or that the observation has been falsified. Therefore, each analysis recording results by observation requires risk assessment to determine the criticality of the data being generated: for example, is a color determination as critical as weighing an analytical reference standard? No. The weighing of an analytical standard to prepare a reference solution that may be used across multiple batch analyses is much more critical than colour determination for a single sample. This criticality is reflected in the MHRA data integrity guidance where there is a bullet point under the section on Designing Systems to Ensure Data Integrity that *states Automated data capture or printers attached to equipment such as balances* [24]. Therefore, it is important where analytical balances are used that there is a printer attached to capture the weighing sequence. Ideally, it would be better if the balance weightings were captured by a Laboratory Execution System (LES), LIMS or a similar laboratory informatics solution and transferred electronically to where the data are required.

Hybrid CDS System with Spreadsheet Calculations

The next example is a chromatography data system used as a hybrid system where the peak area results after checking any and permitted re-integration are printed out and the peak areas are entered into a validated spreadsheet for the calculation of the reportable value. Although a CDS can be installed as a standalone or networked system and data can be stored within a database or in directories in the operating system. Our example in this discussion will be a standalone CDS workstation with files stored in directories not a database.

There are a number of potential data integrity problems with a CDS installed on a standalone workstation. The first is security as in many cases the application needs to be open while the run is in progress and anybody can potentially access the system and make unauthorized changes to the run parameters. Next there is often lower security and a user can access the

Table A6.1 Records Associated with Manual Observation and Hybrid and Electronic Systems

Record	*Observation*	*Hybrid*	*Electronic*
Raw Data	• Written record	• Electronic files of the analysis	• Electronic files of the analysis
Metadata	• Further written data about the sample and analysis, e.g., batch, test, analyst, date, etc.	• Electronic Files for control of the instrument, data acquisition, interpretation and reporting of data. • Identification of who tested the sample, etc. • Audit trail entries of data changes • Further written data about the sample and analysis, e.g., batch, test, etc. • Printouts from the data system	• Electronic files for control of the instrument, data acquisition, interpretation and reporting of data. • Identification of who tested the sample, etc. • Audit trail entries of data changes • Further written data about the sample and analysis, e.g., batch, test, etc.
Processed data	• Not applicable	• Entry into spreadsheet for further calculation of individual values and reportable result • Completed spreadsheet file • Spreadsheet printout	• Interpretation of the raw data • Further metadata and audit trail entries
Information	• Not applicable	• Individual values of aliquots	• Individual values of aliquots
Knowledge	• Reportable Result • Handwritten signatures of tester and reviewer	• Printout of reportable result • Handwritten signatures of tester and reviewer • Linkage to underlying instrument raw data and spreadsheet file	• Reportable result • Electronic signatures of tester and reviewer • Linkage to all data and metadata via application database

workstation clock and make unauthorized changes and even delete data files in the directories without the application audit trail knowing that the files have been deleted.

Owing to the conservative nature of the pharmaceutical industry, the raw data for the system is often defined as paper and the underlying electronic records may be

Level 2 guidance for e-records as raw data. However as discussed earlier in this Appendix, the FDA Level 2 guidance [8] clearly states that the underlying electronic record is the original record not the printed paper.

The analyst will set up the chromatograph for the specific analysis via the CDS and when the chromatographic system is ready begin the analysis and acquire the data. One of the key issues with data integrity and chromatography data systems is the area of integration of the peaks. This was where Able Laboratories began data falsification by integrating standards and samples in different ways to manipulate the reportable result. Therefore, controlled integration and, where appropriate, reintegration of chromatograms is a key requirement for ensuring data integrity in a CDS. The principle of controlled interpretation of data also extends to other laboratory data systems such as spectrometers. There have been 483 citations for failure to have an SOP for manual integration of chromatograms. However, the citation is wrong in the author's opinion, the citation should be for failure to have a procedure for chromatographic integration. This procedure should instruct users how to integrate chromatographic peaks correctly, first automatically and if permissible manually. The problem is that there is no universal definition of manual integration, therefore McDowall [25] has divided the topic into manual intervention and manual integration to ensure that there is an adequate balance between scientific soundness and regulatory compliance.

Manual intervention has two versions:

1. Changing the time settings for one or more peaks to bring them within the time window for a method and all injections are reprocessed the same. No other changes are performed and the peaks areas remain the same.
2. Changing integration settings such a slope setting or minimum area counts in the case where there is excessive detector noise which identifies multiple small peaks as the analyte of interest. All chromatograms are reprocessed the same was but the peak areas of some or all samples and standards may change.

In the author's opinion, manual intervention can be performed by trained analysts on any analytical procedure involving chromatography.

Manual integration should only be permissible in clearly defined situation such as impurity profiling where some peaks may be close to the limit of detection or a disregard limit. Here a chromatographer can manually reposition the baselines of those injections which in his or her professional opinion require changing. Depending on the run, some or all chromatograms will be reintegrated and peak areas will change of the reintegrated peaks. The second person review of both manual intervention and manual integration will be critical in ensuring data integrity of the run.

When the analysis has been completed and any permitted intervention or reintegration has occurred, the chromatograms and any other information required will be printed out from the workstation as per the applicable procedure. The analyst will initial or sign and date the printouts and complete any log books, controlled worksheets or laboratory notebooks required. The analyst will then access the template of the validated spreadsheet and enter the peak areas of all system suitability test (SST) samples, standards and sample injections into the template and save under a new file name. Ideally the new spreadsheet file will be saved in a secure area on the network for protection and backup by the IT department. Furthermore, the file name of the electronic record will be linked to be printout and the handwritten signature of the analyst and reviewer by incorporating it in the header or footer of the printout to comply with §11.70 of 21 CFR 11 [18]. Some people may argue why store the completed spreadsheet file? The answer lies in the same argument for defining the CDS electronic records as the original record not the printout. The FDA has made the it crystal clear that paper printouts from a computerized system are not the original records [8], although focused on chromatography data systems it also applies to other laboratory data systems and spreadsheets.

Second person review of the data, the analytical procedure and the SOPs will be covered in the next section.

Finally, the laboratory must backup the electronic records stored in the hard drive of the standalone workstation. First, as an observation, in a regulated environment this is not a desirable situation as the hard drive is a single point of failure that could result in the loss of records. Second, leaving backup to laboratory staff is to invite failure as this is not their main task and may result in an FDA observation as Ohm Laboratories found out when their failed to back up laboratory CDS records for six months [26].

Overall a single workstation generating and storing regulated laboratory records is not a situation to engender data integrity. As a minimum data should be acquired directly to a secure and resilient server on the company network or ideally the data system should be networked to provider greater secure user accessibility to the functions of the CDS.

Networked CDS using Electronic Signatures

One issue is that the same CDS application software can be installed either on a standalone workstation or as a networked system. McDowall and Burgess have written a four-part series [27–30] looking at the ideal CDS for a regulated laboratory, in this they make 15 recommendations for improvement including the use of a database instead of using directories in the operating system and standalone workstations are should not be used. A CDS must be networked with backup performed by the IT department of the organization rather than left to analytical staff to try to perform.

For any CDS or laboratory system, hybrid or electronic, it is important that the application configuration to ensure that electronic records are protected, the audit trail and other Part 11 functions and the user roles and the corresponding access privileges are documented and set. Once set, the configuration settings become a configuration item and will be subject to change control procedures if any changes are to be made.

For a networked CDS system, to ensure data integrity and avoid conflicts of interest from laboratory based system administrators, it is important to have user account management and configuration settings maintained by the IT department.

When designing electronic ways of working it is important to eliminate spreadsheets from the analytical process and incorporate validated calculations into the CDS. The principle, validate the calculation once and use many times applies. Many laboratories fail to use the investment in a state of the art CDS by perpetuating the use of spreadsheets instead of incorporating their calculations in the chromatography software. For example, many laboratories use their CDS software as an electronic ruler and prefer to manually type the peak areas into a spreadsheet to calculate system suitability test results when these calculations are built into every CDS application as standards. The logic for using a spreadsheet for these calculations borders on lunacy.

The analyst who performs the test should set up the chromatograph and equilibrate the system ready for analysis. While this is happening the sequence file will be set up by entering or copying sample information including sample weights, dilutions, purities, factors, etc. Integration of the resultant chromatogram will follow the same principles for the hybrid system and when the reportable result is calculated, the analyst will electronically sign the report.

Second person review of data is critical for ensuring data integrity and that the procedures for generating, interpreting and integrating the chromatograms and generating the reportable result have been followed. The second person reviewer needs to check that data entered manually from outside the system have been correctly entered (e.g., sample weights, reference standard weights and purities, dilutions, etc.). The right chromatograph, control method, data acquisition method and processing method have all been selected and used. If any changes have been made t control files that they are permitted by the laboratory procedures. Any manual intervention or manual integration that has occurred is permitted by procedure and that the changes are scientifically sound. Ideally the SST, standard and sample injections are all integrated in the same way.

The reviewer also needs to review the audit trail entries associated with the analytical run. The focus here should be on entries that have resulted in deletion of data (if permitted by the system) and modification of data entries or sample numbers in the system can be supported by data from outside the system to justify the changes. Also check if any evaluation samples have been injected and that these have been included in the report. If after these checks are acceptable, the reviewer can electronically sign the report.

In some cases, there may be situations where the reportable result or indeed one or more of the replicate aliquots may be out of trend (OOT), out of expectation (OOE) or out of specification (OOS). All results must be retained and the laboratory OOS procedure should be followed, the latter should be based on the FDA guidance for OOS investigations [4] to decide if there is an assignable cause to invalidate the results or to retest or resample. However, in case of retest or reanalysis of a sample there are stringent conditions to be met.

Records Associated with the Three Example Processes

The records that are generated by the three examples in this Appendix are shown in Table A6.1. As can be seen for the hybrid versus electronic system, the hybrid system is more complex as data are spread across two systems the CDS and the spreadsheet. Managing the same data in a single system is far simpler.

Table A6.2 Ten Compliance Requirements for Laboratory Data Systems [16]

Commandment	*Understanding the Commandment*
1. Management are Responsible	• All levels of management are responsible for quality and compliance in regulated laboratories. • Management set and maintain the ethos, standards and quality expectations of the analytical scientists working there.
2. Use a Networked Data System with a Database	• Laboratory data systems that are file based are not fit for use in a regulated environment as it is easy to delete data, instead use a system with an integrated database. • Standalone workstations are also not fit for purpose, instead network the systems. Furthermore, standalone workstations provide opportunities for loss of data and manipulation of the system clock. • Acquire data without human interaction to a resilient network server and not a local workstation • Restrict access to the network server except via the informatics application • Use the IT department to operate the backup and recovery process
3. Document the System Configuration and Manage all Changes to it	• Ensure that the application is configured (e.g., enable the audit trail, turn on electronic signatures and define user types with associated access privileges) after installation and before completing the user acceptance testing. • Document the software configuration • Change configuration by a formal change management process.
4. Work Electronically and Use Electronic Signatures	• DO NOT USE A DATA SYSTEM AS A HYBRID • Design your work processes to work electronically for greater efficiency and speed [31]. • Validate the system for intended use [22] • Sign the reports electronically • Define electronic records/raw data for the system [23,32] • Keep paper print-outs to a minimum
5. Allocate each User a Unique Identity and Use Adequate Password Strength	• Don't be cheap and save money on user licences, allocate each user a unique user identity. • When a person leaves or no longer requires access, disable the account to ensure that the user identity is not reused. • Ensure that passwords are sufficiently strong and are not shared or written down

(*Continued*)

Table A6.2 (Continued) Ten Compliance Requirements for Laboratory Data Systems [16]

Commandment	*Understanding the Commandment*
6. Separate Roles to Avoid Conflict of Interest	• Use IT to administer the system if possible to avoid conflicts of interest, e.g., ability to change application configuration settings by a laboratory user. • A user with system administrator privileges can be tempted into making unauthorised changes to the system and data.
7. Define Methods that Can and Cannot be Adjusted	• Determine and document which analytical procedures can be adjusted and those which cannot, this control can include the data acquisition, instrument control and integration parameters as deemed necessary.
8. Have an SOP for CDS Integration	• An SOP needs to define which type of method when integration is allowed (coupled with technical controls within the CDS software) and is not allowed. • When integration is allowed what actions are permissible and what are not.
9. Ensure staff are Trained and Competent	• Staff must be trained in the all SOPs applicable to the system • Competence in the SOPs for each data system should be demonstrated.
10. Carry out effective Self-inspections or Internal Audits	• Self-inspections must be independent and focus on ensuring data integrity within a data system. • As such, auditors must focus on the electronic records and working practices within the system rather than any paper records outside of it. • If non-compliances are identified ensure that CAPAs are effective and issues are not repeated. • Frequency will be determined by the risk passed by the system.

Ten Compliance Commandments for Laboratory Data Systems

Although the focus of this Appendix has been on chromatography data systems used as either hybrid or electronic mode, it is important to develop guidance for laboratory data systems in general to ensure the integrity of the data generated, interpreted and analysed. Furthermore, to identify some of the controls that need to be in place to protect the electronic records so that they are trustworthy and reliable. Therefore, based on the warning letters citation summary earlier and the discussions of hybrid and electronic systems above, ten compliance commandments can be drawn up as seen in Table A6.2 for practical implementation for laboratory data systems [16].

Summary

This appendix provides the background to laboratory data integrity and then discusses three examples in common use of creating and managing records: by observation, hybrid and fully electronic working.

To ensure data integrity it is important, wherever possible, to work electronically with validated workflows eliminating the ability to falsify data.

References

1. Burgess, C.L., *Issues related to United States versus Barr Laboratories Inc.*, in *Development and Validation of Analytical Methods*, C.L. Riley and T.W. Rosanske, Eds. Pergamon Press, Oxford, 1996, 352.
2. *Inspection of Pharmaceutical Qualiy Control Laboratories*, Food and Drug Administration, Rockville, MD, 1993.
3. *United States Pharmacopoeia <1010> Outlier Testing*, United States Pharmacopoeia Convention Inc., Rockville, MD.
4. *FDA Guidance for Industry Out of Specification Results*, Food and Drug Administration, Rockville, MD, 2006.
5. *Able Laboratories Form 483 Observations*, 2005; Available from: http://www.fda.gov/downloads/aboutfda/centersoffices/officeofglobalregulatoryoperationsandpolicy/ora/oraelectronicreadingroom/ucm061818.pdf.
6. *Leiner Health Laboratories FDA Warning Letter*, Food and Drug Administration, 2006.
7. Compliance Program Guide 7346.832 Pre-Approval Inspections, in *Chapter 46 New Drug Evaluation*, Food and Drug Administration, Silver Spring, MD, 2010.
8. *Questions and Answers on Current Good Manufacturing Practices, Good Guidance Practices, Level 2 Guidance—Records and Reports*, 2014; Available from: http://www.fda.gov/Drugs/GuidanceComplianceRegulatoryInformation/Guidances/ucm124787.htm.
9. Citations, EudraGMP; European Medicines Agency, Available from: http://eudragmdp.ema.europa.eu/inspections/gmpc/searchGMPNonCompliance.do.
10. *Inspection Tracker*. Health Canada, Available from: http://www.hc-sc.gc.ca/dhp-mps/pubs/compli-conform/tracker-suivi-eng.php.
11. McDowall, R.D., Understanding the layers of data integrity, *Spectroscopy* 31, 4, 2016, In press.
12. *Part 58 Good Laboratory Practice for Non-Clinical Laboratory Studies*, Food and Drug Administration, Rockville, MD, 1978.
13. OECD Principles on Good Laboratory Practice, in *OECD Series on Principles of Good Laboratory Practice and Compliance Monitoring Number 1*, Organisation for Economic Cooperation and Development, Paris, 1995.

14. *OECD Series on Principles of Good Laboratory Practice and Compliance Monitoring Number 10, the Application of the Principles of GLP to Computerised Systems*, Organisation for Economic Cooperation and Development, Paris, 1995.
15. *OECD Series on Principles of Good Laboratory Practice and Compliance Monitoring Draft Number 17, the Application of GLP Principles of Computerised Systems*, Organisation for Ecomomic Cooperation and Development, Paris, 2015.
16. McDowall, R.D., The role of chromatography data systems in fraud and falsification, *LC-GC Europe* 27, 9, 2014, pp. AAA–BBB.
17. *21 CFR 211 Current Good Manufacturing Practice for Finished Pharmaceutical Products*, Food and Drug Administration, Sliver Spring, MD, 2008.
18. *21 CFR 11 Electronic Records; Electronic Signatures, Final Rule*, Food and Drug Administration, Rockville, MD, 1997.
19. *EU GMP Annex 11 Computerised Systems*, European Commission, Brussels, 2011.
20. *Fresenius Kabi Oncology Limited Warning Letter (WL: 320-13-20)*, Food and Drug Administration, Silver Spring, MD, 2013.
21. *Wockhardt Limited Warning Letter (WL 320-13-21)*, Food and Drug Administration, Silver Spring, MD, 2013.
22. *21 CFR Part 211 Current Good Manufacturing Practice for Finished Pharmaceuticals*, Food and Drug Administration, Rockville, MD, 2008.
23. *EU GMP Chapter 4 Documentation*, European Commission, Brussels, 2011.
24. *GMP Data Integrity Definitions and Guidance for Industry*, 2nd Edition, Medicines and Healthcare Products Regulatory Agency, London, 2015.
25. McDowall, R.D., Where can I draw the line? *LC-GC Europe* 28, 6, 2015, pp. AAA–BBB.
26. *FDA Warning Letter Ohm Laboratories*, Food and Drug Administration, 2009.
27. Burgess, C. and McDowall, R.D., The ideal chromatography data system for a regulated laboratory, Part 1: The compliant analytical process, *LC-GC North America* 33, 8, 2015, pp. 554–557.
28. Burgess, C. and McDowall, R.D., The ideal chromatography data system for a regulated laboratory, Part 2: System architecture requirements, *LC-GC North America* 33, 10, 2015, pp. 782–785.
29. Burgess, C. and McDowall, R.D., The ideal chromatography data system for a regulated laboratory, Part 3: Essential chromatographic functions for electronic ways of working, *LC-GC North America* 33, 12, 2015, pp. 914–917.
30. Burgess, C. and McDowall, R.D., The ideal chromatography data system for a regulated laboratory, Part 4: Assuring regulatory compliance. *LC GC North America* 34, 2, 2016, pp. aaa–bbb.
31. McDowall, R.D., *Validation of Chromatography Data Systems: Meeting Business and Regulatory Requirements*, 1st Edition, Royal Society of Chemistry, Cambridge, 2005.
32. *Guidance for Industry, Part 11 Scope and Application*, Food and Drug Administration, Rockville, MD, 2003.

Appendix VII: Electronic Records Integrity in Clinical Systems

Lotta, Greta, and Peter

Markus Roemer

> ICH E 6 Good Clinical Practices: Compliance with this standard (ICH E6) provides public ensurance that the rights, safety, and well-being of trial subjects are protected, consistent with the principles that have their origin in the Declaration of Helsinki, and that the clinical trial data is credible.

Introduction

GMP regulatory authorities have put much emphasis on data integrity (DI) in recent years, not least because they have uncovered serious cases of DI breaches or raw data manipulations. The number of observations and complaints in US FDA Warning Letters with regard to data falsification and fraud has been increasing.

Detailed requirements for audits and inspections of DI have been set in US FDA Compliance Program Guides* and in several European inspection

* US FDA, FDA PAI compliance program guidance, CPG 7346.832, compliance program manual, May 2010. http://www.ipqpubs.com/wp-content/uploads/2010/05/FDA_CPGM_7346.832.pdf.

guidelines. The British MHRA published a GMP Data Integrity Definitions and Guidance for Industry in March 2015.*

In 2011, the European Medicine Agency (EMA) revised EU GMP Chapter 4,† in light of the increasing use of electronic documents within the GMP environment. The regulatory requirements for DI or so-called "data governance systems" (by MHRA) based on a pharmaceutical quality system (PQS) are definitely not new, but nowadays a deeper view and focused investigation is done during all inspections. Some inspections or audits even follow a forensic approach regarding DI verifications.

Basically, the same applies to good clinical practices (GCPs): The regulatory requirements toward DI, also called in a broader view *trail integrity* or *study integrity*, have been in place for many years and an increasing use of electronic systems and applications (i.e., eTMF, eCRF) can be noted too; and it is expected that during inspections DI will or must be challenged more intensively. In addition, inspectors from different agencies are both assigned to GMP and GCP inspections.

However, there is a way for companies to navigate the troubled waters of DI deficiencies by taking some basic behavioral, procedural, and technical steps to significantly improve their quality systems and technical IT systems.

Comparison of GMP and GCP

This section is intended for readers who are more familiar with GMP processes and system validation including IT qualification. It can also be stated that computer system validation initially started in the GMP area in the 1980s, and most of the validation executions are done in this environment. Global companies may combine validation policies and procedures for several areas such as GMP, GDP, GCP, or medical devices, based on the firm's business and product range and setup. Also, the intensive inspection focus on DI started in GMP inspections. Between the GCP and GMP phases, there are also several data and process interfaces or transactions. For example, an investigational medicinal product (IMP) used in a clinical study must be manufactured according GMP rules; the GMP batch release by the European Qualified Person (QP) must include a verification with the requirements of

* MHRA, MHRA GMP data integrity definitions and guidance for industry, March 2015.

† EudraLex, The rules governing medicinal products in the European Union volume 4, Good manufacturing practice, Medicinal products for human and veterinary use, Chapter 4: Documentation, June 2011.

the marketing authorization. The marketing authorization contains GCP data from clinical studies.

Compared to GMP processes, there are some similarities in GCP processes, but especially also for data and document management in an overall view, which will be described later. In the first instance, it is important to understand the overall GCP process, to be able to define a risk-based approach toward process risks and validation including DI. The final goal of a GCP process in terms of information or data is the final clinical study report (CSR), respectively, a trail master file (TMF), which is used for submitting new medicinal products to the regulatory agencies.

A CSR that includes completed case report forms (CRFs) and the comprehensive TMF are comparable to GMP batch processing records; the TMF during the planning stage including, for example, a Sample Case Report Form, instructions for statistical analysis, or shipping records/sample labels for IMPs is comparable to processing or packaging instructions. So it is possible to distinguish in both areas between two document types: instruction type and record/report type (refer to EU GMP Chapter 4—Documentation).

For the subject of DI, which means that data must be credible and accurate, it is important to understand the relationship between predefined instructions and the following data capturing into records and reports, including any changes or deviations, if applicable.

Both document and information types constitute the basis for a quality decision: in GMP for the batch approval (certification) and releasing the batch to the market (patient) and in GCP for transferring the CSR(s) to the submission documents of the electronic Common Technical Document (eCTD; placed into Module 5) and followed by the marketing authorization of the medicinal product by the corresponding authority.

To put it in a simplified manner: In GMP, data is the documented rational for a batch approval (quality decision); in GCP, data is the documented rational for a marketing authorization by an agency.

Where GMP risk is more or less batch oriented, this may affect a dedicated group of patients, and a recall of the batch (or batches) may be required; in GCP, the *entire* medicinal product, respectively, the complete product specification might be highly risky and it may be extremely difficult to detect the risks, in an appropriate time frame.

For example, in January 2014, the European Medicines Agency (EMA) published an announcement based on an inspection by a French agency (ANSM) titled: "Start of a Review Concerning the Conduct of Studies at GVK Biosciences Site in Hyderabad, India."

This inspection by the ANSM revealed data manipulations of electrocardiograms (ECGs) during some studies of medicines that appeared to have taken place over a period of at least 5 years. Their systematic nature, the extended period of time during which they took place, and the number of staff members involved cast doubt on the integrity of the trials conducted at the site generally and on the reliability of the data generated.

As a result, around 700 (700!) pharmaceutical forms and strengths of medicines studied at the Hyderabad CRO site were recommended for suspension in May 2015 after a detailed review and investigation by the EMA.

According to ICH E6, a pharmaceutical company (sponsor) may transfer any or all of the sponsor's trial-related duties and functions to a CRO, but the ultimate responsibility for the quality and integrity of the trial data always resides with the sponsor.

Therefore, it is recommended that *detailed DI assessments* be executed in the scope of CRO selection processes or for any other outsourced activity and to define appropriate *quality agreements* including data management and DI handling. In addition, data reviews and integrity checks should be executed by the sponsor during the study runs.

The case at GVK Biosciences does not only affect the 700 medicines; it turned out that these studies were also run for more than 30 different sponsors (pharmaceutical companies), which were not able to detect the systematic issues regarding data and study integrity. The French agency on medicinal products did that during 5 days on the site for nine different studies.

It seems that for many cases the setup, control, and reviews of data management and handling are very often underestimated in GCP. In addition, IT systems or processes used during clinical studies may be based on many paper-based methods (paper CRF, spreadsheets, dedicated system landscapes), for example, for the data collection, especially for data transferred between different systems, data analysis, and reporting. This should also be made clear by the US FDA "Challenges and Opportunities Report—March 2004," which states: "Often, developers are forced to rely on the tools of the last century to evaluate this century's advances."*

Although this statement is from 2004, the current system landscape and processes (data flows) must be reviewed in detail even nowadays. Each manual process is not only a risk for DI—it also may result in failures,

* US FDA, Challenges and opportunities report—March 2004, http://www.fda.gov/ScienceResearch/SpecialTopics/CriticalPathInitiative/CriticalPathOpportunitiesReports/ucm077262.htm.

slowdowns, barriers, and missed opportunities that occur during product development and clinical studies.

The US FDA Guidance for Industry—Electronic Source Data in Clinical Investigations—states about 10 year later in 2013:

> In an effort to streamline and modernize clinical investigations, this guidance promotes capturing source data in electronic form, and it is intended to assist in ensuring the reliability, quality, integrity, and traceability of data from electronic sources to electronic regulatory submission.*

It must be summarized that working with electronic systems/data must be seen to also streamline and modernize clinical investigations. This implies that clinical studies ideally should be based on a totally paperless approach. The clinical investigation "project" is basically a big-data collection and analysis project.

Admittedly, GCP studies are a complex process or project, where several subject matter experts from different fields must design, control, and verify inputs, processes, and data. This is also why the term "project" was used in the previous sentence; such processes must be based on professional project management methodologies including a well-balanced communication and task plan.

GCP Regulations and DI Requirements

ICH E6 defines good clinical practice as: "A standard for the design, conduct, performance, monitoring, auditing, recording, analyses, and reporting of clinical trials that provides assurance that the data and reported results are credible and accurate, and that the rights, integrity, and confidentiality of trial subjects are protected."

If it cannot be proven beyond a reasonable doubt that the principles for DI are in place and GCP processes are at least designed to avoid data manipulations and/or to prevent accidental errors (data errors), all studies of a site might initially be questioned and marketing authorizations might be suspended.

---

* US FDA, Guidance for industry: Electronic source data in clinical investigations http://www.fda.gov/downloads/Drugs/GuidanceComplianceRegulatoryInformation/Guidances/ucm328691.pdf.

Two major critical areas/steps can be defined regarding GCP DI risks; during the

- *Trial data collection*
- *Statistical evaluation* based on predefined statistical methods

In general, process risks to DI can be defined for any manual input or transfer by operators, and if the concept of segregating duties is not implemented.

Interestingly, different applications and tools including different implementation levels of such applications within the GCP process can be found. *To conclude, the higher the level of automated processes, the lower the risk for poor data integrity.* However, it might be also a question of the right balance between flexibility and transparency. On the other hand, DI does not mean inflexibility, if systems used in GCP provide practical and efficient functions for data management and control, transfer, and even automated reviews and data checks, such as configurable audit trails and user group/access rights management. Some widely used commercial GCP applications and some applications developed in-house by the sponsor or CRO do not (yet) provide such functionalities in a sufficient manner.

Basically, the raw or original data of the study reports are derived from the completed CRFs or other source documents, in accordance with the predefined study protocol. Raw data, which is defined as source data according to ICH E6, *must permit the full reconstruction of the activities* resulting in the generation of the data. Statistical methods should be planned in the study protocol and can be defined as metadata.

ICH E6 chapter 8.3.13 defines *source documents* and *source data*:

> *Source Documents*: To document the existence of the subject and substantiate the integrity of the trial data collected. To include original documents related to the trial, to medical treatment, and history of subject. (Located in files of Investigator/Institution)
>
> *Source Data* are the clinical findings and observations, laboratory and test data, and other information contained in source documents. Source documents are the original records (and certified copies of original records). When applicable, information recorded on CRFs shall match the source data recorded on the source documents.

DI requirements define the ensurance that records are accurate, complete, intact, and maintained. These requirements are basic GCP requirements as defined in ICH E6 and will be described in more detail in the following sections.

In general, the expected and required "quality" of data is identical in GMP and GCP.

The Triad of Data Integrity

According to an MHRA blog* about DI, there are three areas regarding DI that must be considered:

1. *Behavioral:* Based on the quality culture: Impact of organizational culture and senior management behavior on data governance
2. *Procedural:* Based on the quality system and quality agreements between the contract giver (sponsor) and the contract acceptor (investigator/institution)
3. *Technical:* Based on IT system and IT infrastructure setup, processes, and functions (may include validation and qualification for proper verification)

Most of the documents and guidelines written on the subject of DI or validation are very technically oriented. Technology might be a very useful aspect regarding DI solutions, however, it is totally inefficient and useless without the other two aspects. This relationship and correlation is so strong that these three elements are called a "triad" in this book, meaning that all three elements must be fully implemented and each on the highest standards. Any weaknesses in one of these areas will immediately represent the entire quality level; and one of them can therefore be the weakest link of the chain.

The EMA published a "reflection paper on ethical and GCP aspects of clinical trials"† in 2012 and defined a set of useful criteria. The requirements for the study and ethics committees are defined in detail in the guidance

---

* https://mhrainspectorate.blog.gov.uk/2015/06/25/good-manufacturing-practice-gmp-data-integrity-a-new-look-at-an-old-topic-part-1/.

† http://www.ema.europa.eu/docs/en_GB/document_library/Regulatory_and_procedural_guideline/2012/04/WC500125437.pdf.

document. For example, EU regulatory authorities should disregard data obtained in any unethical manner, for example, if the trail protocol was not submitted to the ethics committee. Direct access to the subject's original medical records must be granted to all related parties (ethics committee, national agencies, sponsors, and investigators) for verification of clinical trial procedures and/or data.

In addition, the *transparency* of clinical trials might be questioned and some initiatives demand better ways to verify clinical trial data and how studies were initiated and maintained.

There are several guidelines or standards for ethical behavior. But what are adequate controls over ethical behavior and how can DI be part of it or must it even be part of it? We may ask a couple of questions about that.

Descriptions or diagrams of the electronic data flow (technical aspects) should be part of the trial protocols, data management plans, or investigational plans. Procedural controls should be defined for data entry and management. Such procedural controls must be set up in a vital quality system and driven by a professional project (=study) management approach. But when is a quality system really alive and vital? During quality audits, if observations are found, for example, for training management, how can it be assured that such procedural process controls can really work.

What is the management reaction in case of failures or if the investigation becomes a "flop"? How are the error and fault handled by management—on both sites, at the sponsor and investigator? Some studies simply must be a—commercial—success (project goal). And they might also be a little bit more complex, because the described "triad" must be alive on both sides—the contract giver (=sponsor) and contact acceptor (=investigator, institute, CRO). Basically, this is also a commercial partnership or relationship, possibly lasting many years; but GCP is also following a more scientific approach and a lot of discussions are going around about commercial and scientific conflicts.

What happens if a pharmaceutical company as the sponsor with a size of 10,000 employees starts a study with a CRO with 40 employees? There is no question that, from a monetary point of view, the balance of power seems to be clear. And if the CRO has 40 employees and one single person for IT management including validation and one person for quality management—is a two-page quality agreement document stating one single sentence that "data integrity must be assured by the investigator" sufficient and appropriate?

And on the other hand, during the contract negotiations, some procurement department may try to reduce costs (price dumping) and create massive cost pressure for the entire study, negatively affecting the quality of the study.

We must be very clear about some of these questions and how DI strategies and methodologies might be a solution for them. The risk of the entire pharmaceutical industry losing confidence, trust, and reputation is very high, especially nowadays when IT systems and the entire global world are also getting more complex and transparent. In addition, the current social and media world within our information society has defined a new word—"whistle blower"—which is a person who exposes any kind of information or activity that is deemed illegal or not correct within an organization. If data manipulation cases during clinical investigations became open to the public, the worst scenario would be that this might also have a massive impact on all investigations and medicines. Being in the public eyes there might raise a lot of questions and concerns regarding patient medical treatments, whereas only less than 1% might be affected. Even if this is not well concerted or fair, it would result in a wide patient risk scenario.

Here is a short example of which risks and impacts must also be considered for clinical studies. The National Center for Biotechnology Information, U.S. National Library of Medicine, published a very interesting article titled "Patient Protection in Clinical Trials in India: Some Concerns." It states very clearly that: "There is a danger of focusing on paperwork that documents the accuracy and completeness of clinical trial data."* Reading some more aspects of this article, it must be clear that the responsibility and ethical standards of Western civilization should not stop at its own borders.

Validation of GCP Computerized Systems

All systems (applications) used during clinical studies, for example, for trial data collection, statistical evaluation, and corresponding electronic quality systems, must be validated for the intended purpose. IT applications may not work without an IT infrastructure. Therefore, the IT infrastructure must be qualified. This approach is similar to EU GMP Annex 11 or ISPE GAMP 5. The US FDA requirements of 21 CFR Part 11 also apply to GCP electronic records and signatures.

---

* Srinivasan, S., Patient protection in clinical trails in India: Some concerns, *Perspect Clin Res* 1(3): 101–103.

However, it must be noted that if a system is validated, it does not automatically imply that DI is ensured, and it should not be understood as a single one-off event. Compared to traditional system validations, it might also be very beneficial to follow a multiple approach with at least two steps. First, the functions of the system (e.g., eCRF system) must be verified. A study that is planned to be run on that system "platform" will be configured into the system with study-specific case report forms. This kind of configuration or setup must be validated in the second step, which is study/process-related, and individually in each following study. This approach might be known and is similar to the validation of specific application (work sheets) MS Excel spreadsheets.

It must also be mentioned that for small organizations the validation of applications or the qualification of the IT network might be very complex or even unconvertible. This might be a matter of available resources and needs, and it might not be appropriate from a strategic point of view to build up such detailed and obverse core -business knowledge within small organizations.

Small organizations or even mid-sized companies should not have the expectations that validated systems can be simply bought from vendors and some testing of predefined "validation packages" may lead to success.

In many cases, it turned out that the best results can be achieved when systems (eCRF, eTMF) are hosted by the sponsor in a qualified IT infrastructure and validated systems. Very often, pharmaceutical companies (sponsors) may have more experience and expertise with validation, qualification, and a sufficient number of employees and experts compared to small companies or institutes. In addition, after the finalization of a study, the data are under the control of the sponsor and must not be transferred or migrated back from the investigator in some complicated way. There is also a behavioral aspect that the responsibility for the validation and qualification cannot be outsourced to smaller companies, which may not be empowered to ensure a proper validation execution.

At the end of a study run, data (in paper or electronic form) must be transferred by a coordinated and well-documented handover process to the sponsor/applicant. Generally, these data must include source data and source documents; if such data are transferred electronically, they must be converted or even migrated from one IT infrastructure and applications into a different one. Depending on the level of how different both infrastructures and applications are, this might be a complex handover process, similar to a data migration project, whereas the migration must include "all" data of a study and the data ownership moves from one party to the other. It is not appropriate just to keep source data at the CRO and to exclude it from the handover process, because data also presented in the marketing submission must permit the full reconstruction of results and conclusions.

In 2007, the US FDA published Guidance for Industry—Computerized Systems Used in Clinical Investigations, which states some helpful and important information. For example, a list of recommended standard operating procedures (SOPs) is provided in Appendix A of the FDA Guidance:

Standard operating procedures (SOPs) and documentation pertinent to the use of a computerized system should be made available for use by appropriate study personnel at the clinical site or remotely and for inspection by the FDA. The SOPs should include, but are not limited to, the following processes.

- System setup/installation (including the description and specific use of software, hardware, and physical environment and the relationship)
- System operating manual
- Validation and functionality testing
- Data collection and handling (including data archiving, audit trails, and risk assessment)
- System maintenance (including system decommissioning)
- System security measures
- Change control
- Data backup, recovery, and contingency plans
- Alternative recording methods (in the case of system unavailability)
- Computer user training
- Roles and responsibilities of sponsors, clinical sites, and other parties with respect to the use of computerized systems in the clinical trials

All SOPs should also contain an integral part of the procedural controls of DI and should be implemented into the quality systems and quality agreements between the involved parties.

The Guidance also stated, that:

- The FDA's acceptance of data from clinical trials for decision-making purposes depends on the FDA's ability to verify the *quality and integrity of the data* during FDA on-site inspections and audits (21 CFR 312, 511.1(b), and 812).

- Audit trails or other security methods used to capture electronic record activities should describe when, by whom, and the reason changes were made to the electronic record.

This US FDA guidance for industry is a valuable document, because it gives a clear picture of the requirements and expectations. The given set of SOPs is very similar to the ISPE GAMP recommendations, for example, dchange control, at a backup, and training. In addition, it defines the process of *data collection and handling* as a validation requirement.

Interestingly, there is also a very good definition for audit trails (similar to EU GMP Annex 11), including that activities should be captured:

- When: Date and time including time zone and data/time format
- By whom: Individual's name as unique identifier (first and last name of a person is not sufficient/unique; normally User IDs are biunique)
- Reason for change (if the activity was a data change after initial data entry)

Having validated a lot of systems, we can also state that a lot of systems have problems with the correct functionality of an audit trail. The process might be as follows: A clinical investigator is filling out a case report form electronically. He or she might select different fields and insert patient data and results. At the end, he or she confirms the data entry by pressing the OK button (or similar). The initial entries might be captured by a kind of activity trail (one type of audit trail). The given reason for change can be automatically written/defined by the system as "initial entry." After this first initial entry and corresponding confirmation, this entered data set is solid and fixed, and may represent Version 1 of this data set. Now the clinical investigator might reread the entered information and find out that in one field he or she made a wrong entry by mistake. Within an acceptable time frame, it might be possible to "re-open" the data set for the same clinical investigator to correct his/her first entry. Logically, this correction should result in Version 2 of this data set. By executing the change, the investigator reopens the data set, corrects the corresponding data, and confirms the change by pressing the OK button (again). Now the system cannot create the "reason for change" automatically; after confirmation, the user must be forced to enter the reason for change, for example, by a pop-up window and a mandatory field for entering the reason for change by the user (ideally as a choice list field).

Automatically generated reasons for the change, for example, stating "data was reopened and field ABC was changed," are not precise reasons and do not state the rational why the change was executed.

From a system design and development view, there must be several different audit trail types implemented covering different situations for data entries (activity trail), data changes (the "real" audit trail), and security (administrative audit trails, e.g., login and logout, assignment to user groups and rights, etc.). Such a determination regarding audit trails makes much sense toward DI and security. If a system can handle only one type of audit trail, most probably one of the key functions is missing. On the other hand, it should be clear that, for example, if you log in to a system, you do not need to give a reason for it.

Oversight of Clinical Investigations

The US FDA mentioned in the Guidance for Industry: Oversight of Clinical Investigations, a so called *risk-based approach to monitoring*. It is very important to define that inaccuracies regarding DI can occur either *accidentally* or *maliciously*. The term *data manipulation* should be used only for malicious cases. The term *data error* is used for accidental cases.

Data manipulations can occur during trial data collection or statistical evaluation in favor of positive study results: A clinical investigator might enter data differently than the given input by a patient about adverse reactions. During statistical evaluation, data might be filtered or reduced in an inappropriated way to get more positive trends or results. There might be several steps or ways to manipulate data. Weak system setups or processes may open wider ranges of possibilities for data migration. For example, one weak but very common setup is that the eCTD system is collecting the study data and such data sets are (manually) exported for statistics to electronic spreadsheets (MS Excel) or statistical programs like SAS (Statistical Analysis System). If the Excel sheet and the data transfer are not—at least—validated or automated, they not include a data verification, for example, by checksums and so on, such data can be manipulated very easily. In addition, such setups are also at very high risk for accidental errors.

It should be also noticed that data manipulations can also have a systemic nature and even be accepted, motivated, or at least be tolerated by senior, upper, or quality management. Such data manipulations are a massive compliance issue and will lead to legal consequences. They include the defined "triad" of behavioral, procedural, and technical aspects. It is not really expected that such setups might read a book about DI and compliance—on the other hand, if such business partners are identified, you should definitely avoid doing business with such companies in any context.

Validated systems and processes must try to reduce accidental errors to a minimum level, but validation itself is not able to guarantee a zero error level.

The idea of a "risk-based approach to monitoring" is that it should be possible to identify various types of data errors by statistical techniques. Additional monitoring techniques, such as routine reviews of data as they are submitted, are also mentioned for studies that use electronic CRFs. In addition to this very interesting approach, the guidance states:

> *Although not a monitoring technique, another method of ensuring data quality routinely implemented in eCRFs is the use of electronic prompts in the eCRF to minimize errors and omissions at the time of data entry, particularly if data are entered directly into the eCRF (refer to audit trail types in the validation chapter).*
>
> Source Data Verification
>
> For example, for a particular study, there may be minimal benefit in comparing 100% of the source data for each subject to the CRFs for each study visit. Rather, it may be sufficient to compare the most critical data points for a sample of subjects and study visits as *an indicator of data accuracy.*
>
> Sponsors should *prospectively* identify critical data and processes, then perform a risk assessment to identify and understand the risks that could affect the collection of critical data or the performance of critical processes. Then they should develop a monitoring plan that focuses on the important and likely risks to critical data and processes.

This implies that the validation of the system and the corresponding study design/setup must be based on a documented risk assessment. This risk assessment should be based on the process flow, defining at which stages data entry, data change, and data usage are processed and how the process steps are designed to avoid data errors.

It is important to understand the objectives and results of such a data-oriented risk assessment for GCP studies:

1. Identification of required system or process enhancements (prospective approach *before* the start of a study)
2. Defining data sets, criteria, and frequency of data verifications (prospective approach *during* the study run)
3. Defining data sets, criteria, and frequency (or even tools) for data monitoring (retrospective approach during or at the end of the study run)

This kind of quality risk management (QRM) for GCP data might bring the ICH Q9 and Q10 approaches to mind. These guidelines can also serve as a basis for choosing and applying different risk tools and methodologies (FMEA, risk ranking, fishbone, etc.).

The MHRA has also defined that "auditing is a quality assurance tool that can be used to evaluate the effectiveness of monitoring to ensure human subject protection and data integrity."

Another US FDA Guidance for Industry: Electronic Source Data in Clinical Investigations September 2013 stated the following requirements:

> Adequate controls should be in place to ensure confidence in the reliability, quality, and integrity of the electronic source data.
>
> Sponsors should include (e.g., in the protocol, *data management plan*, or investigational plan) information about the intended use of computerized systems during a clinical investigation, a description of the security measures employed to protect the data, and a description or *diagram of the* electronic data flow.

This implies very clearly that the CSP and the CSR must include a *data management plan* and a *diagram of the electronic data flow*. It should also contain a *complete* list of all computerized systems used during the study (entire data flow). It can be defined as a study-related inventory list, including but not limited to

- System name
- Version, release, or configuration including IT changes, patches, or hotfixes during the study run
  - If changes were executed: impact analysis required
- Vendor of system and qualification status of supplier or service providers
- Validation status including next periodic evaluation
- Issues or problems with systems during study run
- Organizational changes (e.g., administrator)

If, for example, MS Excel spreadsheets were used during the study for statistical evaluations, all spreadsheets should be listed individually.

Generally, source data is defined in case report forms (CRFs), data collection sheets, and/or study questionnaires.

Study Integrity–Trial Integrity–Data Integrity

This defined "diagram of the electronic data flow" would be a very important part of the "data governance system" during a trial/study, which is an important term defined by the MHRA.

Such a data governance system must encompass the CRF design, trial data collection, statistical evaluation, and medical writing until the final study report. It must be described in the study protocol by a professional diagram of the electronic data flow including all involved persons and system interfaces. This might contain the following interfaces:

- Human to system (manual)
- System to human (manual)
- Automated interfaces between systems (by gateways)
- Semiautomated interfaces (e.g., "copy and paste"; macros)

It is definitely not appropriate to understand this data diagram as a network diagram or a technical system drawing (e.g., showing databases, PCs, etc.). The so-called SIPOC methodology might be a very good iterative tool supporting the creation of such a data flow diagram. SIPOC is based on a table form and each column stands for supplier, input, process, output, and customer; it expresses a relationship between supplier and customer, where supplier must be understood as data source and customer as the receiver of data or information.

If such data flow diagrams and a system inventory list are not part of a study protocol and report, it is hard to prove the integrity of the study, trail, or DI. Basically, all three used terms have the same meaning and intention.

Clinical Trial Management

Each individual clinical trial is different, but some basics regarding DI are identical, which will be described or will be assumed in the following:

In general, clinical trial management without computerized systems or tools might be impossible nowadays, simply because of the volume of data and the efforts to keep the information up-to-date.

Also, the results of a clinical trial may be subject to reporting requirements in electronic format as for electronic submissions (market authorization) and reporting (GVP).

For example, according to the MHRA, the trial master file (TMF) must be maintained in an "inspection-ready state" and must be "complete and legible" (MHRA FAQ). Nowadays, the trail master file is usually managed electronically (as electronic records) and is named as eTMF.

A clinical trial management system (CTMS) is a software system or application to manage clinical trials in GCP. The functional scope, system landscape, and system interfaces may vary strongly between different solutions and setups. For example, some may be hosted by a CRO (clinical research organization) or as a cloud solution by the sponsor; some may include eCTD interfaces and Pharmacovigilance & Safety Reporting, and others may also include functionality for electronic transmission of individual case safety reports (ICSRs according ICH E2B).

One of the basic functions and requirements is definitely the data capturing during a study. In general, there are two types of case report forms (CRFs) used in GCP, that is

1. Paper CRF (traditional)
2. Electronic CRF (eCRF)

For example, the majority of these techniques can be performed using CRF data collected either using electronic data capture systems or entered into a database from a paper CRF collected by the CRO or sponsor.

If the source data are provided on paper and manually entered into a database from that paper CRF, it might be recommended to enter such data according a "double data entry" methodology. That means that two individual persons are entering the same data from an individual paper CRF into the database. This approach should reduce the likelihood of wrong data entries. Basically this is also a valid approach regarding risk reduction, but on the other hand it simply doubles working efforts.

Another problem that comes with paper-based CRFs is that paper forms are never that restrictive and precise-like—well-designed—electronic forms. Some handwritten entries by the clinical investigator, usually, for example, medical doctors, are in reality hard to read correctly. A certain degree of misinterpretations are possible with such input in writing. In addition, on some paper-based forms, comments or even changes are placed somewhere in the document or are not clear according good documentation practices.

Problems may also occur with the readability of paper CRFs, if the transfer process of the paper is done by fax.

Another paper CRF approach is based on the usage of scanning technology and automated text recognition (like OCR—optical character recognition) instead of manual entries by users. In addition, such paper CRFs are printed on a special sort of paper (optimized for scanning) and are transferred by postal mail only.

It must be emphasized that technology (fax systems, scanners, OCR software) has improved to a very high quality standard. However, paper-based systems have several disadvantages or drawbacks compared to paperless approaches, if all relevant costs, efforts, and risks are taken into account.

From a DI point of view, it must be stated that working with paper CRFs is always the solution that carries higher risk and more operational problems and issues. Also, it should be clear that other disadvantages are that this setup is a so-called "hybrid system," and changes or corrections of the CRF during a study are much more complex (distribution, withdrawal, etc.).

This also means that archiving must encompass the electronic data *and* the paper CRF (=source data). And in GCP such data as part of a submission and marketing authorisation might be kept for a very long time period!

On the other hand, there are also regulatory expectations that data must be available in an "inspection ready state"; this can be clearly understood that data must be also up-to-date at any time. The paper CRF process is definitely slow compared to a real-time entry to eCRF; the paper CRF might be on the way by post or somewhere on the to-do desk for manual entry.

The other point to consider is that source data must permit the full reconstruction of the activities and that hybrid systems have a "data flow interrupt" between the entered electronic data and the paper CRF. Following the path from the study report down to the initial paper CRF may cost more time.

Designing a "good" CRF—on paper or as an electronic form—is a major challenge that could result in data errors and wrong conclusions. The quality of the clinical trial depends on the case report forms used to capture the information. Each question ("field") may be set up as dual questions, closed or open questions, or "relative" questions. The *scientific integrity* of the trial and the credibility of the data from the trial depend substantially on the trial design. The performance of the trail results in DI. In total, this defines the study integrity.

Without a specific definition, the regulated industry and several system suppliers use “eClinical” to name technologies such as clinical trial management systems or randomization and trial supply management systems of IMPs, commonly using interactive voice response systems (IVRS), interactive web response systems (IWRS), electronic patient diaries, and other applications.

Summary: GCP Data Integrity

There are very strict requirements for DI in GCP. It is absolutely a fundamental part of the study and trial integrity. Several rules and guidelines have demanded DI for many years. In some “newer” guidelines, such DI requirements are explicitly defined; in others, which might be a little bit “older,” such requirements are stated “between the lines.”

Basically, DI in GCP can simply follow the ALCOA principles for good data management. All activities and useful tools and functions must be applied during study planning, execution, and reporting.

The following points should be considered, especially for GCP studies:

- The study protocol or any other planning document must contain a detailed diagram of the electronic data flow.
- The study Protocol or any other planning document must contain a system inventory list of all software used during the trial.
- All systems must be validated, including spreadsheets, statistical programs, and macros and/or interfaces.
- DI awareness training for all involved parties.
- Verification of system SOPs in place including training.
- Selection process and supplier qualification include data management (“priority A”).
- Defining quality agreements with details about DI.
- Validation should include the reconstruction of data process.
- Planning and execution of detailed DI assessments.
- Planning and execution of risk-based approach to monitoring.
- Risk evaluation of technology used (paper CRF vs. eCRF, eTMF management, statistical systems).
- The CSR must contain a conclusion of used systems and data flows, especially in case of changes, corrections, or modifications.

By following these "golden" or basic rules, GCP compliance and DI are ensured and demonstrate clinical trial oversight for designing, conducting, performing, monitoring, auditing, recording, analyzing, and reporting clinical trials. Within GCP, managing clinical trial data appropriately ensures that the data are complete, reliable, and processed correctly, and that DI is preserved. Data management includes all processes and procedures for collecting, handling, filtering, analyzing, and storing/archiving data from study start to completion. Diagrams of the electronic data flows and all related quality assurance measure and activities are also an important part for the transparency of clinical trials.

Appendix VIII: Electronic Records Integrity in Data Warehouse and Business Intelligence*

Introduction

This chapter covers the e-records integrity areas related to data warehouse† (DW) and business intelligence‡ (BI) settings. The data integrity–related definitions used in this chapter are based on a recent MHRA§ guidance document.¶

* López, O., Electronic records integrity in a data warehouse and business intelligence, *Journal of GxP Compliance*, 22, 2, April.

† A data warehouse is a system used for data reporting and analysis. These are central repositories of integrated data from one or more disparate sources.

‡ Business intelligence is an umbrella term that refers to a variety of software applications used to analyze an organization's raw data. BI as a discipline is made up of several related activities, including data mining, online analytical processing, querying, and reporting.

§ MRHA is the Medicines and Healthcare Products Regulatory Agency, the British Medicines and Medical Devices Regulatory Agency.

¶ MHRA, MHRA GMP data integrity definitions and guidance for industry, March 2015.

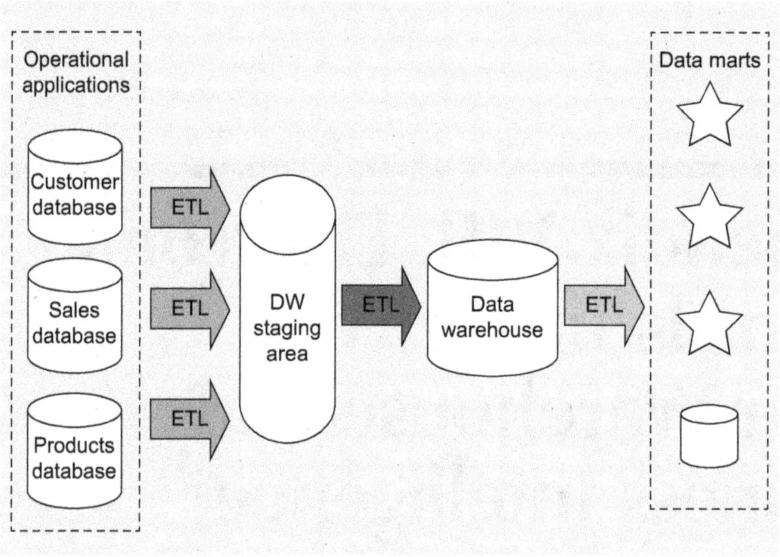

DW/BI environments are the complete end-to-end data warehouse and business intelligent system. The queryable data in the DW/BI system are referred as the data warehouse, and value-add analytics is referred as BI applications.

E-records moving across data warehouses are performed by applications directly interfacing with the source repository and, typically, a secondary repository, called staging areas. These applications are called extract, transform, and load (ETL) systems.*

The raw data† is extracted from its operational application or source repository locations and may be processed/transformed by applying a series of rules or functions. The raw data is converted to data,‡ and then the data is loaded into a final set of tables for the user to access.

BI applications include the entire range of data access methods such as ad hoc queries, dashboards, scorecards, standard reports, ad hoc reports, analytics, process monitoring, data mining, and other BI applications. They leverage the organization's internal and external information assets to

* Extract, transformation, and load (ETL) systems consist of a set of processes by which the operational source data are prepared for the data warehouse. They consist of extracting operational data from source applications, cleaning and data conformance, and delivering the data to the presentation servers, along with ongoing management and support functions.

† Raw data: Original records and documentation, retained in the format in which they were originally generated (i.e., paper or electronic), or as a "true copy" (MHRA).

‡ Data: Information derived or obtained from raw data (e.g., a reported analytical result) (MHRA).

support improved business decision-making. A data mart* is the backend component for achieving BI.

The controls discussed in this chapter ensure that the data in repositories, extracted raw data, transformed data, and loaded data are managed only by the relevant approved controls and/or validated software applications under a controlled infrastructure. These controls provide the trustworthy system† environment required to manage e-records in support to GMPs related decisions.

Principles

This chapter is based on the following essential validation principles:

- Infrastructure or platforms associated with DW/BI are qualified and then documented.
- All records loaded in the DW structures must be stamped with the date/time of the insertion or update. The source of the date/time must be a reliable time stamping service.
- The ETL application should be metadata driven. The application should draw from a repository of information about the tables, columns, mappings, transformations, data quality screens, jobs, and other components.
- Administer role–based security must be established on all data and metadata in the ETL application.
- Secondary data repositories should be used only for data sharing, integration, and reporting.
- E-records in a secondary repository must be physically deleted when the associated e-record retention period in the source system is reached.
- Persisted data‡ should never be modified directly in a secondary repository.
- For data warehouses, the design will cleanse the data by enforcing source system constraints based on business processes within the

---

* A data mart is the access layer of the data warehouse environment that is used to get data out to the users. The data mart is a subset of the data warehouse that is usually oriented to a specific business line or team. Data marts are small slices of the data warehouse.

† López, O., Trustworthy computer systems, *Journal of GxP Compliance* 19, 2, July 2015.

‡ Persisted data: E-records residing in the diverse data warehouses (DW) acquired from a source system(s).

warehouse structure. The business processes will be defined by end users and SMEs. Structures such as data marts will not necessarily enforce such rules.

- Physical and federated data marts will be under a separate schema from the data warehouse schemas.
- Data marts may be in the same database instance as the data warehouse if appropriate, but the default approach will be to keep data marts in an instance separate from the warehouse for upgrade independence.
- Warehouse applications will have open read-only access for database structures that do not contain data considered sensitive. Sensitive data will not have open access and will require additional approvals and restrictions for access according to the security plan.
- Warehouse database structures can be utilized for source system transactional reporting as well as data analysis and general BI. Transactional reporting must not duplicate the reporting capabilities provided by the source system, though, and source system reporting capabilities should be the default option.
- The data warehouse design should be highly normalized while the data mart design should be de-normalized according to consumption needs.

E-Records Life Cycle

Refer to Chapter 3.

E-records can be described according to a life-cycle concept. The e-records life cycle consists of all phases in the life of the e-records from initial generation and recording through processing (including transformation or migration), use, data retention, archive/retrieval, and physical deletion. The life cycle is a needed practice to comprehend any discussion about the controls necessary for properly handling the e-records and ensuring the integrity of those e-records. Failure to address just one element of the e-records life cycle will weaken the effectiveness of the controls implemented elsewhere in the computer system.

From the perspective of DW/BI applications, the typical stages associated with e-records life cycles are creation, access, use and reuse, and physical deletion.

Creation

E-records acquired from operational application or source system repositories are considered raw data.

As applicable, the e-records residing in the diverse DW (data warehouse, data mart, staging area, bolt on, extension and so on) are considered e-records acquired from a source system and considered persisted data.

Access, Use, and Reuse

The raw data acquired from the operational application or source system repositories are transformed and loaded to a data mart in which they can be consumed via BI-related applications.

Physical Deletion

Data in a secondary repository must be deleted when the corresponding record retention for the e-record in the source system is reached.

Persisted data should never be modified directly in a secondary repository. Persisted data are updated as a result of a change in the associated source system. Therefore, secondary data repositories are not required to have an audit trail. If technical limitations require the data to be modified in the secondary data repository, the modification must have traceability to the same change at the corresponding source system.

E-Records Integrity

Consistent with any typical computer system, the required data integrity controls in DW/BI applications can be categorized as follows: data during processing, data storage, data while in transit, and data migration.*

* López, O., A computer data integrity compliance model, *Pharmaceutical Engineering* 35, 2, March/April 2015.

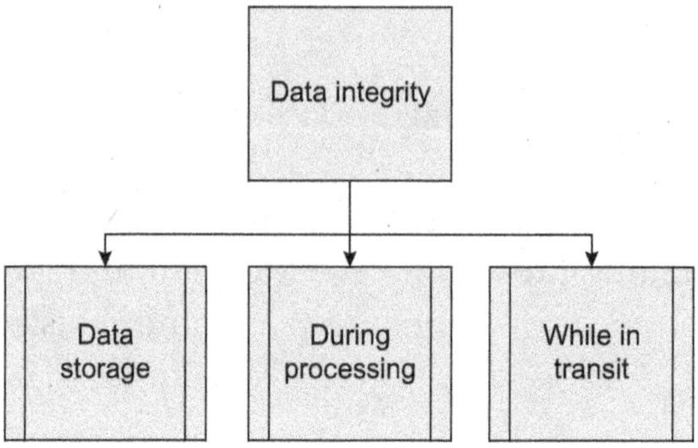

As applicable, these controls must be integrated as part of the associated DW/BI application requirements document.

The controls related to each category just enumerated must be covered in procedural controls and/or specifications.

E-Records Integrity during Processing

For DW/BI applications, the functionality validation/qualification is the foundations to achieve the integrity of the e-records during processing. After deployment, these applications, components, and/or interfaces are maintained following all GMP-related controls applicable to computer systems during the operational and maintenance phases of the SLC.

ETLs are the applications that transform e-records across the warehouse repositories. These applications interface directly with the source repository and, typically, interface as well with the secondary repositories called staging areas. After the e-records reached the staging area, another ETL extract selected e-records and, before loading to the Data Warehouse, these e-records are transformed and, information inserted, updated, and/or deleted.

During the transformation stage, data integrity processing takes place during a series of rules or functions applied to the extracted data. These rules (e.g., operational checks) and functions are applied to prepare the data for loading into the end target (e.g., data mart). The transformation processing must be validated and changes must be controlled and tested.

Some data do not require any transformation at all; such data are known as "direct move" or "pass through" data.

Data Integrity while Data Retained by Computer Storage

Logical and physical protections must be consistent to the criticality of the computer system. For e-records retained by computer storage these protections of the e-records from unauthorized entry as well as the environmental impacts influencing the respective data storage devices..

DW/BI applications have open read-only access for database structures that do not contain data considered sensitive. Sensitive data will not have open access and will require additional approvals and restrictions for access according to the security plan.

To reduce the risk of losing the data in storage and guaranteeing data readiness for the users, periodic backups must be performed. The integrity and accuracy of the backup data and the ability to restore the data should be checked during validation and monitored periodically. In addition, the capacity level of the storage must be monitored.

After completing the specified source system record retention requirements, the respective e-records in the secondary repository must be physically deleted.

Stored data should be checked periodically for accessibility, readability, and accuracy. If changes are implemented to the computer infrastructure and/or DW/BI application, then it is required to ensure and test the ability to retrieve data.

Electronic data storages areas must be qualified by following a process based on an approved validation/qualification procedural control.

As the result of persisted data should never be modified directly in a secondary repository, once raw data had been transferred to the staging area and the data had been transferred to the warehouse and data marts, the raw data in the staging area and, the data in the warehouse and data mart databases should never be directly modified. In the case of a data modification in any warehouse database system, the modification must be performed to the alike operational application source repository data set and the updated data loaded to the staging area using the same automated tool initially used to load data from the source to the storage area. If technical limitations require the data to be modified in the data mart or intermediate database as part of the data warehouse system, the modification must have traceability to the same modification in the source system.

Data while in Transit

The data integrity controls applicable to data while in transit considers the accurate data while transported.

In a DW/BI environment, ETL systems consist of a set of processes by which the operational source data are prepared for the data warehouse.

ETLs consist of extracting operational data from source applications, cleaning and conforming the data, and delivering the data to the presentation servers, along with ongoing management and support functions, such as:

- Data transactions (e.g., insert, update, deletes), business rules, transformation logic
- The reaction to incorrect inputs
- Exception handling
- Algorithm checking
- Recovery of lost or corrupted data

E-records integrity can be impacted by these transformations.

In ETLs, some data do not require any transformation at all; such data are known as "direct move" or "pass through" data. When a transformation is not performed, the key element to consider in ETLs is ensuring that each valid record from the source is loaded to the appropriate target table(s).

As part of the validation of ETLs, data quality assurance testing must be performed and documented. This test consists of running reports using freehand SQL (connecting directly to the DW/BI data warehouse or data mart) to those obtained by running the same report but using the universe as an interface to the data warehouse or data mart. These reports must match.

To minimize the risk associated with the inputs and outputs, the ETL should include appropriate built-in checks for the correct and secure extraction, loading, and processing of the e-records operations.

During operations, the correctness of the data loaded to the data storage area must be periodically reconciled. The technique and tools to be used in the data reconciliation process, the frequency of data reconciliation, the rationale for the choice of subsets of data to reconcile, and the documentation of results of data reconciliation must be defined during the design and implemented according to the specifications. Instructions must be provided to the support team on ETL on data reconciliation requirements.

For critical data entered manually to a DW/BI application, there should be an additional check on the accuracy of the manually entered data. This check may be done by a second operator or by validated electronic means.

One of the built-in checks that must be performed, as applicable, are operational checks to enforce permitted sequencing of steps and events.

During the extract stage, data must be profiled and changes to the captured data analyzed and the extracted system evaluated. This stage is verified and/or tested and controlled via the typical configuration management controls.

During the load stage, the ETL must ensure that each valid e-record from the source is loaded to the appropriate target table(s).

Standard functional requirements applicable to ETLs such as error handling and reporting, record counts, record sums, or any other applicable method must be taken into consideration for continuous control and verify the data integrity during data while in transit.

ETLs are validated based on the standard procedural controls associated with computer systems.

Data Migration

If data are transferred to another data format or database, validation should include verifications that the data are not altered in value and/or meaning during this migration process.

Incidents

Faults, incorrect documentation, data errors, improper operation, and interface errors of computer system components illustrate some of the incidents that can affect the correct operation of a computer system. These incidents are also known as nonconformances.*

Effective monitoring of the operation of a computer system involves users or operators trained in proper operational procedures. This facilitates their ability to recognize unexpected responses and outputs, react to the incident properly, and fully document such incidents to aid in the evaluation and debugging process.

Managed by corrective and preventive actions (CAPA), the initial assessment of the incident includes root cause analysis.†

A data integrity issue characterizes some of the incidents that can affect the correct operation of a DW/BI application. These incidents may become nonconformances.

---

* Nonconformance: A departure from minimum requirements specified in a contract, specification, drawing, or other approved product description or service.

† EudraLex, *The Rules Governing Medicinal Products in the European Union* Volume 4, EU Guidelines for Good Manufacturing Practice for Medicinal Products for Human and Veterinary Use, Chapter 1, Pharmaceutical Quality System, Section 1.4A (xiv), January 2013.

Damaged Electronic Records

There must be a recovery mechanism. The damaged records process provides a mechanism for creating an accurate reproduction of an original record that is discovered to be stained, marred, or otherwise damaged.

When an e-record is discovered to be unreadable, it can be restored from a true copy of the record. If a true copy is not available, look for a trustworthy backup copy of the record and restore from the backup set.

Damaged e-records may be considered an incident and investigated.

Security Features

There must be provisions for e-records security and integrity. The data warehouse must be reasonably secure from intrusion and misuse, and must be adhering to generally accepted security principles.

Because BI applications are geared toward a number of users, it is important to make sure people have read-only access to what they are supposed to see.

At the data mart level, security can reside from the BI application level to the cell level. By and large, all established BI commercial tools have these capabilities. Furthermore, they have a security layer that can interact with common corporate login protocols. There are, however, cases where large corporations have developed their own user authentication mechanism and have a "single sign-on" policy. For these cases, having a seamless integration between the tool and the in-house authentication can require some work.

Summary

This chapter discussed the e-records integrity topics associated with DW/BI environments.

During processing, special attention is provided to the application sequencing and data flows.

The integrity of the e-records retained in computer storages is safeguarded by implementing a comprehensive, logical, and physical security program.

E-records in transit are protected by maintaining the GMP controls to the related infrastructure and validating the ETL transformations.

The migration of data must be verified to ensure the accuracy of the data set that has been migrated.

The above actions provide the proper controls applicable to e-records to ensure the integrity of the e-records throughout the e-records life cycle.

Additional Readings

Kimbal, R., Ross, M., Thornthwaite, W., Mundy, J., Becker, B., *The Data Warehouse—Lifecycle Toolkit,* 2nd Edition, Wiley, Indianapolis, IN, 2008.

López, O., A computer data integrity compliance model, *Pharmaceutical Engineering* 35, 2, 79–85, 2015.

López, O., EU Annex 11 and the integrity of erecs, *Journal of GxP Compliance* 18, 2, 2014.

Appendix IX: Checklist E-Records Integrity

The following are the items to consider in e-records integrity–related verifications.

Documentation to Be Reviewed (As Applicable)

- E-records integrity governance document
- E-records integrity–related risk assessment
  - Identification of the risks associated with the software, infrastructure, e-records, monitoring of interfaces and validation documentation and counter measures to achieve e-records integrity
- Procedural controls
  - E-records management procedure
  - E-records creation
  - E-records modification
    - How the e-records can be changed?
    - Where are the changes of e-records saved? Audit trails?
    - How are the changes to and the history (audit trails) of the e-records protected?
    - How are these changes reviewed (e.g., SOPs)?
  - E-records review
    - E-records retirement
    - E-records security
    - E-records availability
  - Archiving
  - Backups and restoration

  - Business continuity
  - E-records quality control
  - Problem reporting and management
  - Computer system change management
  - Reconciliation
  - Periodic reviews (e-records and metadata)
- System requirements related to the e-records
  - Requirements for e-records security (e.g., backup management, security applied to the folder saving e-records, audit trail e-records.)
  - Management of the revision of the access system
  - Requirements for monitoring of unauthorized access, requirements to restrict access to the system clock and operating system
- Critical e-records
- Inputs (automated and manual), outputs and interfaces
- E-records flow (from point of origin (raw e-records)), manipulation, final repository (e.g., MES), and other activities
  - What is the source of the e-records?
  - How is it managed through different systems for review and approval?
- True copy records/files determination
- Segregation of duties

General Questions

- If the computer system is used in a regulated application, has the system demonstrated to consistently function as expected (validation, control of changes and deviations)?
- What process is used to control changes to systems and programs that can have an effect on the quality of the product, to ensure that those changes receive the proper reviewal and approval with regard to their potential effects before being instituted, and that only authorized personnel can make such changes? Are personnel trained subsequent to making these changes?
- How can computer systems access be limited, in order to protect the records from tampering and prevent the e-records' alteration?
- If passwords are used as a security measure, are there provisions for the periodic changing of those passwords? Are there designees for all critical system operations and emergencies?

- What is the procedure for reviewing and updating security access when a person leaves the department or company? Is their access to the system or are their access codes for the system revoked in a timely fashion?
- What backup systems are in place, such as copies of programs and files, duplicate tapes, or microfilm? Has the retrievability of information from master tapes and backup tapes been verified? Are there procedures in place for disaster recovery, in the event of a power outage, loss of the server and computer systems and so on?
- Type of audit trails.
  - Electronic audit trails
  - Paper audit trails
  - Version control of files
- Timestamping.
  - Timestamping service
  - Periodic synchronization between the stamping service and the local computer clock
  - Limit the access of the computer date and time local function
- E-records Management.
  - What is the source of the e-records entered into the computer?
  - Who enters the e-records?
  - When?
  - Who has access to computer? Security codes?
  - Is the storage area capturing the e-records (raw data*) the final destination? What is the final destination?
  - How are e-records that have previously been entered changed? Audit trails? By whom?
  - How are errors, omissions, and so on, in the received e-records corrected, and how are they documented?

* Original records and documentation, retained in the format in which they were originally generated (i.e., paper or electronic), or as a 'true copy'. A true copy is an exact verified copy of an original record.

Appendix X: Bibliography

Aide-mémoire of German ZLG regarding EU GMP Annex 11nnex 11, September 2013.

Appel, K., How far does Annex 11 go beyond Part 11?, *Pharmaceutical Processing*, September 2011.

APV, The APV guideline "Computerized Systems" based on Annex 11 of the EU-GMP guideline, Version 1.0, April 1996.

ASTM, E 2500—13 Standard Guide for Specification, Design, and Verification of Pharmaceutical and Biopharmaceutical Manufacturing Systems and Equipment, 2013.

Boogaard, P.; Haag, T.; Reid, C.; Rutherford, M.; Wakeham, C., Data integrity, *Pharmaceutical Engineering* special report, 39–67, March/April 2016.

Brown, A., Selecting storage media for long-term preservation, *The National Archives*, DPGN-02, August 2008.

Cappucci, W., Clark, C., Goossens, T., Wyn, S., ISPE GAMP CoP Annex 11 interpretation, *Pharmaceutical Engineering*, Vol 31, Number 4 (July/August), 2011.

CEFIC, Computer validation guide, API Committee of CEFIC, January 2003.

Center for Technology in Government University at Albany, SUNY, Practical tools for electronic records management and preservation, July 1999.

Churchward, D., Good Manufacturing Practice (GMP) data integrity: A new look at an old topic, Part 1 of 3, June 2015.

Churchward, D., Good Manufacturing Practice (GMP) data integrity: A new look at an old topic, Part 2 of 3, July 2015.

Churchward, D., Good Manufacturing Practice (GMP) data integrity: A new look at an old topic, Part 3 of 3, August 2015.

Commission Directive 91/412/EEC, Laying down the principles and guidelines of good manufacturing practice for veterinary medicinal products, July 1991.

Commission Directive 95/46/EC of the European Parliament and of the Council of 24 October 1995 on the protection of individuals with regard to the processing of personal data and on the free movement of such data http://eur-lex.europa.eu/LexUriServ/LexUriServ.do?uri=CELEX:31995L0046:en:HTML

Commission Directive 2003/94/EC, Laying down the principles and guidelines of good manufacturing practice in respect of medicinal products for human use and investigational medicinal products for human use, October 2003.
Council of Europe, Handbook on European data protection law, December 2013.
EC (European Commission), "General data protection regulation (GDPR)," January 2012 (Proposed regulation to replace EU Data Protection Directive 95/46/EC).
EMA/INS/GCP/454280/2010, GCP Inspectors Working Group (GCP IWG), Reflection paper on expectations for electronic source data and data transcribed to electronic data collection tools in clinical trials, August 2010.
EU Annex III to Guidance for the Conduct of Good Clinical Practice Inspections Computer Systems, May 2008. http://ec.europa.eu/health/files/eudralex/vol-10/chap4/annex_iii_to_guidance_for_the_conduct_of_gcp_inspections_-_computer_systems_en.pdf.
EudraLex, The Rule Governing Medicinal Products in the European Union, Volume 4 EU Good manufacturing practice (GMP) medicinal products for human and veterinary use, Chapter 9: Self inspections, 2001.
EudraLex, The Rules Governing Medicinal Products in the European Union, Volume 4, EU guidelines to good manufacturing practice, medicinal products for human and veterinary use, Annex 16—Certification by a qualified person and batch release, 2001.
EudraLex, The Rules Governing Medicinal Products in the European Union Volume 4, Good manufacturing practice, medicinal products for human and veterinary use, Chapter 3: Premises and equipment, 2007.
EudraLex, The Rules Governing Medicinal Products in the European Union Volume 4, Good manufacturing practice, medicinal products for human and veterinary use: Glossary, 2007.
EudraLex. The Rules Governing Medicinal Products in the European Union, Volume 4, EU guidelines for good manufacturing practices for medicinal products for human and veterinary use, Annex 20—Quality risk management, February 2008.
EudraLex, The Rules Governing Medicinal Products in the European Union Volume 4, Good manufacturing practice, medicinal products for human and veterinary use, Chapter 4: Documentation, June 2011.
EudraLex, The Rules Governing Medicinal Products in the European Union, Volume 4, EU guidelines to good manufacturing practice, medicinal products for human and veterinary use Part 1, Annex 11: Computerized systems, June 2011. http://ec.europa.eu/health/files/eudralex/vol-4/annex11_01-2011_en.pdf.
EudraLex, The Rules Governing Medicinal Products in the European Union Volume 4, Good manufacturing practice, medicinal products for human and veterinary use, Chapter 7: Outsourced activities, January 2013.
EudraLex, The Rules Governing Medicinal Products in the European Union, Volume 4, EU guidelines to good manufacturing practice, medicinal products for human and veterinary use: Glossary, February 2013.
EudraLex, The Rule Governing Medicinal Products in the European Union, Volume 4, EU guidelines for good manufacturing practices for medicinal products for human and veterinary use, Part 1, Chapter 2: Personnel, February 2014.

EudraLex, The Rules Governing Medicinal Products in the European Union, Volume 4, EU guidelines to good manufacturing Practice, Medicinal Products for Human and Veterinary Use, Annex 15: Validation and qualification, October 2015.

European Agencies Agency, Questions and Answers: Good manufacturing practice, EU GMP guide annexes: Supplementary requirements: Annex 11: Computerised systems, http://www.ema.europa.eu/ema/index.jsp?curl=pages/regulation/general/gmp_q_a.jsp&mid=WC0b01ac058006e06c#section8

European Directorate for the Quality of Medicine and Healthcare, OMCL validation of computerised systems core documents, May 2009. (http://www.edqm.eu/ medias/fichiers/Validation_of_Computerised_Systems_Core_Document.pdf)

European Medicines Agency (EMA), Reflection paper on the expectations for electronic source documents used in clinical trials, August 2010.

European Medicines Agency (EMA), Q&A: Good Manufacturing Practices (GMP), February 2011.

George, J. G., Jr., E. J. Subak, Jr., and M. L. Wyrick, Validation key practices for computer systems used in regulated operations, *Pharmaceutical Technology*, pp. 74–98, June 1997.

GHTF, Implementation of risk management principles and activities within a Quality Management System, May 2005.

GMP Journal, Q&As on Annex 11 (1–4) at the computer validation in Mannheim, Germany, in June 2011, Issue 7, October/November 2011.

GMP Journal, Q&As on Annex 11 (5–11) at the computer validation in Mannheim, Germany, in June 2011, Issue 8, April/May 2012.

GMP Journal, Q&As on Annex 11 (12–16) at the computer validation in Mannheim, Germany, in June 2011, Issue 9, October/November 2012.

ICH Harmonized Tripartite Guideline, Good clinical practice, E6, June 1996.

ICH Harmonized Tripartite Guideline, Good manufacturing practice guidance for active pharmaceutical ingredients, Q7, November 2000.

ICH Harmonized Tripartite Guideline, Quality risk management, Q9, November 2005.

ICH Harmonized Tripartite Guideline, Pharmaceutical quality systems, Q10, June 2008.

IDA Programme of the European Commission, Model requirements for the management of electronic records, www.cornwell.co.uk/moreq.html, October 2002.

ISO 12207:1995,* Information technology: Software life cycle processes, 1995.

ISO 11799: 2003(E) Information and documentation: Document storage requirements for archive and library materials.

ISO 13485:2012, Medical devices: Quality management systems—Requirements for regulatory purposes.

* Note: The 1995 revision is not the most recent version.

ISO/IEC 1799:2005, Information technology: Security techniques—Code of practice for information security management.

ISO/IEC 27001:2013, Information technology: Security techniques—Information security management systems—Requirements.

ISPE, GAMP® COP, Considerations for a corporate data integrity program, 2016.

ISPE, GAMP® good practice guide: A risk-based approach to compliant electronic records and signatures, 2005.

ISPE, GAMP® good practice guide: Electronic data archiving, 2007.

ISPE, GAMP® good practice guide: Global information systems control and compliance—Appendix 2—Data management considerations, 2005.

ISPE, GAMP® good practice guide: IT control and compliance, International Society of Pharmaceutical Engineering, Tampa FL, 2005.

ISPE, GAMP® good practice guide: Risk-based approach to operation of GXP computerized systems, 2010.

ISPE, GAMP®/ISPE, Risk assessment for use of automated systems supporting manufacturing process: Functional risk, *Pharmaceutical Engineering*, May/Jun 2003.

ISPE GAMP®, A risk approach to compliant GxP computerized systems, *International Society for Pharmaceutical Engineering (ISPE)*, Fifth Edition, February 2008.

ISPE GAMP Forum, Risk assessment for use of automated systems supporting manufacturing processes: Part 2—Risk to records, *Pharmaceutical Engineering*, Vol. 23, No. 6, November/December 2003.

ISPE/PDA, Good practice and compliance for electronic records and signatures. Part 1 Good Electronic Records Management (GERM). July 2002.

ITIL Service Design, *Section 5.2: Management of Data and Information*, 2011 Edition.

Journal for GMP and Regulatory Affairs, Q&As on Annex 11, Issue 8, April/May 2012.

López, O., "A Computer Data Integrity Compliance Model", Pharmaceutical Engineering, Volume 35 Number 2, March/April 2015.

López, O., "A Historical View of 21 CFR 211.68," Journal of GxP Compliance, Volume 15, Issue 2 (Spring), 2011.

López, O., An easy to understand guide to Annex 11, *Premier Validation*, Cork, Ireland, 2011, http://www.askaboutvalidation.com/1938-an-easy-to-understand-guide-to-annex-11.

López, O., Annex 11: Progress in EU computer systems guidelines, *Pharmaceutical Technology Europe*, Vol 23, Issue 6 (June), 2011. http://www.pharmtech.com/pharmtech/article/articleDetail.jsp?id=725378

López, O., Annex 11 and 21 CFR Part 11: Comparisons for international compliance, *MasterCotrol*, January 2012. http://www.mastercontrol.com/newsletter/annex-11–21-cfr-part-11-comparison.html.

López, O., *Computer Infrastructure Qualification for FDA Regulated Industries*, PDA and DHI Publishing, LLC. 2006.

López, O., Computer systems validation, in *Encyclopedia of Pharmaceutical Science and Technology*, Fourth Edition, Taylor and Francis: New York, Published online: 23 Aug 2013; pp. 615–619.

López, O., *Computer Technologies Security Part I: Key Points in the Contained Domain*, Sue Horwood Publishing Limited, West Sussex, London, 2002.

López, O., Electronic records lifecycle, *Journal of GxP Compliance*, Vol 19, Number 4, November 2015.

López, O., EU Annex 11 and the integrity of erecs, *Journal of GxP Compliance*, Vol 18, Number 2, May 2014.

López, O., *EU Annex 11 Guide to Computer Validation Compliance for the Worldwide Health Agency GMP*, CRC Press, Boca Raton, FL, March 2015.

López, O., Hardware/software suppliers qualification, in *21 CFR Part 11: Complete Guide to International Computer Validation Compliance for the Pharmaceutical Industry*, Eds., Interpharm/CRC, Boca Raton, Florida 1st edition, 2004.

López, O., Maintaining the validated state in computer systems. *Journal of GxP Compliance*, Vol. 17, Number 2, August 2013.

López, O., Overview of technologies supporting security requirements in 21 CFR Part 11: Part I, *Pharmaceutical Technology*, February 2002.

López, O., Overview of technologies supporting security requirements in 21 CFR Part 11: Part II, *Pharmaceutical Technology*, March 2002.

López, O., Requirements for electronic records contained in 21 *CFR* 211, *Pharmaceutical Technology*, Vol. 36, No. 7, July 2012.

López, O., Requirements management, *Journal of Validation Technology*, May 2011.

López, O., Trustworthy computer systems, *Journal of GxP Compliance*, Vol 19, No 2, July 2015.

McCormick, K., Regulatory framework: EMEA, ISPE, 2009.

McCormick, K., Regulatory framework: PIC/S and ICH, ISPE, 2009.

McDowall, R. D., Comparison of FDA and EU regulations for audit trails, *Scientific Computing*, January 2014, http://www.scientificcomputing.com/article/2014/01/comparison-fda-and eu-regulations-audit-trails.

McDowall, R. D., Computer validation: Do all roads lead to Annex 11?, *Spectroscopy*, Vol 29, Number 12, December 2014.

McDowall, R. D., Ensuring data integrity in a regulated environment, *Scientific Computing*, March/April 2011, https://www.scientificcomputing.com/article/2011/05/ensuring-data-integrity-regulated-environment.

McDowall, R. D., Maintaining laboratory computer validation: How to conduct periodic reviews?, European Compliance Academy (ECA), GMP News, April 2012, http://www.gmp-compliance.org/pa4.cgi?src=eca_new_news_print_data.htm&nr=3085.

McDowall, R. D., The new GMP Annex 11 and Chapter 4 is Europe's answer to Part 11, European Compliance Academy (ECA), GMP News, January 2011, http://www.gmp-compliance.org/eca_news_2381_6886,6885,6738,6739,6934.html.

McDowall, R. D. and Ratcliff, J., How important is data integrity to regulatory bodies?, *Pharmaceutical Technology*, Vol. 40, No. 3, March 2016.

Mell, P., and Grance, T., The NIST definition of cloud computing, NIST Special Publication 800-145 National Institute of Standards and Technology, Gaithersburg, Maryland 2011.

MHRA, Good laboratory practice: Guidance on archiving, March 2006.

MHRA, MHRA expectation regarding self inspection and data integrity, May 2014.

MHRA, MHRA GMP data integrity definitions and guidance for industry, March 2015.

MHRA, GMP/GDP consultative committee note of meeting, October 2015. (https://www.gov.uk/government/uploads/system/uploads/attachment_data/file/483846/GMP-GDP_CC_minutes_Oct_2015_FINAL.pdf)

MHRA, GCP inspections metrics report, GCP inspectorate, February 2016.

NIST, *An Introduction to Computer Security: The NIST Handbook*, Chapter 7, Computer Security Risk Management (Special Publication 800-12), 2007.

NIST, Guide for conducting risk assessments, 800-30 Rev 1, September 2012.

OECD, The application of GLP principles to computerized systems OECD Guidance Document (Draft), September 2014.

PDA, Technical Report No. 31, Validation and qualification of computerized laboratory data acquisition systems, *PDA Journal of Pharmaceutical Science and Technology*, Vol. 53 Number 4, Section 4.5, September 1999.

PDA, Technical Report No. 32, Auditing of supplier providing computer products and services for regulated pharmaceutical operations, *PDA Journal of Pharmaceutical Science and Technology*, Release 2.0, Vol. 58, Number 5, Sep/Oct 2004.

PI 011-3, Good practices for computerised systems in regulated "GXP" environments, Pharmaceutical Inspection Co-operation Scheme (PIC/S), September 2007.

Pressman, R. S., *Software Engineering: A Practitioner's Approach*, McGraw Hill, 2010.

Roemer, M., New Annex 11: Enabling innovation, *Pharmaceutical Technology*, June 2011.

Safe Harbor US: EU Agreement on Meeting Directive 95/46/EC http://www.export.gov/safeharbor/index.asp.

Schmitt, S., Data integrity, *Pharmaceutical Technology*, Vol 38, Number 7, July 2014.

Schmitt, S., *Data Integrity: FDA and Global Regulatory Guidance*, IVT, October 2014.

Stenbraten, A., Cost-effective Compliance: Practical solutions for computerised Systems, paper presented at the ISPE Brussels Conference, GAMP: Cost Effective Compliance, 2011-09-19/20.

Stokes, D., Compliant cloud computing: Managing the risks, *Pharmaceutical Engineering*, Vol 33, Number 4, 1–11, 2013.

Stokes, T., Management's view to controlling computer systems, *GMP Review*, Vol 10, Number 2, July 2011.

TGA, Australian Code of Good Manufacturing Practice for human blood and blood components, human tissues and human cellular therapy products, Version 1.0 April 2013.

US FDA, 21 CFR Part 11, Electronic records; electronic signatures; final rule, *Federal Register*, Vol 62, Number 54, 13429, March 1997.

US FDA, General principles of software validation; final guidance for industry and FDA staff, CDRH and CBER, January 2002.

US FDA, Guidance for industry: Electronic records; electronic signatures—Scope and application, August 2003.

US FDA, Guidance for industry: Computerized systems in clinical investigations, May 2007.

US FDA, FDA PAI compliance program guidance, CPG 7346.832, Compliance program manual, May 2010. http://www.ipqpubs.com/wp-content/uploads/2010/05/FDA_CPGM_7346.832.pdf.

US FDA, Guidance for industry: Blood establishment computer system validation in the user's facility, April 2013.

US FDA, Guidance for industry: Electronic source data in clinical investigations, September 2013.

US FDA, 21 CFR Part 58, Good laboratory practice for non-clinical laboratory studies, April 2015.

US FDA, 21 CFR Part 110, Current good manufacturing practice in manufacturing, packing, or holding human food, April 2015.

US FDA, 21 CFR Part 312, Investigational new drug application, April 2015.

US FDA, 21 CFR Part 606, Current good manufacturing practice for blood and blood components, April 2015.

US FDA, 21 CFR Part 803, Medical device reporting, April 2015.

US FDA, 21 CFR 1271, Human cells, tissues, and cellular and tissue-based products, April 2015.

US FDA, Guidance for industry: Data integrity and compliance with CGMP guidance for industry, April 2016.

Wechsler, J., Data integrity key to GMP compliance, *Pharmaceutical Technology*, September 2014.

WHO, Guidance on good data and record management practices, QAS/15.624, September 2015 (Draft).

WHO, Technical Report Series No. 937, Annex 4. Appendix 5, Validation of computerized systems, 2006.

WHO, Technical Report Series No. 981, Annex 2, WHO guidelines on quality risk management, 2013.

Wingate, G., Validating automated manufacturing and laboratory applications: Putting principles into practice, Taylor & Francis, 1997.

Yves, S., New Annex 11, evolution and consequences, www.pharma-mag.com, January/February, 2012.

Index

A

Accuracy checks, 62, 188
Active Pharmaceutical Ingredients (APIs), 78–86
Ad hoc reports, 182
Agência Nacional de Vigilância Sanitária (ANVISA), 81–82, 107, 111, 113–114
ANVISA. *see* Agência Nacional de Vigilância Sanitária (ANVISA)
APIs. *see* Active Pharmaceutical Ingredients (APIs)
Application-dependent algorithms, 181–182
Archiving, electronic records, 132, 148, 170–172
ASEAN. *see* Association of Southeast Asian Nations (ASEAN)
Association of Southeast Asian Nations (ASEAN), 106, 110, 112–113
Audit trails, 67–68, 179–181
Authorized personnel, and electronic records, 159
Automated manufacturing system, 51–52

B

Backup storage principles, electronic records handling, 61, 148
BPaaS. *see* Business Process as a Service (BPaaS)
Built-in checks, 186–187
Business continuity, and electronic records, 149, 157
Business Process as a Service (BPaaS), 194
Business requirements, and MHRA, 125–126

C

CAPA. *see* Corrective and preventive actions (CAPA)
CD-P-TS. *see* European Committee on Blood Transfusion (CD-P-TS)
Cell controller, primary concern of, 51
CFDA. *see* China Food & Drug Administration (CFDA)
CFR. *see* 21 Code of Federal Regulations (CFR) part 211
CGMPs. *see* Current good manufacturing practices (cGMPs)
China Food & Drug Administration (CFDA), 88
Chromatography data systems (CDS), 303–304
  hybrid CDS system with spreadsheet calculations, 311–315
  networked CDS using electronic signatures, 315–316
Clinical systems, data integrity in
  clinical trial management, 336–339
  GCP regulations and DI requirements, 325–327
  GMP *vs.* GCP, 322–325
  oversight of investigations, 333–336
  overview, 321–322
  study and trial, 336

triad of, 327–329
validation of GCP computerized systems, 329–333
Clinical trial management, 336–339
Clinical trial management system (CTMS), 337
Cloud computing, and electronic records, 193–199
Code of Federal Regulations (CFR). *see* 21 Code of Federal Regulations (CFR) part 211
Community of Practice (CoP), 106
Computer system retirement, 131, 151–152
Computer systems life cycles, 44–45
Computer systems validation, and MHRA, 124
Conseil Européen des Fédérations de l'Industrie Chimique (CEFIC), 85
Contract manufacturers, and electronic records, 189–190
Controls, electronic records
accuracy checks, 188
audit trails, 179–181
and authorized personnel, 159
built-in checks, 186–187
and business continuity, 157
electronic signature, 181
handling system life cycle, 69–74
and incident management, 158
operational checks, 181–182
periodic (or continuous) reviews, 158–159
printouts/reports, 182–184
qualification of IT infrastructure, 185–186
requirements document, 159–160
risk management, 160–162
and security, 162–166
time stamping, 166–167
CoP. *see* Community of Practice (CoP)
Corrective and preventive actions (CAPA), 158
Creation stage, e-records life cycle, 40, 345
CTMS. *see* Clinical trial management system (CTMS)
Current good manufacturing practices (cGMPs), 59, 158, 180, 185, 189

D

Data collection and handling, 332
Data criticality and risk, 274–275
Data error, 333
Data governance. *see* Governance, e-records
Data integrity. *see* Integrity, e-records
Data manipulation, 333
Data migration, 42, 129–130, 172–173, 349
Data quality, and integrity, 275–288
Data storage principles, electronic records handling, 61, 150, 173–175
Data terminology, 48–50
Data transformation, 42–43
Data warehouse (DW)/business intelligence (BI)
damaged e-records, 350
data migration, 349
data while in transit, 347–349
life cycle, 344–345
monitoring, 349
overview, 341–343
principles, 343–344
during processing, 346
retained by computer storage, 346–347
security features, 350
Demilitarized zone (DMZ), 174
Destruction. *see* Life cycle, e-records
Digital timestamping service (DTS), 166–167
DMZ. *see* Demilitarized zone (DMZ)
DTS. *see* Digital timestamping service (DTS)
DW/BI. *see* Data warehouse (DW)/business intelligence (BI)

E

EC. *see* European Commission (EC)
ECGs. *see* Electrocardiograms (ECGs)
Electrocardiograms (ECGs), 324
Electronic records (e-records)
archiving, 170–172
and MHRA, 132
and cloud computing, 193–199
21 Code of Federal Regulations (CFR) part 211

access authorization principles, 60
accuracy check, 62
data input/output and storage/backup principles, 61
and contract manufacturers, 189–190
controls
accuracy checks, 188
audit trails, 179–181
and authorized personnel, 159
built-in checks, 186–187
and business continuity, 157
electronic signature, 181
and incident management, 158
operational checks, 181–182
and periodic (or continuous) reviews, 158–159
printouts/reports, 182–184
qualification of IT infrastructure, 185–186
requirements document, 159–160
risk management, 160–162
and security, 162–166
time stamping, 166–167
definitions
automated manufacturing system, 51–52
data terminology, 48–50
MHRA, 53–55
primary records, 55
raw data, 55–56
European Medicines Agency (EMA)
access, use, and reuse, 65–69
controls based on system life cycle, 69–74
creation, 64–65
physical deletion, 69
file integrity checking, 175–176
governance
integrity guidelines, 138
integrity plan, 136–138
integrity policy, 136
integrity strategy, 135
organization, 138–141
overview, 133–135
handling, 176–177
life cycle
access, use, and reuse, 40–42
and computer systems, 44–45
creation, 40
data migration, 42
physical deletion, 43
transformation, 42–43
migration, 172–173
procedural controls
integrity, 144–147
maintenance activities, 153–155
operational activities, 147–153
overview, 143–144
self-inspections, 202–204
storage, 173–175
Electronic records remediation project, 204–205
corrective action planning, 209–210
evaluating controls, 208–209
overview, 207–208
process activities, 210–212
execution, 211
interpretation, 211
new/upgrades to systems/ components, 212
suppliers qualification program, 212
training, 211
report, 212
Electronic signatures, 181
networked CDS using, 315–316
EMA. *see* European Medicines Agency (EMA) Annex 11
E-records. *see* Electronic records (e-records)
European Commission (EC), 202
European Committee on Blood Transfusion (CD-P-TS), 89
European Medicines Agency (EMA) Annex 11, 47, 86–87, 109, 112, 181, 183, 299
access, use, and reuse, 65–69
controls based on system life cycle, 69–74
creation, 64–65
overview, 63–64
physical deletion, 69
and trustworthy computer systems, 106
Extract, transform, and load (ETL) systems, 342–343, 346–349

F

FDA. *see* Food and Drug Administration (FDA)
Federal Information Processing Standards Publication (FIPS PUB), 166
File integrity checking, 175–176
FIPS PUB. *see* Federal Information Processing Standards Publication (FIPS PUB)
Food and Drug Administration (FDA), 93–95, 109, 112, 181, 299

G

GCP. *see* Good clinical practice (GCP)
GLP. *see* Good laboratory practice (GLP)
GMP. *see* Good manufacturing practice (GMP)
Good clinical practice (GCP), 290–295, 322
  GMP *vs.*, 322–325
  regulations and DI requirements, 325–327
  validation of computerized systems, 329–333
Good laboratory practice (GLP), 295–299
  regulations and guidance, 303
Good manufacturing practice (GMP), 143, 175, 179–182, 201
  data integrity
    data criticality and risk, 274–275
    and data quality, 275–288
  vs. GCP, 322–325
  regulations and guidelines, 86–98, 302
    API, 78–86
    overview, 77
Good Manufacturing Practices Audit Guideline for Pharmaceutical Excipients, 203
Governance, e-records
  integrity guidelines, 138
  integrity plan, 136–138
  integrity policy, 136
  integrity strategy, 135
  and MHRA, 123–124
  organization, 138–141
  overview, 133–135
GXP regulations, and data integrity, 302–309
  equipment citations, 304–306
  GLP regulations and guidance, 303
  GMP regulations and guidance, 302
  illustrating laboratory issues, 303–304
  and laboratory controls, 306–307
  and laboratory records, 307
  test analysis, 307–309

H

Heads of Medicines Agencies (HMA), 121
Health Products and Food Branch Inspectorate (HPFBI), 83, 87, 106, 110, 112–113
HMA. *see* Heads of Medicines Agencies (HMA)
HPFBI. *see* Health Products and Food Branch Inspectorate (HPFBI)
Hybrid system, 338

I

IaaS. *see* Infrastructure as a Service (IaaS)
Incident management, and electronic records, 158
Infrastructure as a Service (IaaS), 193, 194
Inspection trends, 5–37
Integration, transformation of data, 42–43
Integrity, e-records, 65
  checklist, 353–355
  in clinical systems
    clinical trial management, 336–339
    GCP regulations and DI requirements, 325–327
    GMP *vs.* GCP, 322–325
    oversight of investigations, 333–336
    overview, 321–322
    study and trial, 336
    triad of, 327–329
    validation of GCP computerized systems, 329–333
  data warehouse (DW)/business intelligence (BI)
    damaged e-records, 350
    data migration, 349

data while in transit, 347–349
life cycle, 344–345
monitoring, 349
overview, 341–343
principles, 343–344
during processing, 346
retained by computer storage, 346–347
security features, 350
GMP and MHRA
data criticality and risk, 274–275
data quality and, 275–288
guidelines, 138
in non-clinical laboratories
data generation and reporting, 309–318
GXP regulations, 302–309
overview, 299–301
sample analysis, 301–302
plan, 136–138
policy, 136
strategy, 135
Interactive voice response systems (IVRS), 339
Interactive web response systems (IWRS), 339
Internal audits. *see* Self-inspections
International Conference on Harmonization of Technical Requirements for Registration of Pharmaceuticals for Human Use (ICH), 83, 107, 110, 113
International Pharmaceutical Excipients Council (IPEC), 203
IPEC. *see* International Pharmaceutical Excipients Council (IPEC)
IVRS. *see* Interactive voice response systems (IVRS)
IWRS. *see* Interactive web response systems (IWRS)

L

Laboratory data generation and reporting, 309–318
hybrid CDS system with spreadsheet calculations, 311–315
networked CDS using electronic signatures, 315–316
by observation, 309–311
ten compliance commandments, 318
and three example processes, 316–318
Life cycle, e-records
access, use, and reuse, 40–42
and computer systems, 44–45
creation, 40
data migration, 42
and DW/BI, 344–345
overview, 39–40
physical deletion, 43
transformation, 42–43

M

Maintenance activities, e-records, 153–155
change control, 154
checks, 154–155
verification and revalidation, 153–154
Marketing authorization, 55
Medical and Health Products Regulatory Agency (MHRA), 41, 47, 53–55, 201
and business requirements, 125–126
and computer system retirement, 131
and computer systems validation, 124
and data governance, 123–124
data integrity
data criticality and risk, 274–275
and data quality, 275–288
and data migration, 129–130
and e-records archiving, 132
and e-records migration, 131
operational stage, 130–131
overview, 121–122
and quality risk management, 126–128
MHLW. *see* Ministry of Health, Labor and Welfare (MHLW)
MHRA. *see* Medical and Health Products Regulatory Agency (MHRA)
Migration, of electronic records, 42, 129–130, 172–173, 349
Ministry of Health, Labor and Welfare (MHLW), 107
Monitoring, DW/BI, 349

N

National Administration of Medicines, Food and Medical Technology, 78
National Institute of Standards and Technology (NIST), 193
NIST. *see* National Institute of Standards and Technology (NIST)
Non-clinical laboratories, data integrity in data generation and reporting, 309–318
  hybrid CDS system with spreadsheet calculations, 311–315
  networked CDS using electronic signatures, 315–316
  by observation, 309–311
  ten compliance commandments, 318
  and three example processes, 316–318
 GXP regulations, 302–309
  equipment citations, 304–306
  GLP regulations and guidance, 303
  GMP regulations and guidance, 302
  illustrating laboratory issues, 303–304
  and laboratory controls, 306–307
  and laboratory records, 307
  test analysis, 307–309
 overview, 299–301
 sample analysis, 301–302
Nonconformances, 158

O

OOS. *see* Out of Specification (OOS)
Operational activities, e-records, 147–153
 archiving, 148
 back-ups, 148
 business continuity, 149
 infrastructure maintenance, 150
 and MHRA, 130–131
 problem management, 151
 problem reporting, 151
 quality control, 149–150
 restoring, 152
 retirement, 151–152
 risk management, 152
 security, 152–153
 storage, 150
 training, 153
Operational checks, 181–182
Out of Specification (OOS), 300
Over-rides, transformation of data, 42–43

P

PaaS. *see* Platform as a Service (PaaS)
Periodic (or continuous) reviews, 158–159
Physical deletion, 43, 69, 345
Physical to Virtual (P2V), 171
PIC/S PI-011-3, 106, 110, 112–113
Platform as a Service (PaaS), 193, 194
Primary records, 55
Printouts, electronic records, 182–184
Problem management, e-records, 151
Problem reporting, e-records, 151
Procedural controls, e-records
 integrity, 144–147
 maintenance activities, 153–155
  change control, 154
  checks, 154–155
  verification and revalidation, 153–154
 operational activities, 147–153
  archiving, 148
  back-ups, 148
  business continuity, 149
  infrastructure maintenance, 150
  problem management, 151
  problem reporting, 151
  quality control, 149–150
  restoring, 152
  retirement, 151–152
  risk management, 152
  security, 152–153
  storage, 150
  training, 153
 overview, 143–144
P2V. *see* Physical to Virtual (P2V)

Q

QRM. *see* Quality risk management (QRM)
Qualification of IT infrastructure, 185–186
Quality control, e-records, 149–150, 299
Quality risk management (QRM), 126–128, 335

R

Raw data, records retention on, 55–56
Regulatory cross match, 256–271
Reports, electronic records, 182–184
Requirements document, 159–160
Restoring, e-records, 152
Risk-based approach to monitoring, 333
Risk management, 126–128, 152, 160–162, 274–275

S

SaaS. *see* Software as a Service (SaaS)
SCADA. *See* Supervisory control and data acquisition
Secure Hash Algorithm 1 (SHA-1), 176
Security, and electronic records, 114–116, 152–153, 162–166, 350
Self-inspections
  e-records, 202–204
    remediation, 204–205
  overview, 201–202
Service-level agreement (SLA), 190, 195
Service-level commitment (SLC), 179, 211
SFDA. *see* State Food and Drug Administration (SFDA)
SHA-1. *see* Secure Hash Algorithm 1 (SHA-1)
SIPOC methodology, 336
SLA. *see* Service-level agreement (SLA)
SLC. *see* Service-level commitment (SLC); System life cycle (SLC)
Software as a Service (SaaS), 193, 194
SOP. *see* Standard operating procedure (SOP)
Source data, 326
Source documents, 326
SST. *see* System suitability test (SST)
Standard operating procedure (SOP), 180, 331
Standards for Security Categorization of Federal Information and Information Systems, 166
State Food and Drug Administration (SFDA), 106, 110, 112
Storage, of electronic records, 150, 173–175, 346–347
Supervisory control and data acquisition (SCADA), 52
Suppliers qualification program, 212
System life cycle (SLC), 162, 195
System suitability test (SST), 311

T

Technology emulation, 171
21 Code of Federal Regulations (CFR) part 211, 181
  access authorization principles, 60
  accuracy check, 62
  data input/output and storage/backup principles, 61
TGA. *see* Therapeutic Goods Administration (TGA)
Therapeutic Goods Administration (TGA), 78, 80, 106, 109, 112
Time stamping controls, 166–167
TMF. *see* Trial master file (TMF)
Transformation, of data, 42–43
Trial master file (TMF), 337
Trustworthy computer systems
  availability, reliability, and operational checks
    ANVISA, 111
    ASEAN, 110
    EMA and TGA, 109
    FDA, 109
    HPFBI, 110
    ICH, 110
    ISO 9000-3, 109
    overview, 107–109
    PIC/S PI-011-3, 110
    SFDA, 110
    WHO, 110
  description, 102–103
  efficacy/validation of, 103–111
    ANVISA, 107
    Association of Southeast Asian Nations (ASEAN), 106
    European Medicines Agency (EMA) Annex 11, 106
    FDA, 105
    HPFBI, 106
    ICH, 107

ISO 9000-3, 105
MHLW, 107
PIC/S PI-011-3, 106
State Food and Drug Administration (SFDA), 106
Therapeutic Goods Administration (TGA), 106
WHO, 107
infrastructure, 116–118
overview, 101–102
secure from intrusion and misuse, 111–114
ANVISA, 113–114
ASEAN, 112–113
EMA, 112
FDA, 112
HPFBI, 112–113
ICH, 113
ISO 9000-3, 112
PIC/S PI-011-3, 112–113
SFDA, 112
TGA, 112
WHO, 113
security principles, 114–116

U

US FDA. *See* US Food and Drug Administration
US Food and Drug Administration (US FDA), 59

W

WHO. *see* World Health Organization (WHO)
World Health Organization (WHO), 96–98, 107, 110, 113, 134, 299